Handbook of Eye Surgery

Handbook of Eye Surgery

Editor: Joanne Galbraith

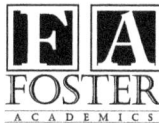

FA
FOSTER
ACADEMICS

www.fosteracademics.com

www.fosteracademics.com

FA
FOSTER
ACADEMICS

Cataloging-in-Publication Data

Handbook of eye surgery / edited by Joanne Galbraith.
    p. cm.
Includes bibliographical references and index.
ISBN 978-1-63242-943-8
1. Eye--Surgery. 2. Eye--Diseases--Treatment. 3. Ophthalmology. I. Galbraith, Joanne.
RE80 .H36 2020
617.71--dc23

Foster Academics,
118-35 Queens Blvd., Suite 400,
Forest Hills, NY 11375, USA

ISBN 978-1-63242-943-8 (Hardback)

Contents

Preface

Surgery performed on an eye or its adnexa by an ophthalmologist is called an eye surgery or ocular surgery. Local anesthesia and topical anesthesia are commonly used during the process of eye surgery. There are various forms of eye surgeries like oculoplastic surgery, eye muscle surgery, corneal surgery, refractive surgery, vitreo-retinal surgery, etc. Extreme care is required before, during and after the surgery procedure to minimize as well as prevent further damage. Eye removal surgeries include enucleation, evisceration and exenteration. These procedures are performed to reduce pain in a blind eye or to treat malignant orbital tumors. This book is compiled in such a manner, that it will provide in-depth knowledge about the practice of eye surgery. The various studies that are constantly contributing towards advancing technologies and the evolution of this field are examined in detail. Ophthalmologists and students actively engaged in this field will find this book full of crucial and unexplored concepts.

This book is the end result of constructive efforts and intensive research done by experts in this field. The aim of this book is to enlighten the readers with recent information in this area of research. The information provided in this profound book would serve as a valuable reference to students and researchers in this field.

At the end, I would like to thank all the authors for devoting their precious time and providing their valuable contribution to this book. I would also like to express my gratitude to my fellow colleagues who encouraged me throughout the process.

Editor

The Effect of Steep Trendelenburg Positioning on Retinal Structure and Function during Robotic-Assisted Laparoscopic Procedures

Kazuyuki Hirooka [iD],[1] Kaori Ukegawa,[1] Eri Nitta [iD],[1] Nobufumi Ueda,[2] Yushi Hayashida,[2] Hiromi Hirama,[2] Rikiya Taoka,[2] Yuma Sakura,[2] Mari Yamasaki,[2] Hiroyuki Tsunemori,[2] Mikio Sugimoto,[2] and Yoshiyuki Kakehi[2]

[1]Department of Ophthalmology, Kagawa University Faculty of Medicine, 1750-1 Ikenobe, Miki, Kagawa 761-0793, Japan
[2]Department of Urology, Kagawa University Faculty of Medicine, 1750-1 Ikenobe, Miki, Kagawa 761-0793, Japan

Correspondence should be addressed to Kazuyuki Hirooka; kazuyk@med.kagawa-u.ac.jp

Academic Editor: Michele Figus

Purpose. Robotic-assisted laparoscopic radical prostatectomy (RALP) has become a standard treatment choice for localized prostate cancer. RALP requires a steep Trendelenburg position, which leads to a significant increase in intraocular pressure (IOP). This study evaluated the effect on the retinal structure and function in patients undergoing RALP. *Methods.* Standard automated perimetry (SAP) and optical coherence tomography (OCT) were performed in 20 males scheduled for RALP at 1 month and 1 day before the operation and at 1 and 3 months after the operation. IOP measurements were made in the supine position at 5 min after intubation under general anesthesia (T1), at 6 discrete time points (5, 30, 60, 120, 180, and 240 min; T2-7), and at 5 min after returning to a horizontal supine position (T8). Serial retinal nerve fiber layer (RNFL) thicknesses and visual field progression were assessed using the guided progression analysis software program. RNFL thickness progression and visual field progression were evaluated by event analysis. *Results.* Average IOP (mmHg) for each time point was as follows: $T1 = 12.3 \pm 2.6$, $T2 = 20.4 \pm 4.2$, $T3 = 23.3 \pm 3.8$, $T4 = 24.0 \pm 3.2$, $T5 = 24.3 \pm 3.4$, $T6 = 27.1 \pm 7.2$, $T7 = 29.8 \pm 8.7$, and $T8 = 20.1 \pm 4.4$. During RALP, IOP significantly increased. There was no progression of the visual field and RNFL thickness after surgery or any other ocular complications found. *Conclusions.* Although IOP significantly increased during RALP, there were no significant changes in the retinal structure and function between the pre- and postoperation observations.

1. Introduction

Prostate cancer is one of the most common cancers in men. Although there are several treatment options, radical prostatectomy is a standard treatment for clinically localized prostate cancer. After introduction of robotic-assisted laparoscopic radical prostatectomy (RALP), it has spread rapidly in the world. As compared to the radical prostatectomy, there are several benefits associated with RALP, including reduced blood loss, fewer perioperative complications, improved functional outcomes, and a faster return to work [1–3].

RALP requires the use of a steep Trendelenburg position in which patients are placed in a supine position with their feet positioned above their head at an angle of inclination of 25 to 30 degrees. However, an increased intraocular pressure (IOP) has been reported to occur during surgeries when using the steep Trendelenburg position [4–8]. After refractive surgeries, it has also been reported that increases in the IOP during the operation can potentially lead to complications such as glaucoma and ischemic optic neuropathy [9, 10]. Hoshikawa et al. previously reported that despite finding a significantly increased IOP during the RALP procedure, they did not observe any significant changes in the retinal nerve fiber layer (RNFL) thickness or visual acuity [5]. In contrast, Taketani et al. recently reported OCT-detected visual field defects at 1 week after surgery, even though they found no abnormal findings in the fundus, RNFL thickness, or optic disc morphology, with the visual field returning to normal within 3 months after the surgeries in all cases [7]. It should be noted, however, that since perimetry is a psychophysical test, this technique will be limited by the "noise" of the variability, which is dependent upon the nature of the changes in the visual system, the testing situation, and the patient's condition [11]. Changes outside the limits of the short-term variability can be identified by guided progression analysis (GPA), which is a statistical method that uses the analysis of variance [12].

The aim of our current study was to investigate the influence of RALP on the retinal function and structure through the use of GPA software in patients without pre-existing ocular disease.

2. Materials and Methods

2.1. Patients. This single-center, prospective, nonrandomized study was conducted in accordance with the principles outlined in the Declaration of Helsinki. The Ethics Committee of Kagawa University Faculty of Medicine approved the study protocol. After explanation of the study protocol, each subject provided written informed consent. Between March and September of 2016 at Kagawa University Hospital, we enrolled a total of 24 consecutive male patients who underwent the RALP procedure. Enrolled patients were evaluated at our Ophthalmology Department at 1 month and 1 day prior to the operation and at 1 and 3 months after the operation. Since local visual field defects were recovering to normal within 3 months after the operation in the previous study [7], we evaluated glaucomatous progression until 3 months after the operation. Each of the subjects underwent ophthalmic evaluations at both of the visits. The examinations performed included dilated fundus examination with stereoscopic biomicroscopy of the optic nerve head using slit-lamp and indirect ophthalmoscopy, IOP testing, and visual acuity testing with refraction. Subjects also underwent gonioscopic examinations, which were performed and evaluated by the Shaffer classification. Subjects with previous abnormal visual field test results, ocular hypertension (IOP >21 mmHg), or the history of any kind of neurologic disease, retinal laser procedure, retinal pathology, or retinal surgery were excluded from the study. All subjects underwent visual field and optical coherence tomography (OCT) testing.

2.2. Cirrus HD-OCT RNFL Thickness and Optic Disc Morphology. Cirrus HD-OCT (Carl Zeiss Meditec, Dublin, CA), which is based on the use of spectral domain technology, was used to obtain all measurements by using an optic disc cube that was generated from a 3-dimensional data set. Each data set was composed of 200 A-scans from each of 200 B-scans that were obtained over a $6\,mm^2$ area that was centered on the optic disc. The methods for measuring and analyzing the RNFL thickness have been previously described elsewhere in detail [4]. The cube is used to create an RNFL thickness map, with the software then determining the center of the disc. Using this data set, the software subsequently extracts a circumpapillary circle (1.73 mm radius). To be included in the analysis of the current study, the images were required to have signal

strengths of at least 6. The RNFL thickness deviation and the RNFL thickness change maps were automatically determined by the OCT instrument, with the data then exported to a computer for the purpose of analyzing the progression pattern of the RNFL defects. The RNFL thickness deviation map, which was composed of 50×50 pixels, was used to visualize the RNFL defects. When RNFL measurements were below 95% of the percentile range for a particular pixel, yellow was used to code the pixel, while red was used if it was below 99%.

RNFL measurements were performed in each of the subjects at 1 month and 1 day prior to the operation and at 1 and 3 months after the operation. The RNFL thickness change map is one of the components of the GPA software (Carl Zeiss Meditec). This software provides event-based analysis of the RNFL progression based on the serial RNFL thickness maps. Furthermore, as the baseline and follow-up OCT images are automatically aligned and registered, this guarantees that changes at the same pixel locations can be measured. However, in order to generate a GPA report, a minimum of four patient visits is required. Once the images have been obtained and analyzed, the GPA program overlays the images and then compares the serial RNFL thickness versus that obtained during the duration of the follow-up. The event analysis of the GPA was used to assess the RNFL thickness progression. Data obtained from the first two exams were averaged and used as the baseline values. Once the series of RNFL thickness measurements were completed, the baseline RNFL thickness values were compared to the final measurement values via the use of the GPA software. In the current study, the RNFL thickness was defined as having progressed when the RNFL Thickness Map Progression indicated a "likely loss" or "possible loss."

2.3. Visual Field Examination. Each subject underwent standard visual field testing at 1 month and 1 day prior to the operation and at 1 and 3 months after the operation. The visual field testing was performed using static automated white-on-white threshold perimetry (Humphrey Field Analyzer II; Carl Zeiss Meditec, Dublin, CA) with the 30-2 SITA (Swedish Interactive Threshold Algorithm) standard test. Visual fields were only defined as being reliable if the fixation losses and the false-positive and false-negative rates were less than 20%. Only reliable test data were used in our current analyses. When a cluster of three or more points in a pattern deviation plot within a single hemifield with a P value < 5% was observed, it was defined as an abnormal visual field. In accordance with the Anderson and Patella criteria, one of these points had to have a P value < 1% in order to have the data acceptable [13].

The visual field data determined during the series of follow-up examinations were compared to the patients' baseline visual field data using the GPA software. Data from the first two exams were averaged and used for the baseline values, with the progression evaluation performed relative to the baseline. To evaluate the progression, a database of stable glaucoma patients who were tested over a very short period of time was compared to the observed modifications of the threshold. Fluctuations related to the eccentricity and advancing disease were taken into account for all of the evaluations. To determine if progression had occurred, consecutive visual field tests performed at the same locations (≥ 3) were examined. In line with the results of a prior study [14], when 2 locations exhibited progression, the GPA printouts defined this as "possible progression," while "likely progression" was defined when there were 3 locations.

2.4. General Anesthesia Procedures. A standardized anesthesia protocol for the drugs was employed during the surgical procedures, with all patients anesthetized with $2-4\,\mu g/ml$ propofol or 3–5% desflurane. All patients additionally received a continuous infusion of $0.1-1.0\,\mu g/kg/min$ remifentanil in order to maintain the blood pressure, heart rate, and bispectral index. For pain relief, patients were given remifentanil and fentanyl, while rocuronium was used for muscle relaxation. Mechanical ventilation of the lung was used in order to maintain the end-tidal carbon dioxide ($ETCO_2$) concentration at 30–40 mmHg.

A Tono-Pen XL handheld tonometer (Medtronic, Jacksonville, FL) was used to perform the IOP measurements in both eyes of each patient on the day of the operation. Prior to each measurement, the tonometer was calibrated in accordance with the guidelines of the manufacturer. If the variability between sequential measurements exceeded 5%, the measurements were repeated. Measurements of the IOP were performed at 5 min after intubation of the patients who were under systemic anesthesia (T1) and in a supine position, at 6 discrete time points (5, 30, 60, 120, 180, and 240 min; T2-7) after the head was lowered 30 degrees, and at 5 min after returning the patients to a horizontal supine position (T8). The same examiner performed all of the IOP measurements in each subject.

2.5. Statistical Analysis. Dunnett's multiple comparison test was used for all of the data analyses. All statistical analyses were performed using SPSS version 19.0 (IBM, New York, NY). A P value less than 0.05 was considered to be statistically significant. Data are presented as the mean ± standard deviation.

3. Results

Open angles (grade 3 and 4 according to the Shaffer grading system) were observed in all of the patients. After the ophthalmologic examinations, a total of 4 patients with glaucomatous optic disc cupping were excluded. As a result, a total of 40 eyes of 20 subjects, a mean age of 66.9 ± 4.4 years (range, 59 to 72 years), were included in the study. The mean IOP was 15.1 ± 2.0 mmHg at the first visit. The mean visual acuity was -0.09 ± 0.13 log MAR.

Mean operation time was 274.4 ± 52.2 min (range: 196–376 min). Mean blood loss was 173.3 ± 158.9 ml (range: 0–452 ml). Mean blood pressure was $109.7 \pm 12.0/64.5 \pm 9.3$ mmHg at T3, $110.0 \pm 11.8/66.1 \pm 10.5$ mmHg at T4, $111.1 \pm 12.0/67.9 \pm 7.3$ mmHg at T5, $100.3 \pm 15.5/59.7 \pm 10.1$ mmHg at T6, and $101.4 \pm 11.4/58.2 \pm 11.5$ mmHg at T7. Mean IOP was $12.3 \pm$

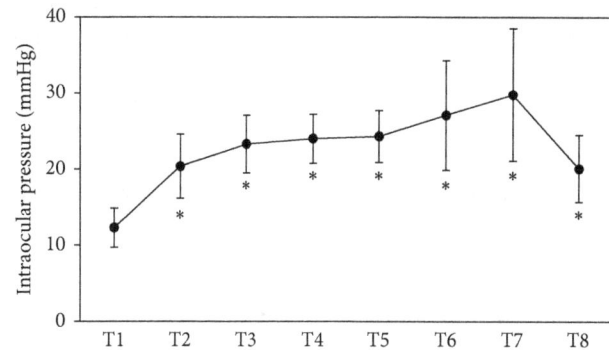

FIGURE 1: Intraocular pressure (IOP) at each time point. IOP was increased during RALP. $^*P < 0.001$ compared with T1.

TABLE 1: Retinal nerve fiber layer thickness and visual field at each measure points.

	Average RNFLT (μm)	P value	Average MD (dB)	P value
1 M before	90.5 ± 10.4		-0.89 ± 1.08	
1 D before	91.0 ± 10.0		-0.85 ± 0.74	
1 M after	91.3 ± 10.2	0.98	-0.54 ± 1.09	0.21
3 M after	91.3 ± 10.2	0.96	-0.40 ± 0.72	0.06

M: month; D: day; RNFLT: retinal nerve fiber layer thickness; MD: mean deviation; P value is compared with 1 D before.

2.6 mmHg (range: 8–21 mmHg; $n = 40$) at T1, 20.4 ± 4.2 mmHg (range: 13–30 mmHg; $n = 40$) at T2, 23.3 ± 3.8 mmHg (range: 16–33 mmHg; $n = 40$) at T3, 24.0 ± 3.2 mmHg (range: 18–30 mmHg; $n = 40$) at T4, 24.3 ± 3.4 mmHg (range: 19–33 mmHg; $n = 38$) at T5, 27.1 ± 7.2 mmHg (range: 20–53 mmHg; $n = 24$) at T6, 29.8 ± 8.7 mmHg (range: 23–49 mmHg; $n = 8$) at T7, and 20.1 ± 4.4 mmHg (range: 12–31 mmHg; $n = 40$) at T8 (Figure 1). IOP was significantly increased at all points (T2-8) as compared to T1 ($P < 0.001$).

No abnormal findings were observed before and after RALP for the peripapillary RNFL thickness. After the RALP, there was no progression observed for the RNFL thickness, with a mean RNFL thickness of $90.5 \pm 10.4\,\mu$m at 1 month before surgery, $91.0 \pm 10.0\,\mu$m at 1 day before surgery, $91.3 \pm 10.2\,\mu$m at 1 month after surgery, and $90.9 \pm 10.2\,\mu$m at 3 months after surgery, respectively (Table 1).

No abnormal findings were observed for the visual fields before and after RALP, and there was no visual field progression after the procedure. Mean deviation (MD) was -0.89 ± 1.08 dB at 1 month before surgery, -0.85 ± 0.74 dB at 1 day before surgery, -0.54 ± 1.09 dB at 1 month after surgery, and -0.40 ± 0.72 dB at 3 months after surgery, respectively (Table 1).

4. Discussion

Despite reports of increases in the IOP during the surgery in normal subjects, our current study demonstrated that there were no changes in the values for the visual field and RNFL thickness observed at 1 month and 1 day prior to the RALP procedure and at 1 and 3 months after the RALP procedure. In addition, we used the GPA software to evaluate the effect of the steep Trendelenburg positioning on the visual structure and function. To the best of our knowledge, this is the first study to use statistical analysis to examine the effect of the steep Trendelenburg positioning on the visual structure and function.

Of particular interest is the significant range of IOP elevation that was noted between the patients for each of the measurement time points. At 180 minutes into the procedure, readings of 20 to 53 mmHg were observed, with 9 of 40 eyes found to be above 30 mmHg during the surgery. None of the patients in this study experienced any ocular complications related to the observed increase in the IOP. However, it should be noted that since this study examined patients with healthy eyes, drastic IOP elevations in individuals with glaucomatous eye would most likely be more severe and could potentially impact the vision.

Taketani et al. previously examined patients without any abnormal findings in their optic nerve head and retina at 1 week after surgery and reported that local visual field defects were detected in 7 of 50 eyes in the lower hemifield, with the visual field eventually recovering to normal within 3 months after the surgery [7]. In the current study, however, we observed a normal visual field in every subject at every measurement time point. Even so, since we did not examine the visual field until 1 month after surgery, the possibility exists that we could have missed some subjects who had an abnormal visual field. Another possible explanation for this discrepancy is that visual field defect might be short-term variability in the study of Taketani et al.

Weber et al. previously reported on the development of posterior ischemic optic neuropathy in a 62-year-old patient who lost 1200 ml of blood during a 6 h 35 min RALP procedure [15]. In the current study, the blood loss in our patients was relatively small (mean of 173 ml and maximum of 452 ml), and there was a relatively short operation time (mean of 274 min and maximum of 376 min). Thus, it could be possible that the visual impairment observed in these types of cases is due to a massive blood loss or longer operation time.

As each patient can have a different blood loss and operation time, it is important to evaluate RNFL thicknesses and the visual field progression. However, in order to determine the progression of the RNFL thickness and visual field in each patient, it is necessary to measure the event analysis at least 4 times or if using trend analysis, then 5 times. To the best of our knowledge, this is the first report that has evaluated the RNFL thicknesses and visual field progression using not only the difference of the mean average before and after the operation but also the difference before and after the operation in each patient.

Glaucoma is a neurodegenerative disease of the optic nerve. Although characterized by accelerated retinal ganglion cell (RGC) death, subsequent axonal loss and optic nerve damage, and eventual visual field loss, patients may present with various stages ranging from undetectable to asymptomatic to symptomatic disease [16]. Kerrigan-Baumrind et al. estimated that, in order for standard automated perimetry (SAP) to determine a statistically significant abnormality, a patient would need to have lost at least 23–35% of their RGCs [17]. Functional changes may be

detected in many patients prior to any structural changes. However, a structural abnormality of the optic nerve head (ONH) and RNFL is observed in many cases and can be used for an earlier detection of the manifestation of glaucoma [18]. As objective quantification of the structural characteristics of the ONH and RNFL is now possible through the use of OCT, it is feasible to detect glaucoma at an early stage [19]. Thus, in order to help better understand the mechanism of this neurodegenerative disease, it is important that further OCT and SAP evaluations of the effect of the steep Trendelenburg positioning on the retinal structure and function be undertaken.

There were a few limitations for our current study. First, we found no deleterious effect on the retinal function and structure at 1 and 3 months after surgery in the eyes of our healthy subjects. However, given the level of IOP elevation and the length of follow-up in the current study, a larger number of subjects with longer follow-ups are required in order to determine the potential risk to ocular health from glaucomatous changes. Another limitation is that glaucoma or ocular hypertension patients were excluded from the analysis in the current study. Previous studies have reported that eyes with glaucoma or ocular hypertension do exhibit greater IOP fluctuations in conjunction with postural changes [20–22]. At the present time, we are yet to discover what effect the steep Trendelenburg positioning has on the retinal structure and function in glaucoma or ocular hypertension patients while undergoing the RALP procedure. Another potential limitation of the current study is that the sample size was small.

In conclusion, we demonstrated that there was a significantly increased IOP during the RALP procedure. Despite this IOP increase, there were no significant postoperative changes in the retinal structure and function and there were no complications observed in patients without preexisting ocular diseases.

Conflicts of Interest

The authors have no conflicts of interest.

Acknowledgments

This work was supported by a Grant-in-Aid for Scientific Research from the Ministry of Education, Culture, Sports, Science, and Technology of Japan (26462689).

References

[1] V. Ficarra, G. Novara, S. Fracalanza et al., "A prospective, nonrandomized trial comparing robot-assisted laparoscopic and retropublic radical prostatectomy in one European institution," *BJU International*, vol. 104, no. 4, pp. 534–539, 2009.

[2] A. Tewari, P. Sooriakumaran, D. A. Bloch, U. Seshadri-Kreaden, A. E. Hebert, and P. Wiklund, "Positive surgical margin and perioperative complication rates of primary surgical treatments

for prostate cancer; a systematic review and meta-analysis comparing retropublic, laparoscopic, and robotic prostatectomy," *European Urology*, vol. 62, no. 1, pp. 1–15, 2012.

[3] A. J. Epstein, P. W. Groeneveld, M. O. Harhay, F. Yang, and D. Polsky, "Impact of minimally invasive surgery on medical spending and employee absenteeism," *JAMA Surgery*, vol. 148, no. 7, pp. 641–647, 2013.

[4] H. Awad, S. Santilli, M. Ohr et al., "The effects of steep Trendelenburg positioning on intraocular pressure during robotic radical prostatectomy," *Anesthesia & Analgesia*, vol. 109, no. 2, pp. 473–478, 2009.

[5] Y. Hoshikawa, N. Tsutsumi, K. Ohkoshi et al., "The effect of steep Trendelenburg positioning on intraocular pressure and visual function during robotic-assisted radical prostatectomy," *British Journal of Ophthalmology*, vol. 98, no. 3, pp. 305–308, 2014.

[6] O. Raz, T. W. Boesel, M. Arianayagam et al., "The effect of the modified Z Trendelenburg position on intraocular pressure during robotic assisted laparoscopic radical prostatectomy: a randomized, controlled study," *Journal of Urology*, vol. 193, no. 4, pp. 1213–1219, 2015.

[7] Y. Taketani, C. Mayama, N. Suzuki et al., "Transient but significant visual field defects after robot-assisted laparoscopic radical prostatectomy in deep Trendelenburg position," *PLoS One*, vol. 10, no. 4, Article ID e0123361, 2015.

[8] T. J. Mondzelewski, J. W. Schmitz, M. S. Christman et al., "Intraocular pressure during robotic-assisted laparoscopic procedures utilizing steep Trendelenburg positioning," *Journal of Glaucoma*, vol. 24, no. 6, pp. 399–404, 2015.

[9] D. M. Bushley, V. C. Parmley, and P. Paglen, "Visual field defect associated with laser in situ keratomileusis," *American Journal of Ophthalmology*, vol. 129, no. 5, pp. 668–671, 2000.

[10] H. S. Weiss, R. S. Rubinfeld, and J. F. Anderschat, "Case reports and small case series: LASIK-associated visual field loss in a glaucoma suspect," *Archives of Ophthalmology*, vol. 119, no. 5, pp. 774–775, 2001.

[11] J. Flammer, S. M. Drance, and M. Zulauf, "Differential light threshold. Short- and long-term fluctuation in patients with glaucoma, normal controls, and patients with suspected glaucoma," *Archives of Ophthalmology*, vol. 102, no. 5, pp. 704–706, 1984.

[12] P. H. Artes, N. O'Leary, M. T. Nicolela, B. C. Chauhan, and D. P. Crabb, "Visual field progression in glaucoma: what is the specificity of the guided progression analysis?," *Ophthalmology*, vol. 121, no. 10, pp. 2023–2027, 2014.

[13] D. R. Anderson and V. M. Patella, *Automated Static Perimetry*, Mosby, St. Louis, MO, USA, 1999.

[14] R. N. Weinreb and P. T. Khaw, "Primary open angle glaucoma," *The Lancet*, vol. 363, no. 9422, pp. 1711–1720, 2004.

[15] E. D. Weber, M. H. Colyer, R. L. Lesser, and P. S. Subramanian, "Posterior ischemic optic neuropathy after minimally invasive prostatectomy," *Journal of Neuro-Ophthalmology*, vol. 27, no. 4, pp. 285–287, 2007.

[16] A. Heijl, M. C. Leske, B. Bengtsson, B. Bengtsson, M. Hussein, and Early Manifest Glaucoma Trial Group, "Measuring visual field progression in the Early Manifest Glaucoma Trial," *Acta Ophthalmologica Scandinavica*, vol. 81, no. 3, pp. 286–293, 2003.

[17] L. A. Kerrigan-Baumrind, H. A. Quigley, M. E. Pease, D. F. Kerrigan, and R. S. Mitchell, "Number of ganglion cells in glaucoma eyes compared with threshold visual field tests in the same persons," *Investigative Ophthalmology and Visual Science*, vol. 41, no. 3, pp. 741–748, 2000.

[18] M. A. Kass, D. K. Heuer, E. J. Higginbotham et al., "The ocular hypertension treatment study: a randomized trial determines that topical ocular hypotensive medication delays or prevents the onset of primary open-angle glaucoma," *Archives of Ophthalmology*, vol. 120, no. 6, pp. 701–713, 2002.

[19] G. J. Jaffe and J. Caprioli, "Optical coherence tomography to detect and manage retinal disease and glaucoma," *American Journal of Ophthalmology*, vol. 137, no. 1, pp. 156–169, 2004.

[20] S. Tsukahara and T. Sasaki, "Postural change of IOP in normal persons and in patients with primary-open angle glaucoma and low-tension glaucoma," *British Journal of Ophthalmology*, vol. 68, no. 6, pp. 389–392, 1984.

[21] K. Hirooka and F. Shiraga, "Relationship between postural change of the intraocular pressure and visual field loss in primary open-angle glaucoma," *Journal of Glaucoma*, vol. 12, no. 4, pp. 379–382, 2003.

[22] T. Kiuchi, Y. Motoyama, and T. Oshika, "Relationship of progression of visual field damage to postural changes in intraocular pressure in patients with normal-tension glaucoma," *Ophthalmology*, vol. 113, no. 12, pp. 2150–2155, 2006.

Comparison of Visual Outcome and Morphologic Change between Different Surgical Techniques in Idiopathic Epiretinal Membrane Surgery

Yo-Chen Chang ⓘ,[1,2,3] Chia-Ling Lee,[1] Kuo-Jen Chen ⓘ,[3] Li-Yi Chiu ⓘ,[1] Tzu-En Kao ⓘ,[1] Pei-Kang Liu ⓘ,[1,4] Kwou-Yeung Wu ⓘ,[1,2] and Wen-Chuan Wu ⓘ[1,2]

[1]Department of Ophthalmology, Kaohsiung Medical University Hospital, Kaohsiung 80708, Taiwan
[2]Department of Ophthalmology, School of Medicine, Kaohsiung Medical University, Kaohsiung 80708, Taiwan
[3]Department of Ophthalmology, Kaohsiung Municipal Hsiao-Kang Hospital, Kaohsiung Medical University, Kaohsiung 81267, Taiwan
[4]Department of Ophthalmology, Yuan's General Hospital, Kaohsiung, Taiwan

Correspondence should be addressed to Wen-Chuan Wu; wcwu.oph@gmail.com

Academic Editor: Marcel Menke

Purpose. To investigate the morphological and functional outcomes of idiopathic epiretinal membrane (ERM) surgery between three different surgical techniques: ERM peeling only, whole-piece ILM peeling, and maculorrhexis ILM peeling. *Patients and Methods.* This is a retrospective, consecutive, and comparative study enrolling 60 patients from Kaohsiung Medical University Hospital, Kaohsiung, Taiwan. Surgery performed between July 2011 and June 2012 was done with ERM peeling only (group I). ERM peeling and ILM peeling as a whole piece (group II) were performed between July 2012 and July 2013. Surgery performed between August 2013 and December 2014 was done with maculorrhexis ILM peeling (group III). Main outcome measures include visual acuity change (BCVA) and central foveal thickness (CFT). *Results.* At 12 months postoperation, the mean BCVA in group III was significantly better than in group I and group II. Comparison of CFT reduction between the three groups revealed significantly more reduction in group III than in group II at all postoperative follow-up periods. Eyes with restoration of foveal depression were observed in 52.6% in group I, 52.4% in group III, but only 20% of eyes in group II. None of the eyes in both ILM peeling groups encountered recurrence of macular pucker formation. *Conclusion.* All three techniques can achieve visual acuity improvement and macular thickness reduction. Maculorrhexis ILM peeling achieves more rapid improvement of visual function, better final visual outcome, and a higher rate of normal foveal contour than whole-piece ILM peeling.

1. Introduction

Idiopathic epiretinal membrane (ERM) is a disorder occurring in the vitreomacular interface that can cause visual impairment [1]. The clinical manifestation of an ERM can be completely asymptomatic or profoundly symptomatic with metamorphopsia, micropsia or macropsia, decreased visual acuity (VA), and loss of central vision. In 1978, Machemer first applied pars plana vitrectomy (PPV) and membrane peeling to remove ERM. From now on, it has become a well-established procedure for the removal of ERM with good results [2]. Surgical removal of the

membranes in symptomatic patients can reduce metamorphopsia and improve visual acuity in approximately 70–90% of cases [3–5]. However, the recurrence of ERM has been reported in 10% to 21% of eyes with membrane peeling [6–8]. The possible pathogenesis of ERM regrowth is thought to be due to incomplete ERM removal and the presence of residual myofibroblasts [9, 10]. Recently, in order to prevent the recurrence of ERM, internal limiting membrane (ILM) peeling has been applied in ERM surgery. Compared with ERM peeling only, conventional whole-piece ILM peeling after ERM peeling can achieve comparable visual improvement and reduced ERM recurrence [11, 12]. However,

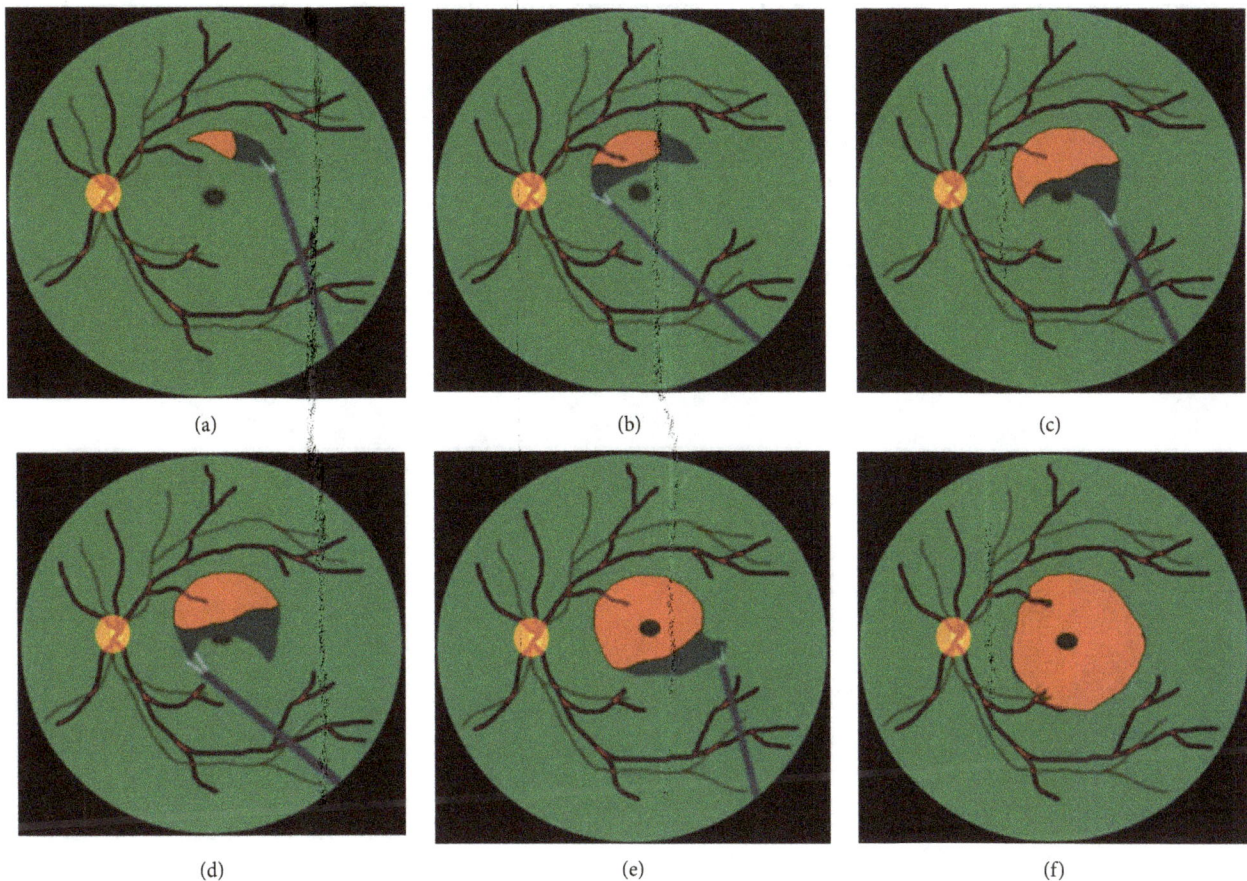

FIGURE 1: Schematic drawing of whole-piece internal limiting membrane (ILM) peeling. (a) After indocyanine green (ICG) staining, first create an ILM flap with 25-gauge forceps near the vascular arcade. (b, c) Expand the flap from both sides. (d, e) Peel off the ILM as a large whole piece passing through the fovea. (f) Constantly adjust the force to keep the flap large enough and prevent its immature rupture near the fovea.

remaining thickened macula postoperatively and formation of postoperative central or eccentric macular hole have been reported [11, 13]. In order to prevent the above complications, we used a modification of ILM peeling technique named "maculorrhexis ILM peeling" to improve the surgical outcome for patients with ERM.

2. Patients and Methods

The present study is a retrospective, consecutive case series. Between January 2012 and December 2014, we enrolled patients who were diagnosed as idiopathic ERM. The research adhered to the tenets of the Declaration of Helsinki 1964. Spectral-domain optical coherence tomography (SD-OCT; Heidelberg Retina Angiograph 2, Heidelberg Engineering, Heidelberg, Germany) was used to confirm the presence of ERM. Patients with the history of ocular diseases (i.e., retinal vascular occlusion, high myopia, glaucoma, neoplastic, or chronic inflammatory disorders), cases with spontaneous peeling of ILM during ERM peeling, and those with systemic diseases (uncontrolled hypertension or diabetes) were excluded. Preoperatively, a complete ophthalmic and medical history was obtained, and a detailed examination including best-corrected visual acuity (BCVA) measured by Snellen chart, intraocular pressure, fundus examination by fundus photography, indirect binocular ophthalmoscopy, and SD-OCT was performed. All patients underwent 25-gauge PPV and epiretinal membrane peeling assisted with triamcinolone and high-magnification viewing system. If the posterior vitreous detachment (PVD) was not already present, it was induced by active suction of ocutome above the optic disc. Surgeries before July 2012 were done with PPV and ERM peeling only. Indocyanine green- (ICG-) assisted ILM peeling as a whole piece was performed after ERM peeling between July 2012 and July 2013 (Figure 1). Surgeries after July 2013 were performed with the newly developed maculorrhexis ILM peeling technique (Figure 2) [14]. For eyes undergoing ILM peeling, an intravitreal injection with indocyanine green, which was mixed as per the bottle instructions with sterile water then diluted in a 1:24 ratio with 5% glucose water, was performed to make the internal limiting membrane (ILM) more visible. Concomitant cataract surgery was performed on phakic patients. After surgery, comprehensive ophthalmic examination including SD-OCT was performed 1, 3, 6, 9, and 12 months postoperatively. For better comparison of visual outcome between the groups, the visual acuity measured at preoperative and each postoperative follow-up visit was converted to the logarithm of the minimum angle of resolution (logMAR).

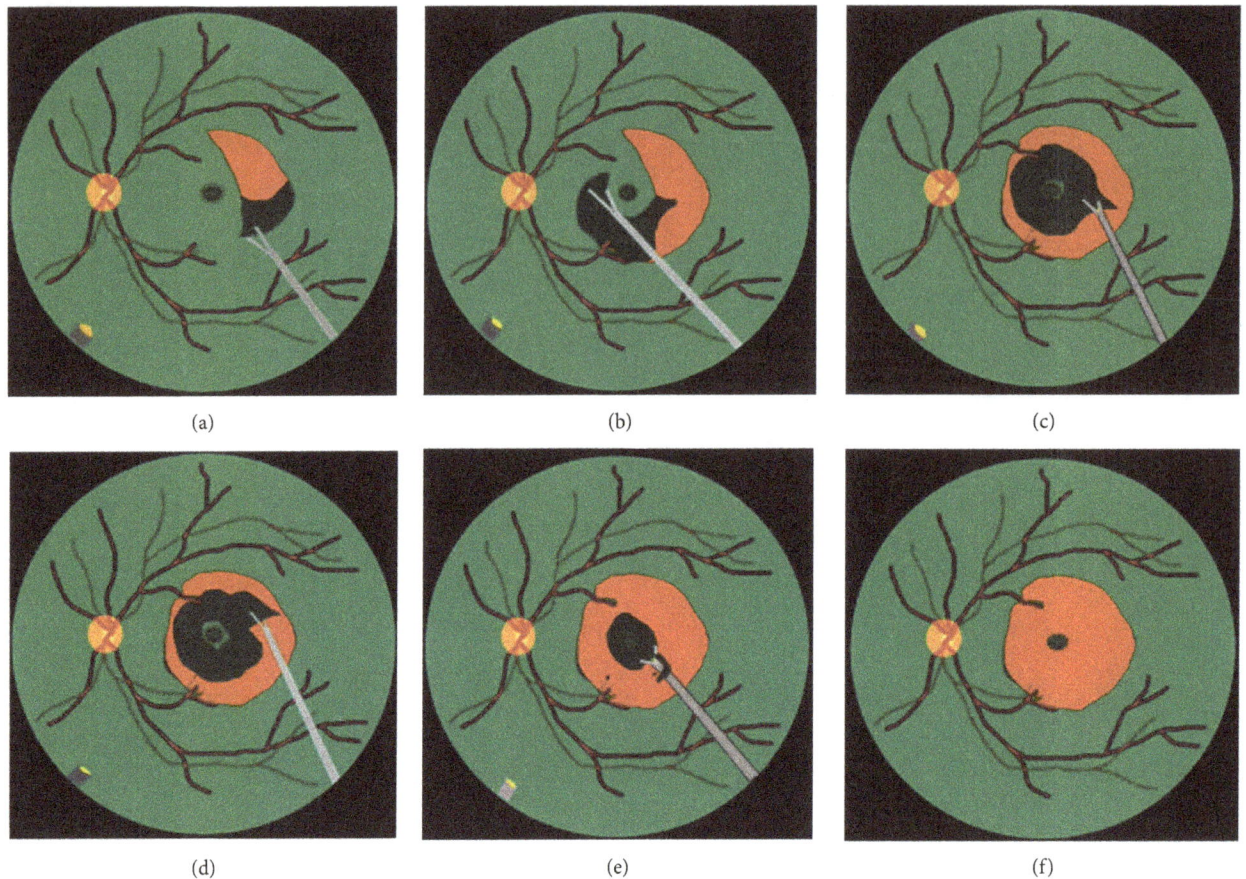

FIGURE 2: Schematic drawing of maculorrhexis ILM peeling. (a) After ICG staining, first create an ILM flap with 25-gauge forceps near the vascular arcade. (b) Proceed with ILM peeling in a circular fashion, caution must be taken not to peel off the central foveal area. (c, d, e) After finishing peeling of peripheral round of ILM, paracentral ILM was also gently peeled in a circular fashion. (f) When the circle is nearly complete, the ILM on the fovea is peeled off gently.

2.1. Statistical Analysis. All data were analyzed by the Fisher's exact test and Student's *t*-test, using SPSS statistical software (version 13.0; SPSS Inc., Chicago, IL, USA). A difference at $p < 0.05$ was considered to be statistically significant.

3. Results

3.1. Preoperative Demographic Data. A total of 60 eyes in 60 patients were included in the present study. The mean age was 64.4 ± 7.6 years. There were 19 eyes that underwent ERM removal only (group I), 20 eyes underwent ERM removal and whole-piece ILM peeling (group II), and 21 eyes underwent ERM removal with maculorrhexis ILM peeling (group III). Eight eyes in group I, 8 eyes in group II, and 10 eyes in group III were phakic prior to surgery. The mean preoperative logMAR BCVA and central foveal thickness (CFT) for the total 60 eyes were 0.79 ± 0.42 and $491.5 \pm 114.8\,\mu m$, respectively. The major characteristics for these three groups were similar and without significant difference. The patient details for group I, group II, and group III are listed in Table 1.

3.2. Temporal Change of CFT. The mean preoperative CFT was $480.7 \pm 102.6\,\mu m$ for group I, $501.7 \pm 132.7\,\mu m$ for group II, and $491.4 \pm 111.6\,\mu m$ for group III (Table 1). Significant

differences in CFT were not found between these three groups. The mean CFT at 1 month after surgery decreased by 115.1 ± 99.8 to $365.6 \pm 113.3\,\mu m$ for group I, by only 44.3 ± 98.3 to $457.4 \pm 86\,\mu m$ for group II, and by 137.0 ± 100.4 to $354.5 \pm 64.8\,\mu m$ for group III, ($p = 0.007$, group I versus group II; $p < 0.001$, group II versus group III; $p = 0.7$, group I versus group III). At 6 months, the mean CFT decreased by 154.5 ± 93.9 to $326.2 \pm 63.3\,\mu m$ for group I, by 137.1 ± 112.4 to $364.6 \pm 82.2\,\mu m$ for group II, and by 206.3 ± 118.6 to $285.1 \pm 32.0\,\mu m$ for group III ($p = 0.112$, group I versus group II; $p < 0.001$ group II versus group III; $p = 0.012$ group I versus group III). At 12 months, the mean CFT decreased by 174.6 ± 107.7 to $306.1 \pm 71.5\,\mu m$ for group I, by 163.1 ± 121.1 to $338.6 \pm 73.8\,\mu m$ for group II, and by 228.7 ± 115.9 to $262.7 \pm 25.7\,\mu m$ for group III ($p = 0.171$, group I versus group II; $p < 0.001$, group II versus group III; $p = 0.013$, group I versus group III). The CFT differed significantly between group I and group II at 1 and 3 months after surgery ($p < 0.05$). The mean CFT was significantly higher in group II than it was in group III at 1, 3, 6, 9, and 12 months of follow-up. The mean change in CFT and mean CFT over the course after surgery was shown in Figure 3.

3.3. Temporal Change of Visual Acuity. Before surgery, the mean BCVA was 0.79 ± 0.40, 0.82 ± 0.48, and 0.77 ± 0.39

TABLE 1: Preoperative demographics of patients in three groups.

	Total ($n = 60$)	Group I ($n = 19$)	Group II ($n = 20$)	Group III ($n = 21$)	p I versus II	p II versus III	p I versus III
Age (yrs)	64.4 ± 7.6	65.7 ± 7.4	64.0 ± 8.1	63.4 ± 7.4	0.489	0.815	0.329
M/F	25/35	8/11	9/11	8/13	1.000	0.756	1.000
Phakia	26 (43.3%)	8 (42.1%)	8 (40%)	10 (47.6%)	1.000	0.756	0.761
LogMAR	0.79 ± 0.42	0.80 ± 0.40	0.82 ± 0.48	0.77 ± 0.40	0.859	0.700	0.827
CFT (μm)	491.5 ± 114.8	480.1 ± 102.6	501.7 ± 13.27	491.4 ± 111.6	0.585	0.790	0.754

CFT: central foveal thickness; ERM: epiretinal membrane; F: female; Group I: ERM removal without ILM peeling; Group II: ERM removal and whole-piece ILM peeling; Group III: ERM removal and maculorrhexis ILM peeling; ILM: internal limiting membrane; LogMAR: logarithm of the minimum angle of resolution; M: male; yrs: years.

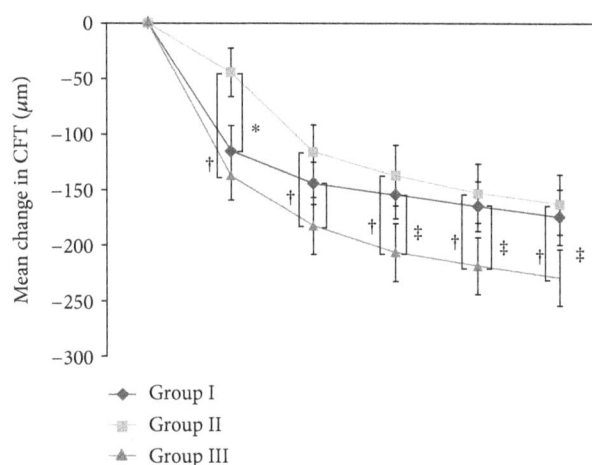

		Follow-up (months)				
	Baseline	1 M	3 M	6 M	9 M	12 M
CFT of group I	480.7	365.6	336.6	326.2	315.7	306.1
CFT of group II	501.7	457.4	385.9	364.6	348.6	338.6
CFT of group III	491.4	354.5	309.0	285.1	273.2	262.7
P (I versus II)	0.585	*0.007*	*0.044*	0.112	0.166	0.171
P (II versus III)	0.790	*<0.001*	*<0.001*	*<0.001*	*<0.001*	*<0.001*
P (I versus III)	0.754	0.702	0.108	*0.012*	*0.011*	*0.012*

FIGURE 3: Temporal change of central foveal thickness (CFT) postoperatively. The reduction in CFT differed significantly between group I and group II during the first month after surgery. The reduction in CFT differed significantly between group II and group III at 1, 3, 6, 9, and 12 months of follow-up. The table below the graph shows the absolute values of the mean CFT for each follow-up visit (group I: ERM removal without ILM peeling; group II: ERM removal and whole-piece ILM peeling; group III: ERM removal and maculorrhexis ILM peeling; * indicates $p < 0.05$ compared between group I and group II at each follow-up visit; † indicates $p < 0.05$ compared between group II and group III at each follow-up visit; ‡ indicates $p < 0.05$ compared between group I and group III at each follow-up visit).

logMAR in group I, group II, and group III, respectively. The preoperative BCVA was similar, and no significant difference between these three patient groups was observed (Table 1). In all three groups, the BCVA improved significantly postoperatively. At 1 month, the line improvement increased by 2.9 ± 3.4, 1.1 ± 3.2, and 3.1 ± 3.0 lines from preoperation in group I, group II, and group III, respectively ($p = 0.094$, group I versus group II; $p = 0.841$, group I versus group III; $p = 0.049$, group II versus group III). At 6 months, the mean line improvement increased by 3.8 ± 4.0, 4.8 ± 3.8, and 5.3 ± 3.6 lines from preoperation in group I, group II, and group III, respectively. At 12 months, the mean BCVA was increased by 4.0 ± 4.3, 5.2 ± 4.2, and 6.1 ± 3.3 lines from preoperation

in group I, group II, and group III, respectively. At 12 months, the mean logMAR BCVA improved to 0.39 ± 0.43, 0.30 ± 0.13, and 0.16 ± 0.27 in group I, group II, and group III, respectively. ($p = 0.403$, group I versus group II; $p = 0.048$, group I versus group III; $p = 0.041$, group II versus group III). The logMAR BCVA in group III was significantly better than that in group I and group II at 12 months postoperatively. Figure 4 illustrates the line improvement in BCVA and mean logMAR BCVA of these three groups over the course of the study.

3.4. Morphology of Fovea and Recurrence of Epiretinal Membrane. We defined a normal foveal contour on OCT as

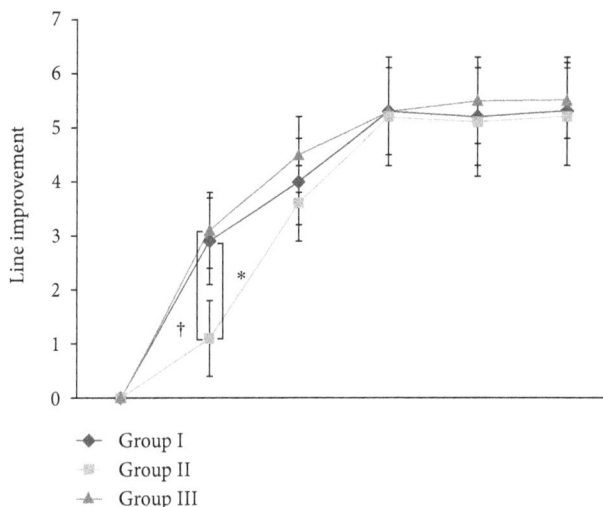

LogMAR BCVA	Follow-up (months)					
	Baseline	1 M	3 M	6 M	9 M	12 M
Group I	0.79	0.51	0.39	0.42	0.40	0.39
Group II	0.82	0.71	0.46	0.35	0.32	0.30
Group III	0.77	0.46	0.32	0.24	0.20	0.16
P between I & II	0.859	0.101	0.550	0.315	0.360	0.403
P between II & II	0.700	0.060	0.168	0.267	0.136	0.041
P between I & II	0.827	0.679	0.498	0.184	0.084	0.048

FIGURE 4: Temporal change of BCVA by line after surgery. At 1 month, the mean line improvement increased more rapidly in group I and group III than in group II. However, 6 months and thereafter, the postoperative line improvement and BCVA were similar and became stable in all three groups. The table below the graph shows the absolute value of the mean logMAR BCVA for each follow-up visit (Group I: ERM removal without ILM peeling; Group II: ERM removal and whole-piece ILM peeling; Group III: ERM removal with maculorrhexis ILM peeling; * indicates $p < 0.05$ compared between group I and group II at each follow-up visit; † indicates $p < 0.05$ compared between group II and group III at each follow-up visit).

TABLE 2: Postoperative morphology of macula by SD-OCT.

	Group I number of eyes (%)	Group II number of eyes (%)	Group III number of eyes (%)	p I versus II	p II versus III	p I versus III
With foveal depression	10 (52.6%)	4 (20%)	11 (52.4%)	0.047	0.048	1.000
DONFL formation	0 (0%)	10 (50%)	7 (33.3%)	0.001	0.444	0.019
ERM recurrence	4 (21.1%)	0 (0%)	0 (0%)	0.047	1.000	0.042

DONFL: dissociated optic nerve fiber layer; ERM: epiretinal membrane; Group I: ERM removal without ILM peeling; Group II: ERM removal and whole-piece ILM peeling; Group III: ERM removal and ILM maculorrhexis; ILM: internal limiting membrane; SD-OCT: spectral-domain optical coherence tomography.

the retinal thickness at the center of the fovea was 50 μm or more thinner than that of the retina 1 mm away from the foveola, accompanied by a foveal depression without evident intraretinal edema [11]. At 12 months postoperation, normal foveal contour with a foveal depression was found in 10 eyes (52.6%) in group I, only 4 eyes (20%) in group II, and 11 eyes (52.4%) in group III (Table 2). Two representative cases are illustrated in Figures 5 and 6. A dissociated optic nerve fiber layer (DONFL) appearance is defined as arcuate retinal striae along the optic nerve fibers in the macular region, which is slightly darker than the surrounding retina [15]. Postoperative occurrence of DONFL was found in none of the eyes in group I, 10 eyes (50%) in group II, and 7 eyes (33.3%) in

group III (Table 2). The external limiting membrane (ELM) and ellipsoid zone (EZ) were evaluated in all three groups. In the preoperative assessment, preservation of ELM was observed in 11 eyes (57.9%) in group I, 13 eyes (65%) in group II, and 13 eyes (61.9%) in group III, respectively. At one month postoperatively, numbers of eyes with intact ELM were still 11 eyes (57.9%) in group I, slightly decreased to 10 eyes in group II, and still 13 eyes (61.9%) in group III. Thereafter, the numbers of eyes with intact ELM continued to increase. At 6 months, preservation of ELM was observed in 19 eyes (100%) in group I, 18 eyes (90%) in group II, and 21 eyes (100%) in group III, respectively. All eyes in group II with intact ELM were observed at 9 months postoperatively

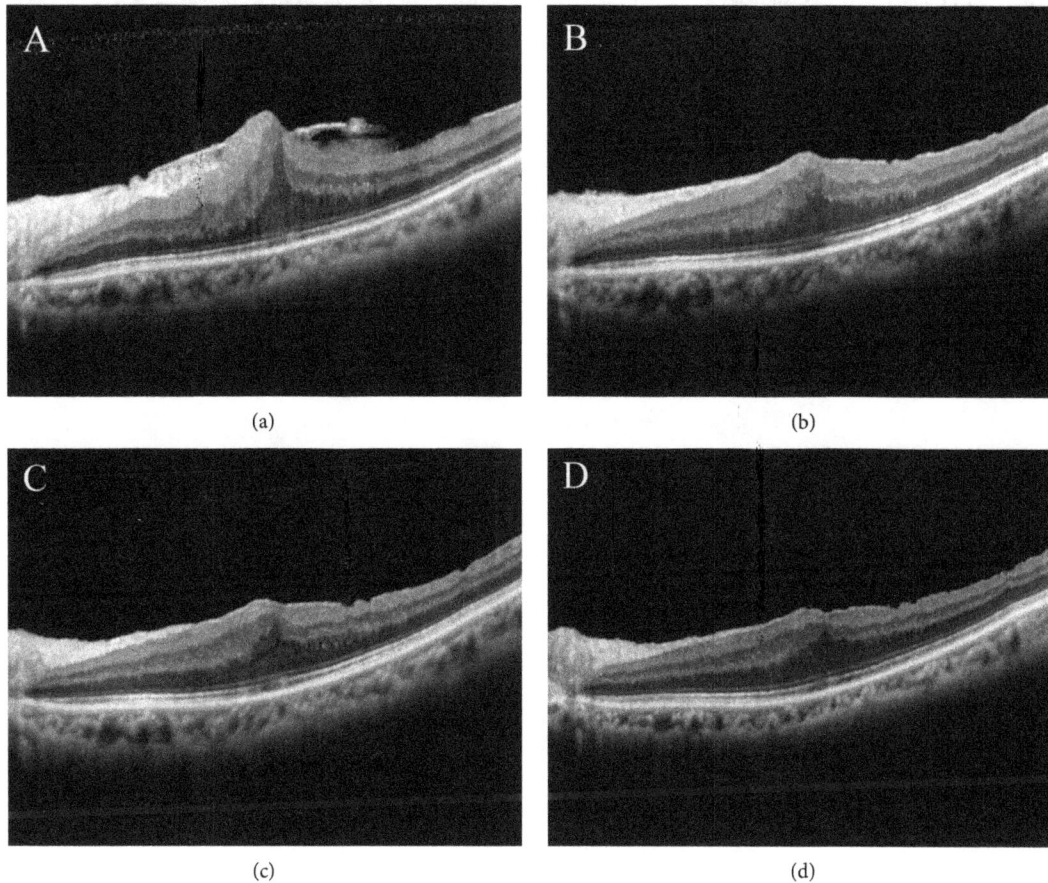

FIGURE 5: Pre- and postoperative OCT findings in a patient with ERM receiving vitrectomy, membrane peeling, and whole-piece internal limiting membrane peeling. Preoperative image shows an ERM overlying the macula. The CFT and BCVA were 659 μm and 20/100, respectively (a). The CFT decreased to 484 μm one month postoperatively (b). At six months after operation, the CFT was 422 μm (c). At 12 months after operation, the CFT decreased to 382 μm and the BCVA improved to 20/30. However, foveal depression was not observed (d).

(Table 3). With regard to EZ, 12 eyes (63.2%) in group I, 13 eyes (65%) in group II, and 14 eyes (66.7%) in group III showed a normal EZ preoperatively. At 1 month after surgery, still 12 eyes (63.2%) in group I, slightly decreased to 10 eyes (50%) in group II, and still 14 eyes (66.7%) in group III showed intact EZ. At 9 months, preservation of ELM was observed in 19 eyes (100%) in group I, 18 eyes (90%) in group II, and 21 eyes (100%) in group III, respectively. At 12 months, preservation of EZ was observed in all eyes in these three groups (Table 3). ERM recurrence is defined as OCT-based evidence of macular pucker formation. Using this definition, a recurrence within 12 months following surgery was found in 4/19 eyes (21.1%) in group I. However, none of the eyes in group II or group III showed evidence of recurrent ERM during the follow-up period (Table 2).

4. Discussion

For patients with symptomatic ERM, pars plana vitrectomy with membrane peeling is a useful technique, and favorable outcome can be achieved in most patients [2–6]. Nevertheless, the recurrence of ERM has been reported in 10% to 21% of eyes with membrane peeling [6–8]. In recent years, conventional whole-piece ILM peeling after ERM peeling

can achieve comparable visual improvement and reduced ERM recurrence [11, 12]. Nevertheless, remaining thickened macula postoperatively has been reported [11, 13].

According to our results, the CFT decreased significantly after surgery in all three groups. In the early postoperative period, the CFT decreased relatively slowly and the mean CFT was significantly higher in eyes undergoing whole-piece ILM peeling compared to eyes undergoing maculorrhexis ILM peeling. Furthermore, postoperative OCT showed that loss of the normal foveal contour with macular thickening was more frequently seen in the whole-piece ILM peeling group than it was in the maculorrhexis ILM peeling group and ERM peeling-alone group. The reason for this finding in the present study remains unclear. The possible explanation may be due to the impact on Müller cells by different ILM peeling methods. The outer portion of the ILM is built by the Müller cell footplates. During ILM peeling, the Müller cell footplates might suffer some degree of damage. In addition, in the foveola, the specialized Müller cell formed an inverted cone-shaped zone that constitutes the base of the fovea, serves as a plug that binds the photoreceptor cells, and gives support for the structure [16, 17]. Furthermore, the Müller cells also maintain the arrangement of nerve fiber bundles being close to each other [18]. Therefore,

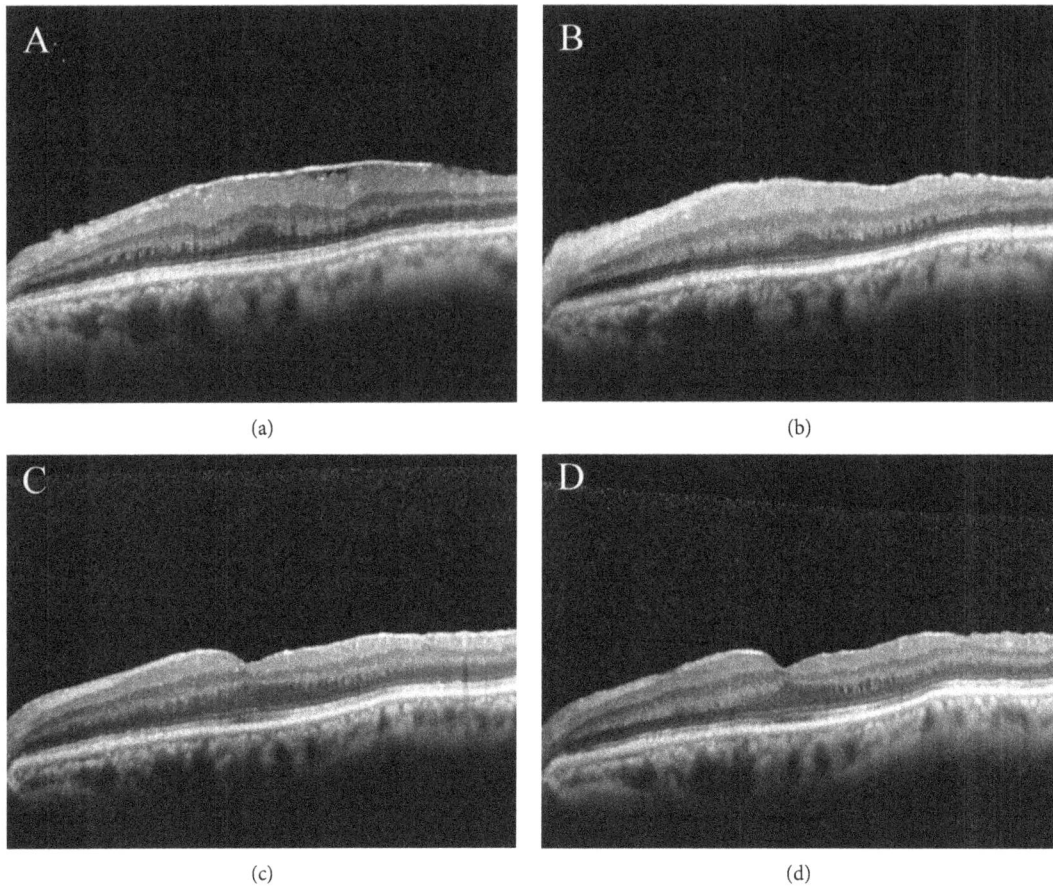

(a)

(b)

(c)

(d)

FIGURE 6: Pre- and postoperative OCT findings in a patient with ERM receiving vitrectomy, membrane peeling, and maculorrhexis ILM peeling. Preoperative image shows an ERM overlying the macula. The CFT and BCVA were 448 μm and 20/80, respectively (a). The CFT decreased to 425 μm one month postoperatively (b). At six months after operation, the CFT was 306 μm and foveal depression was observed (c). At 12 months after operation, the foveal depression still remained. The CFT further decreased to 289 μm, and the BCVA improved to 20/20 (d).

TABLE 3: Pre- and postoperative characteristics of ELM and EZ.

	Baseline		1 M		3 M		6 M		9 M		12 M	
	ELM(+)	EZ(+)	ELM(+)	EZ(+)	ELM(+)	EZ(+)	ELM(+)	EZ(+)	ELM(+)	EZ(+)	ELM(+)	EZ(+)
I (19)	11	12	11	12	15	14	19	17	19	19	19	19
II (20)	13	13	10	10	14	14	18	17	20	18	20	20
III (21)	13	14	13	14	16	16	21	19	21	21	21	21
p value												
I versus II	0.899	0.905	0.863	0.613	0.785	0.798	0.491	0.676	1	0.491	1	1
II versus III	0.837	0.88	0.651	0.444	0.925	0.925	0.447	0.954	1	0.447	1	1
I versus III	0.7986	0.816	0.796	0.816	0.835	0.855	1	0.916	1	1	1	1

ELM(+): preservation of external limiting membrane; EZ(+): preservation of ellipsoid zone; Group I: ERM removal without ILM peeling; Group II: ERM removal and whole-piece ILM peeling; Group III: ERM removal and ILM maculorrhexis; M: month.

ILM peeling may cause loss of structural support in the fovea and may lead to damage to the nerve fibers. In order to reduce damage to the retina, especially to the Müller cells, we developed maculorrhexis ILM peeling where the ILM is grasped away from the central fovea and peeled off in a circular fashion which is parallel to the arrangement of nerve fiber bundle. We believe that by using this method, the shearing on Müller cells can be decreased and therefore remodeling of the intraretinal structure might be facilitated.

Many investigators have made a lot of efforts to determine etiologies of macular DONFL after ILM peeling. In the present study, postoperative DONFL was observed in none of the eyes in group I, 10 eyes (50%) in group II, and 7 eyes (33.3%) in group III. Our results suggest that this characteristic appearance was related to ILM peeling itself. Ito et al. reported that DONFL occurred in 50% of eyes with ILM peeling and they found that no functional abnormalities were observed, suggesting that DONFL was probably due to a dehiscence of the nerve fiber layer rather than a true defect of nerve fiber [19].

In our study, the integrity of the outer retina was assessed by SD-OCT. In the first month, compared to preoperative data, the number of eyes with intact ELM and EZ was decreased in group II while the number of eyes with intact ELM and EZ remained static in group I and group III. However, these two layers recovered over time and were fully recovered in all patients of three groups after 12 months. De Novelli et al. found that in the first month, in the group that had the ILM removed, there was an increase in the discontinuity of the EZ. They postulated that conventional removal of the ILM may cause additional surgical trauma [20]. However, by using maculorrhexis ILM peeling method, the number of eyes with intact ELM and EZ wasn't decreased at one month postoperatively. The reason for this finding maybe due to the ILM peeling method of circular fashion might place less damaging tension on retina.

In the present study, the recurrence of ERM is significantly lower in patients undergoing ILM peeling compared with those without ILM peeling. From literature review, recurrence of ERM ranges from 10% to 56% after the removal of ERM alone and from 0% to 9% after peeling of both the ERM and ILM [8, 21–23]. When the ILM persists after ERM peeling, this residual ILM acts as a scaffold for cell proliferation leading to ERM recurrence [24]. Therefore, we believe that ILM peeling could not only eliminate residual ERM but also remove the scaffold allowing proliferation of myofibroblasts.

According to our present results, there were significant improvements of BCVA in the ERM peeling only (group I), whole-piece ILM peeling (group II), and the maculorrhexis ILM peeling (group III) groups after ERM surgery. One month postoperatively, the line improvement of BCVA in group I and group III was similar with 2.9 and 3.1 lines, respectively. Both groups were superior to only 1.1 line improvement in group II. We postulate that the early rapid visual improvement in eyes undergoing maculorrhexis ILM peeling might be due to fewer insults to retinal structure. At 12 months postoperation, the BCVA in group III was significantly better than in group I and group II. Previous studies also showed both ERM peeling only and ILM peeling can achieve significant and similar visual improvement postoperatively [22, 25, 26]. Our results were consistent with theirs. However, even better visual outcome can be achieved by using maculorrhexis ILM peeling method.

In summary, our preliminary data of combined 25-gauge vitrectomy, ERM peeling, and ICG-assisted maculorrhexis ILM peeling showed relatively rapid improvement of visual function, better final visual outcome, and normal foveal contour and avoid recurrence of macular pucker in patients with idiopathic ERM. The limitation of our study included relative small number of patients and no randomization. Therefore, these results had to be confirmed by a large prospective and randomized trial.

Disclosure

This paper was presented in part at the 31st Asia-Pacific Academy of Ophthalmology Congress (APAO 2016) in March 2016, Taipei, Taiwan.

Conflicts of Interest

None of the authors have proprietary interest in any material used in this study.

Acknowledgments

The authors are thankful for the help from the Statistical Analysis Laboratory, Department of Medical Research, Kaohsiung Medical University Hospital, Kaohsiung Medical University.

References

[1] T. M. Johnson and M. W. Johnson, "Epiretinal membrane," in *Ophthalmology, Ed 3*, M. Yanoff and J. S. Duker, Eds., pp. 686-687, Elsevier, Netherlands, 2004.

[2] R. Machemer, "The surgical removal of epiretinal macular membranes," *Klinische Monatsblätter für Augenheilkunde*, vol. 173, no. 1, pp. 36–42, 1973.

[3] R. R. Margherio, M. S. Cox Jr, M. T. Trese, P. L. Murphy, J. Johnson, and L. A. Minor, "Removal of epimacular membranes," *Ophthalmology*, vol. 92, no. 8, pp. 1075–1083, 1985.

[4] S. de Bustros, J. T. Thompson, R. G. Michels, T. A. Rice, and B. M. Glaser, "Vitrectomy for idiopathic epiretinal membranes causing macular pucker," *British Journal of Ophthalmology*, vol. 72, no. 9, pp. 692–695, 1988.

[5] P. Y. Lee, K. C. Cheng, and W. C. Wu, "Anatomic and functional outcome after surgical removal of idiopathic macular epiretinal membrane," *The Kaohsiung Journal of Medical Sciences*, vol. 27, no. 7, pp. 268–275, 2011.

[6] R. Grewing and U. Mester, "Results of surgery for epiretinal membranes and their recurrences," *British Journal of Ophthalmology*, vol. 80, no. 4, pp. 323–326, 1996.

[7] G. Donati, A. D. Kapetanios, and C. J. Pournaras, "Complications of surgery for epiretinal membranes," *Graefe's Archive for Clinical and Experimental Ophthalmology*, vol. 236, no. 10, pp. 739–746, 1998.

[8] D. W. Park, P. U. Dugel, J. Garda et al., "Macular pucker removal with and without internal limiting membrane peeling: pilot study," *Ophthalmology*, vol. 110, no. 1, pp. 62–64, 2003.

[9] C. P. Wilkinson, "Recurrent macular pucker," *American Journal of Ophthalmology*, vol. 88, no. 6, pp. 1029–1031, 1979.

[10] A. M. Maguire, W. E. Smiddy, S. K. Nanda, R. G. Michels, Z. de la Cruz, and W. Richard Green, "Clinicopathologic correlation of recurrent epiretinal membranes after previous surgical removal," *Retina*, vol. 10, no. 3, pp. 213–222, 1990.

[11] J. W. Lee and I. T. Kim, "Outcomes of idiopathic macular epiretinal membrane removal with and without internal limiting membrane peeling: a comparative study," *Japanese Journal of Ophthalmology*, vol. 54, no. 2, pp. 129–134, 2010.

[12] J. J. Jung, Q. V. Hoang, M. L. Ridley-Lane, D. B. Sebrow, E. Dhrami-Gavazi, and S. Chang, "Long-term retrospective analysis of visual acuity and optical coherence topographic changes after single versus double peeling during vitrectomy

for macular epiretinal membranes," *Retina*, vol. 36, no. 11, pp. 2101–2109, 2016.

[13] F. Amouyal, S. U. Shah, C. K. Pan, S. D. Schwartz, and J. P. Hubschman, "Morphologic features and evolution of inner retinal dimples on optical coherence tomography after internal limiting membrane peeling," *Retina*, vol. 34, no. 10, pp. 2096–2102, 2014.

[14] C. L. Lee, W. C. Wu, K. J. Chen, L. Y. Chiu, K. Y. Wu, and Y. C. Chang, "Modified internal limiting membrane peeling technique (maculorrhexis) for myopic foveoschisis surgery," *Acta Ophthalmologica*, vol. 95, no. 2, pp. e128–e131, 2017.

[15] R. Gelman, W. Stevenson, C. P. Ponce, D. Agarwal, and J. B. Christoforidis, "Retinal damage induced by internal limiting membrane removal," *Journal of Ophthalmology*, vol. 2015, Article ID 939748, 10 pages, 2015.

[16] E. Yamda, "Some structural features of the fovea centralis in the human retina," *Archives of Ophthalmology*, vol. 82, no. 2, pp. 151–159, 1969.

[17] J. D. M. Gass, "Müller cell cone, an overlooked part of the anatomy of the fovea centralis: hypotheses concerning its role in the pathogenesis of macular hole and foveomacular retinoschisis," *Archives of Ophthalmology*, vol. 117, no. 6, pp. 821–823, 1999.

[18] H. Holländer, F. Makarov, Z. Dreher, D. van Driel, T. Chan-Ling, and J. Stone, "Structure of the macroglia of the retina: sharing and division of labour between astrocytes and Müller cells," *Journal of Comparative Neurology*, vol. 313, no. 4, pp. 587–603, 1991.

[19] Y. Ito, H. Terasaki, A. Takahashi, T. Yamakoshi, M. Kondo, and M. Nakamura, "Dissociated optic nerve fiber layer appearance after internal limiting membrane peeling for idiopathic macular holes," *Ophthalmology*, vol. 112, no. 8, pp. 1415–1420, 2005.

[20] F. J. De Novelli, M. Goldbaum, M. L. R. Monteiro, F. B. Aggio, and W. Y. Takahashi, "Surgical removal of epiretinal membrane with and without removal of internal limiting membrane: comparative study of visual acuity, features of optical coherence tomography, and recurrence rate," *Retina*, p. 1, 2017.

[21] R. Sorcinelli, "Surgical management of epiretinal membrane with indocyanine-green-assisted peeling," *Ophthalmologica*, vol. 217, no. 2, pp. 107–110, 2003.

[22] A. K. H. Kwok, T. Y. Y. Lai, and K. S. C. Yuen, "Epiretinal membrane surgery with or without internal limiting membrane peeling," *Clinical & Experimental Ophthalmology*, vol. 33, no. 4, pp. 379–385, 2005.

[23] H. S. Walia, G. K. Shah, and S. M. Hariprasad, "ILM peeling a vital intervention for many vitreoretinal disorders," *Ophthalmic Surgery, Lasers and Imaging Retina*, vol. 45, no. 2, pp. 92–96, 2014.

[24] H. Shimada, H. Nakashizuka, T. Hattori, R. Mori, Y. Mizutani, and M. Yuzawa, "Double staining with brilliant blue G and double peeling for epiretinal membranes," *Ophthalmology*, vol. 116, no. 7, pp. 1370–1376, 2009.

[25] E. H. Bovey, S. Uffer, and F. Achache, "Surgery for epimacular membrane: impact of retinal internal limiting membrane removal on functional outcome," *Retina*, vol. 24, no. 5, pp. 728–735, 2004.

[26] S. Chang, E. M. Gregory-Roberts, S. Park, K. Laud, S. D. Smith, and Q. V. Hoang, "Double peeling during vitrectomy for macular pucker: the Charles L. Schepens lecture," *JAMA Ophthalmology*, vol. 131, no. 4, pp. 525–530, 2013.

3

The Effect of NSAID Pretreatment on Aqueous Humor Prostaglandin E_2 Concentration in Eyes Undergoing Femtosecond Laser-Assisted Capsulotomy

Vasilios F. Diakonis ⓘ,[1,3] **Apostolos G. Anagnostopoulos** ⓘ,[1] **Angeliki Moutsiopoulou,**[2] **Nilufer Yesilirmak,**[1] **Florence Cabot,**[1] **Daniel P. Waren,**[1] **Terrence P. O'Brien,**[1] **Sonia H. Yoo** ⓘ,[1] **Robert J. Weinstock,**[3] **and Kendall E. Donaldson**[1]

[1]*Bascom Palmer Eye Institute, University of Miami Miller School of Medicine, Miami, FL, USA*
[2]*Department of Chemistry, University of Miami, Miami, FL, USA*
[3]*The Eye Institute of West Florida, Largo, FL, USA*

Correspondence should be addressed to Vasilios F. Diakonis; diakonis@gmail.com

Academic Editor: Lisa Toto

Purpose. To assess aqueous humor concentration of prostaglandin E_2 (PGE_2) after capsulotomy creation using a femtosecond laser (FLAC) in patients pretreated with short-term topical ketorolac versus patients without pretreatment. *Methods.* This prospective study comprised consecutive patients scheduled to undergo cataract surgery using a femtosecond laser platform to perform only capsulotomies. An identical protocol for preoperative mydriasis was used for all the eyes included in the study, while aqueous humor was extracted from the anterior chamber of all patients immediately after the initial side port incision. ELISA was performed to quantify aqueous humor PGE_2. The patients were divided into 2 groups; in group 1, the patients received short-term topical ketorolac preoperatively, while the patients in group 2 did not receive NSAID pretreatment. *Results.* Twenty eyes of 20 patients were included in the study (10 eyes in each group). Mean concentration of aqueous humor PGE_2 after FLAC was 392.16 ± 162.00 pg/ml and 622.63 ± 331.84 pg/ml for groups 1 and 2, respectively. A statistically significant difference in aqueous humor PGE_2 concentration between the two groups ($p < 0.05$) was demonstrated, with the eyes that received ketorolac pretreatment demonstrating a lower concentration of PGE_2. *Conclusion.* Short-term topical use of ketorolac prior to FLAC seems to prevent excessive release of PGE_2 in the anterior chamber of the eyes that received NSAID pretreatment when compared to the eyes that did not receive NSAIDs preoperatively.

1. Introduction

Cataract surgery requires sufficient mydriasis, to facilitate capsulorhexis or capsulotomy, phacoemulsification, and finally intraocular lens insertion. Even though all patients undergoing cataract surgery receive preoperatively topical mydriatic agents, intraoperative pupillary miosis may occur due to the release of inflammatory mediators (prostaglandins) or due to iris surgical trauma [1] Miotic pupils during cataract surgery have been associated with increased complication rates during cataract surgery, leading in some cases in visual loss [2, 3].

The pretreatment with femtosecond laser-assisted cataract surgery (FLACS) platforms during cataract surgery has been associated with pupillary miosis [4–6]; the latter has been attributed to the increase of inflammatory mediator (prostaglandins) concentration in the anterior chamber (AC) after FLACS [7, 8]. Recent studies have demonstrated that short-term topical NSAIDs as a pretreatment prior to FLACS results in less prostaglandin release in the AC [9], and also NSAID pretreatment seems to induce significantly less pupillary miosis when compared to the eyes that did not receive NSAID prior to FLACS [10, 11]. The patients in the study assessing prostaglandin quantification in the AC received both capsulotomy and lens fragmentation during FLACS [9], while the NSAID used was diclofenac [9].

The following study will assess aqueous humor prostaglandin E2 (PGE$_2$) concentrations after FLAC (lens fragmentation may influence the inflammatory response and hence prostaglandin production due to cataract density disparities between the eyes) in patients who were pretreated with topical ketorolac compared with patients who did not receive NSAID pretreatment.

2. Methods

2.1. Patient Population. This prospective, randomized, observational case series included 20 consecutive patients (one eye was included per patient, 14 were male and 16 female, aged 68.34 ± 8.65 years (range, 50–90 years)) undergoing cataract surgery using FLACS between July 2015 and July 2016. FLACS pretreatment included the creation of only the capsulotomy, using the Catalys (Abbott Medical Optics Inc., Santa Ana, California, USA) laser platform. The interface utilized in all cases was the Liquid Optics Interface, 14.0 mm inner diameter (Abbott Medical Optics Inc., Santa Ana, California, USA). An identical protocol for preoperative mydriasis was used for all the eyes, while pupil diameter was evaluated before FLACS. The patients were divided into 2 groups; in group 1 (10 eyes) the patients received short-term topical NSAIDs preoperatively (ketorolac, 4 times per day for 3 days prior to cataract extraction), while the patients in group 2 (10 eyes) did not receive NSAID pretreatment. Furthermore, intraoperative grading of capsulotomy creation was performed as follows: type 1 (complete treatment pattern or free floating), type 2 (microadhesions), type 3 (incomplete treatment pattern), and type 4 (complete pattern, but not continuous), as described by a previous study [11].

All patients were informed of the risks and benefits prior to cataract surgery, and they gave written informed consent in accordance with institutional guidelines and the Declaration of Helsinki for human research. Prior to the study, an institutional review board approval was obtained.

2.2. Inclusion and Exclusion Criteria. Patients included in the study had an unremarkable ocular history. Glaucoma patients receiving topical treatment or patients with any other ocular or systemic disease involving the eyes such as inflammatory eye disease, pseudoexfoliation, diabetes mellitus, history of treatment with an α-adrenergic-antagonist, history of poor pupillary dilation (less than 6.0 mm), previous ocular surgery or trauma, or rheumatic disease were excluded from the study.

2.3. Cataract Surgery Technique. Preoperative mydriasis was performed using topical 1.0% tropicamide (Alcon Inc., Lake Forest, IL, USA) eye drops and 2.5% phenylephrine (Paragon BioTeck Inc., Portland, OR, USA) eye drops, instilled three times (every 10 minutes) within 1 hour prior to FLACS (the last application of topical mydriatics was instilled 15 minutes prior to surgery). All procedures were performed

under topical anesthesia; a 5.0 mm in diameter femtosecond capsulotomy was performed in all cases, while corneal incisions and lens fragmentation was not performed in any case. Clear corneal incisions were performed manually, followed by standard phacoemulsification (Centurion, Alcon, Fort Worth, TX, USA). The capsulotomy settings were identical for all cases: the pattern was circular with a 5.0 mm diameter centered at the pupil and the incision depth was 600 microns. The horizontal and vertical spot spacings were 5 and 10 microns, respectively, while the pulse energy was 4 microjoules.

Five minutes after capsulotomy creation and prior to traditional phacoemulsification, a 1.15 mm paracentesis port was made, and aqueous humor was collected in a syringe (a volume of 100 microliters or more was considered to be an adequate sample); all aqueous humor samples were immediately stored in $-80°C$ and were only again in room temperature conditions prior to performing ELISA. No intraoperative complications were noted in any of the cases included in the study, while an intraocular lens was placed in the capsular bag in all cases.

Postoperatively, all patients received the same treatment regimen: a combination of an antibiotic, steroid, and nonsteroidal anti-inflammatory agent.

2.4. ELISA Assessment. All aqueous humor samples from both groups were assessed by the same investigator with the same standard preparation to avoid interuser or plate variability. PGE$_2$ concentrations were determined using a commercially available PGE$_2$ Parameter Assay Kit (R&D Systems, Minneapolis, MN) according to the manufacturer's instructions. Measurements were performed using a microplate reader (Clariostar Monochromator Microplate Reader, BMG LABTECH, Ortenberg, Germany).

2.5. Statistical Analysis. Comparisons between groups were performed using Student's *t*-test. Statistical analysis was performed using the SPSS statistical package (version 22; IBM Software). A P value of 0.05 or less was considered statistically significant in our analyses.

3. Results

Twenty eyes (10 eyes per group) of 20 patients were included in the study ((20 patients, one eye was included per patient, 14 were male and 16 female, aged 68.34 ± 8.65 years (range, 50–90 years)). There was no statistically significant difference between the 2 groups in terms of age ($p > 0.05$). All femtosecond laser-assisted capsulotomies in both groups were graded as type 1 (complete capsulotomies or free floating).

Mean concentration of aqueous humor PGE$_2$ after FLAC was 392.16 ± 162.00 pg/ml (range: from 202.04 to 713.71 pg/ml) and 622.63 ± 331.84 pg/ml (range: from 310.09 to 1469.74 pg/ml) for groups 1 and 2, respectively. There was a statistically significant difference in aqueous humor PGE$_2$ concentration between the two groups ($p = 0.03$), with the eyes that received ketorolac pretreatment demonstrating lower concentrations of PGE_2.

4. Discussion

Previous studies have shown that FLACS pretreatment results in significant pupillary miosis [4–6]. A published study from our department that evaluated the effect of 3 femtosecond laser platforms after FLACS pretreatment on pupil diameter also revealed significant pupillary miosis which was independent to the laser platform used [6], It is hypothesized that pupillary miosis is associated with prostaglandin release in the AC and with the dissipation of laser energy around the iris tissue [5, 6]. In support of the above theories, a study by Schultz et al. [7] reported significant increase of prostaglandins in the aqueous humor after FLACS. Furthermore, a study by Jong et al. [8] associated pupillary miosis with the with the patient's age [8] and the total time of laser application, while suction time (of the patient interface) did not seem to effect pupil diameter [8].

The use of topical NSAIDs prior to cataract surgery has been regularly used as the standard of care to minimize pupillary miosis during surgery since the mid 1980s. It seems that the intraocular manipulations during cataract surgery cause breakdown of the blood-aqueous barrier promoting an inflammatory cascade with the release of prostaglandins by ciliary body [12–15]. The topical use of NSAIDs inhibits the synthesis of prostaglandins in the AC and thereby minimizes the likelihood of pupillary miosis [16–18]. A recent study from our institute demonstrated that patients receiving a 3-day topical regimen of ketorolac prior to FLAC better retained their mydriasis after the laser treatment [10]. Furthermore, a study by Schultz et al. showed that the use of topical NSAIDs (diclofenac) prior to FLACS reduced prostaglandin release in the AC [9]. In the study mentioned above, the authors performed FLACS treatment that included capsulotomy creation and lens fragmentation, while diclofenac was used as an NSAID agent treatment at the day of surgery [9], while in our previous study, only FLACS capsulotomy was performed (to better control the study parameters) and ketorolac was used prior to surgery [10].

The current study evaluated aqueous humor concentration of PGE_2 after FLAC (only capsulotomy was performed), using the same laser platform and the same settings for capsulotomy creation in all eyes included. This study approach was designed to control the effects of laser energy dissipation in the AC (only femtosecond capsulotomy which seems to be the main inducer of prostaglandin release [19]) avoiding the possible implications that cataract density disparities that could influence prostaglandin release (increase the variables of the current study). Furthermore, ketorolac was used and its topical application commenced 3 days prior to cataract surgery (4 times per day) in contrast to the Schultz et al. study where diclofenac was used one day prior to cataract surgery; a recent study by Kiss et al. utilized nepafenac one day prior to FLACS and demonstrated significant reduction of prostaglandin concentration in the aqueous humor when compared even with manual cataract surgery [20]. Our study demonstrated that short-term (3 days prior to FLAC, we utilized 3 days of NSAID as we followed the standard protocol used in our department for the preoperative regimen, and as mentioned above, other studies demonstrate that the shorter preoperative regimen seems equally efficacious to ours) topical use of ketorolac prior to FLAC seems to prevent excessive release of PGE_2 in the anterior chamber of the eyes that received NSAID pretreatment when compared to the eyes that did not receive NSAIDs. These findings were similar to the published study by Schultz et al.; these two studies suggest that any FLACS treatment may lead to increased PGE_2 levels in the AC and subsequently to pupil miosis. Finally, the use of different NSAID agents either immediately prior to cataract surgery or for a few days prior to surgery seems to well control the release of PGE_2 in the AC.

Our findings reveal that even capsulotomy creation which secures short laser time exposure, minimal laser energy utilization, and short suction time by the patient interface in patients with no comorbidities may cause a significant increase in PGE_2 levels in the AC. Furthermore, a 3-day pretreatment with topical ketorolac prior to FLACS seems to significantly inhibit FLACS-induced PGE_2 release in the AC when compared with patients who did not receive a NSAID pretreatment. There was a difference between the findings of this study and the study by Schultz et al. in terms of the actual concentration values of PGE_2, with our study demonstrating much higher concentrations in both the NSAID and no NSAID group. This may be attributed to the ELISA kit used which could have different sensitivity; furthermore, this could be a result of different dilution the aqueous humor samples underwent in these two studies prior to ELISA. Finally, the concentration differences quantified by different ELISA kits could be attributed to their specificity and more specifically to the cross-reactivity they demonstrate.

The current study is limited by the small sample of eyes included and the fact that we did not include more groups to assess other NSAID agents. Despite the above limitations, we demonstrate that a 3-day (4 times per day) topical use of an NSAID agent (ketorolac) prior to FLAC seems to prevent excessive release of PGE_2 in the anterior chamber. Additionally, the eyes that did not receive topical NSAID pretreatment demonstrated higher concentrations of prostaglandins on the AC when compared with the eyes that received the NSAID prior to FLACS that could potentially lead to significant pupillary miosis. It is suggested that patients undergoing any type of FLACS treatment prior to cataract surgery to receive a course of topical NSAID regimen to avoid pupillary miosis and miosis-related complications.

Conflicts of Interest

Sonia H. Yoo and Kendall E. Donaldson serve as speakers and consultants for ALCON and Abbott Medical Optics. Dr. Diakonis received a scholarship (2014) from the Hellenic Society of Intraocular Implants and Refractive Surgery for fellowship training.

References

[1] B. Lundberg and A. Behndig, "The mydriatic effect of intracameral epinine hydrochloride," *Investigative Opthalmology and Visual Science*, vol. 50, no. 11, pp. 5336–5338, 2009.

[2] H. Hashemi, M. A. Seyedian, and M. Mohammadpour, "Small pupil and cataract surgery," *Current Opinion in Ophthalmology*, vol. 26, no. 1, pp. 3–9, 2015.

[3] G. Carifi, M. H. Miller, C. Pitsas et al., "Complications and outcomes of phacoemulsification cataract surgery complicated by anterior capsule tear," *American Journal of Ophthalmology*, vol. 159, no. 3, pp. 463–469, 2015.

[4] Z. Nagy, A. Takacs, T. Filkorn, and M. Sarayba, "Initial clinical evaluation of an intraocular femtosecond laser in cataract surgery," *Journal of Refractive Surgery*, vol. 25, no. 12, pp. 1053–1060, 2009.

[5] S. J. Bali, C. Hogde, M. Lawless, T. V. Roberts, and G. Sutton, "Early experience with the femtosecond laser for cataract surgery," *Ophthalmology*, vol. 119, no. 5, pp. 891–899, 2012.

[6] V. F. Diakonis, N. Yesilirmak, I. O. Sayed-Ahmed et al., "Effects of femtosecond laser-assisted cataract pretreatment on pupil diameter: a comparison between three laser platforms," *Journal of Refractive Surgery*, vol. 32, no. 2, pp. 84–88, 2016.

[7] T. Schultz, S. C. Joachim, M. Kuehn, and H. B. Dick, "Changes in prostaglandin levels in patients in patients undergoing femtosecond laser assisted cataract surgery," *Journal of Refractive Surgery*, vol. 29, no. 11, pp. 742–747, 2013.

[8] H. J. Jong, Y. H. Kyu, D. C. Sung, and J. Choun-Ki, "Pupil-size alterations by photodisruption during femtosecond laser-assisted cataract surgery," *Journal of Cataract and Refractive Surgery*, vol. 41, no. 2, pp. 278–285, 2015.

[9] T. Schultz, S. C. Joachim, M. Szuler, M. Stellbogen, and H. B. Dick, "NSAID pretreatment inhibits prostaglandin release in femtosecond laser-assisted cataract surgery," *Journal of Refractive Surgery*, vol. 31, no. 12, pp. 791–794, 2015.

[10] V. F. Diakonis, G. A. Kontadakis, A. G. Anagnostopoulos et al., "Effects of short-term preoperative topical ketorolac on pupil diameter in eyes undergoing femtosecond laser-assisted capsulotomy," *Journal of Refractive Surgery*, vol. 33, no. 4, pp. 230–234, 2017.

[11] Z. Z. Nagy, A. I. Takacs, T. Filkorn et al., "Complications of femtosecond laser-assisted cataract surgery," *Journal of Cataract and Refractive Surgery*, vol. 40, no. 1, pp. 20–28, 2014.

[12] P. Bhattacherjee and K. E. Eakins, "Inhibition of the prostaglandin synthetase systems in ocular tissues by indomethacin," *British Journal of Pharmacology*, vol. 50, no. 2, pp. 227–230, 1974.

[13] N. Ambache and H. C. Brummer, "A Simple chemical procedure for distinguishing E from F prostaglandins with application to tissue extracts," *British Journal of Pharmacology and Chemotherapy*, vol. 33, no. 1, pp. 162–170, 1968.

[14] N. Ambache, L. Kavanagh, and J. Whiting, "Effect of mechanical stimulation on rabbits eyes: release of active substance in anterior chamber perfusates," *Journal of Physiology*, vol. 176, no. 3, pp. 378–408, 1965.

[15] E. Anggard and B. Samuelsson, "Smooth muscle stimulating lipids in sheep iris: the identification of prostaglandin F2," *Biochemical Pharmacology*, vol. 13, no. 2, pp. 281–283, 1964.

[16] R. Srinivasan and Madhavaranga, "Topical ketorolac tromethamine 0.5% versus diclofenac sodium 0.1% to inhibit miosis during cataract surgery," *Journal of Cataract and Refractive Surgery*, vol. 28, no. 3, pp. 517–520, 2002.

[17] E. D. Donnenfeld, H. D. Perry, J. R. Wittpenn, R. Solomon, A. Nattis, and T. Chou, "Preoperative ketorolac tromethamine 0.4% in phacoemulsification outcomes: pharmacokinetic-response curve," *Journal of Cataract and Refractive Surgery*, vol. 32, no. 9, pp. 1474–1482, 2006.

[18] S. J. Kim, A. J. Flach, and L. M. Jampol, "Nonsteroidal anti-inflammatory drugs in ophthalmology," *Survey of Ophthalmology*, vol. 55, no. 2, pp. 108–133, 2010.

[19] T. Schultz, S. C. Joachim, M. Stellbogen, and H. B. Disk, "Prostaglandin release during femtosecond laser-assisted cataract surgery: main inducer," *Journal of Refractive Surgery*, vol. 31, no. 2, pp. 78–81, 2015.

[20] H. J. Kiss, A. I. Takacs, K. Kranitz et al., "One-day use of preoperative topical nonsteroidal anti-inflammatory drug prevents intraoperative prostaglandin level elevation during femtosecond laser-assisted cataract surgery," *Current Eye Research*, vol. 41, no. 8, pp. 1064–1067, 2016.

4

Challenges and Complication Management in Novel Artificial Iris Implantation

Christian S. Mayer ⓘ,[1,2] **Andrea E. Laubichler,**[1] **Ramin Khoramnia,**[2] **Tamer Tandogan,**[2] **Philipp Prahs,**[3] **Daniel Zapp,**[1] **and Lukas Reznicek**[1]

[1]*Department of Ophthalmology, Technical University of Munich, Munich, Germany*
[2]*Department of Ophthalmology, University of Heidelberg, Heidelberg, Germany*
[3]*Department of Ophthalmology, University of Regensburg, Regensburg, Germany*

Correspondence should be addressed to Christian S. Mayer; augenarzt.mayer@gmx.de

Academic Editor: Tamer A. Macky

Purpose. Evaluation of postoperative artificial iris prosthesis-related complications. *Design.* Retrospective cohort study. *Methods.* Fifty-one consecutive patients underwent pupillary reconstruction using an artificial iris implant made from silicone between 2011 and 2015. Quantity and quality of complications were subclassified into three groups including mild, moderate, and severe complications. Their management and the learning curve were evaluated. *Results.* In total, 13 (25.5%) of 51 included artificial iris implantations showed unexpected events in various degrees: mild complications: recurrent bleeding ($n = 1$, 2.0%), slight but stable iris deviation ($n = 1$, 2.0%), capsular fibrosis ($n = 2$, 3.9%); moderate complications: suture cutting through the residual iris ($n = 1$, 2.0%), glaucoma ($n = 3$, 5.9%), and corneal decompensation ($n = 3$, 5.9%); severe complications: artificial iris suture loosening ($n = 2$, 3.9%) and dislocation ($n = 3$, 5.9%), synechiae ($n = 2$, 3.9%), glaucoma ($n = 2$, 3.9%), and corneal decompensation ($n = 5$, 9.8%) with the need for surgery, cystoid macular edema ($n = 3$, 5.9%) and retinal detachment ($n = 1$, 2.0%). The complication rate decreased from 83.3% (5 of 6 implantations) in the first year to 13.3% (2 of 15 implantations) in the 4th year. Nineteen of 45 evaluated patients showed a significant gain in best-corrected visual acuity (BCVA) from 1.09 ± 0.56 logMAR to 0.54 ± 0.48 logMAR ($p < 0.001$), and 13 of 45 eyes had a significant BCVA loss from 0.48 ± 0.39 logMAR to 0.93 ± 0.41 logMAR after surgery ($p < 0.001$). *Conclusions.* The artificial iris is a feasible option in the treatment of iris defects with a wide spectrum of postoperative complications. The significant reduction of complications after twelve implantations implicates that the procedure is not to be recommended in low volume settings.

1. Introduction

Patients with iris defects suffer from severe visual impairment with especially increased glare sensitivity and cosmetic disturbances. In addition to those iris defects, these eyes show corneal and scleral scars, aphakia, retinal changes, and glaucoma depending on the initial trauma. Furthermore, iris atrophy and pupil size can deteriorate the visual function of an increase of higher order aberrations [1]. In the past, various types of artificial iris implants were used to address those iris defects [2–7]. Most of them were rigid, needed large incisions, and were not satisfying for the patients.

A custom-made, flexible silicone iris implant is a relatively new and promising additional option for the surgical treatment of iris defects [8–10]. The ArtificialIris® (HumanOptics) is a foldable, custom-tailored iris prosthesis made of flexible, biocompatible silicone. This device received the Conformité Européenne (CE) conformity marking for products sold within the European Economic Area approval for Europe in 2011 and received a Food and Drug Administration (FDA) approval procedure in the United States recently. Several surgeons have presented different cases or small case series of pupil and iris reconstruction using this novel type of silicone iris implant with good results [10–16]. In a previous publication, we were able to present good functional outcomes in pupillary reconstruction after artificial iris implantation in a larger series with 36 eyes [17]. The presented ArtificialIris must not be confused with the

BrightOcular iris prosthesis (Stellar Devices). Numerous publications evaluating that device report concerns [18, 19] with only few good results [7].

There are still very few published studies addressing complications associated with the implant or the implantation procedure itself [13, 20, 21]. There is currently a need to investigate potential complications and pitfalls in this relatively new and rising therapeutic method in a larger amount of patients.

The purpose of this retrospective cohort study was to describe the learning curve of the implantation surgery, limitations, pitfalls, and associated unexpected events and their potential solutions for the use of this iris prosthesis.

2. Materials and Methods

Fifty-one silicone iris prostheses (ArtificialIris®, Human-Optics, Erlangen, Germany) were implanted at the eye clinic of the Technical University of Munich between June 2011 and December 2015 (Table 1).

The number and quality of complications associated with the implantation procedure or the implant itself were investigated for all included 51 patients with a follow-up time of at least 3 months to a maximum of 4 years.

Informed consent was obtained from all participants. The study was conducted according to the tenets of the Declaration of Helsinki, and approval by the Institutional Review Board was obtained.

The type of implantation procedure depended on the preexisting alterations in the affected eyes [22, 23]. In our cohort, all patients received either a complete ($n = 49$) or a sector-shaped ($n = 2$) iris prosthesis. The custom-made implant was fixed in the ciliary sulcus without sutures in case of a preexisting intracapsular intraocular lens, implanted in the capsular bag together with a new intraocular lens or sutured to the sclera with or without an attached intraocular lens. In two cases, an artificial iris segment was sutured directly in the sectoral iris defect. At the end of surgery, all patients were pseudophakic. Details of the implantation procedure are described elsewhere [17, 23]. All implantations were performed by one single surgeon without any notable intraoperative complications.

Postoperative changes, abnormalities, complications, and unexpected events associated with the artificial iris implantation were noted in standardized full ophthalmic examinations. The development of best-corrected visual acuity (BCVA, Snellen chart) was classified into three groups: BCVA improvement (>2 lines), unchanged BCVA (±2 lines), and decrease in BCVA (>2 lines). The unexpected events and complications during the follow-up period were grouped into "none" (postoperative uneventful course of disease), "mild" (unexpected events requiring noninvasive intervention *with* full recovery), "moderate" (unexpected events requiring noninvasive intervention *without* full recovery), and "severe" (unexpected or expected events resulting in any surgical intervention).

In addition, the complications were evaluated in regard to ocular hyper- and hypotension, suture fixation-associated

TABLE 1: Patients' characteristics and descriptive data.

Number of subjects	$n = 51$
Age (years)	52.9 ± 16.0
Gender	
Male	22 (68.8%)
Female	10 (31.2%)
Iris defects resulting from	
Congenital coloboma	3 (9.3%)
Persistent mydriasis	9 (28.1%)
Traumatic loss of iris tissue	21 (65.6%)
Additional history information	
Preexisting glaucoma	6 (11.8%)
Preexisting corneal impairment (scars or decompensation)	5 (9.8%)
Time period between diagnosis and surgery (years)	12.0 ± 15.7
Follow-up time (months)	13.6 ± 10.9

problems, and misalignment and (sub-)luxation of the artificial iris.

Imaging documentation was performed with photography (Canon 600D SLR including a 100 mm Macro-Objective, Canon Europe LTD, United Kingdom UB11 1ET, and Topcon OneDigiPro 3HD Slit Lamp, Oakland, NJ 07436) and video capturing (Zeiss Lumera 700 ophthalmic microscope Callisto System, Carl Zeiss AG, Oberkochen, Germany).

3. Results

In this retrospective analysis, we were able to evaluate the complications of 51 patients, who had received an artificial iris implantation performed by one single surgeon in a university eye clinic setting between 2011 and 2015. Thirty-four (66.7%) were male and 17 (33.3%) were female. Mean age was 52.9 ± 16.0 years. The iris defects were due to congenital coloboma ($n = 3$; 6.8%), persistent mydriasis ($n = 14$; 27.4%), traumatic loss of iris tissue ($n = 31$; 60.8%), and miscellaneous ($n = 3$; 6.8%). Additional history information revealed preexisting glaucoma in 6 (11.8%) and preexisting corneal impairment (scars or decompensation) in 5 (9.8%) patients. The mean postoperative follow-up period is 13.4 months (min. 3 months and max. 50 months). The postoperative history includes a variety of individual complications ranging from none over moderate intraocular pressure rise for a few days up to a prosthesis explantation due to chronic inflammation and decompensation of the corneal endothelium. Thirty-eight procedures (74.5%) had an uneventful follow-up after artificial iris implantation.

The overall complication rate after surgery included 13 out of 51 patients (25.5%), and the complications were further subclassified into mild, moderate, and severe.

Mild complications manifested in recurrent bleeding into the anterior chamber and secondary rise of the intraocular pressure (IOP) ($n = 1$, 2.0%) with spontaneous solution after 2 months, slight but stable artificial iris deviation ($n = 1$, 2.0%), and capsular fibrosis ($n = 2$, 3.9%) treated with laser-assisted capsulotomy.

Moderate complications were found in sutures cutting through the residual iris tissue ($n = 1$, 2.0%) forming a secondary pupil without the need for intervention (Figure 1), onset of glaucoma ($n = 3$, 5.9%) that could be controlled with topical antiglaucomatous medication, and corneal decompensation ($n = 3$, 5.9%).

Severe complications were artificial iris suture loosening and dislocation with the necessity of surgical revision: Immediate postoperative subluxation of the artificial iris was detected in 3 cases (5.9%) of our collective (Figures 2 and 3).

All cases of significant misalignment and (sub)luxation of the artificial iris needed refixation of the implant. The subluxated irides were reattached with a u-type double-armed suture without significant tension to prevent a repeated cutting through (Figure 2(e); Supplementary Video, available here).

Formation of posterior synechiae requiring synechiolysis occurred in 3.9% ($n = 2$). Severe ocular hypertension was observed in one case with severe pigment dispersion syndrome (Figures 4(a) and 4(b)) and in another case a new onset of glaucoma with the need for shunt surgery with Ahmed® glaucoma valves ($n = 2$, 3.9%). Ocular hypotension after surgery was without exception transient for few days only.

Corneal complications occurred in 9.8% ($n = 5$): Corneal decompensation resulted in perforating keratoplasty in 3 cases (5.9%) or amniotic membrane transplantation in 2 cases (3.9%). One of these cases developed an unexpected corneal decompensation one year after implantation surgery (Figure 5).

Initially, the BCVA in this case had recovered to 20/20 after the artificial iris implantation surgery. Furthermore, this patient developed a macular edema with corneal decompensation and consecutive vision decrease to 20/200 one year after the implant procedure. BCVA did not improve despite medical and surgical (amniotic membrane transplantation) treatment. Consecutively, the artificial iris had to be explanted one year after implantation.

A formation of cystoid macular edema ($n = 3$, 5.9%) required intravitreal steroid application, and one case of retinal detachment ($n = 1$, 2.0%) needed vitrectomy with silicone oil filling. The summary of the unexpected events is shown in Table 2.

In the first year (2011), we found 5 complications in 6 implantation procedures (83.3%), and in the second year (2012), we had 3 documented unexpected events in 7 surgeries (42.9%). In the following years, there were 3 complications in 12 procedures (25.0%, 2013), none in 11 (2014), and 2 in 15 procedures (13.3%, 2015).

Overall, 46.2% of all complications occurred within the first 3 postoperative months, whereas 53.8% occurred after that time period. The surgical learning curve with complications versus number of operations can be seen in Figure 6.

We were able to analyze the BCVA development (preoperative versus postoperative) in 45 out of 51 patients. The BCVA increased significantly (more than 2 lines of a Snellen projection chart) in 19 patients (42.2%) from initially 1.09 ± 0.56 logMAR to 0.54 ± 0.48 logMAR after surgery ($p < 0.001$). In 13 eyes (28.9%), the BCVA remained unchanged (0.47 ± 0.54 logMAR to 0.45 ± 0.55 logMAR) after surgery ($p = 0.502$), and in 13 eyes (28.9%), the BCVA decreased significantly from 0.48 ± 0.39 logMAR to 0.93 ± 0.41 logMAR after surgery ($p < 0.001$) (Figure 7).

4. Discussion

The initial complication rate after artificial iris implantation in the first year is very high (83.3%) due to case mix of rather complicated cases, an unfamiliar implant device, and relatively few and not standardized cases. We were able to show that, roughly after two years, the complication rate decreases indirectly proportional to the increasing experience and the learning effect of the surgeon (Figure 6). Our data suggest a dozen of artificial iris implantations be performed by one surgeon in order to achieve a certain level of standardization with an acceptable complication rate over time. Further investigations will show a possible increase of late-onset complications in eyes with currently short follow-up periods at present.

Best-corrected visual acuity (BCVA) improvement is not a primary goal for the implantation of an artificial iris. Affected eyes often have multiple alterations and a reduced BCVA prognosis. Increase of the BCVA after surgery in 19 patients (42.2%) may result from cataract extraction and/or IOL implantation or by reconstruction of a new pupil with resulting enhanced depth of focus. Nevertheless, the data show that, in 28.9% of the evaluated eyes, BCVA was reduced after implantation of the artificial iris. Therefore, patients should be advised prior to surgery that artificial iris implantation has a potential risk to reduce the patients' vision due to the procedure itself.

The local postoperative therapy with steroids and antibiotics is similar to the therapy in other intraocular procedures. In principle, there is no contraindication for a use of dilating eyedrops in case of intraocular inflammation, although there is no effect on the fixed pupil diameter. However, it may help to reduce the inflammatory reaction due to inhibited ciliary body motility. Another positive effect when dilating the pupil is the fact that there is potentially less pigment dissolving from the residual iris and consecutively a lower risk for secondary pigmentary glaucoma.

In this case with moderate recurrent bleeding into the anterior chamber and secondary rise of the intraocular pressure, the used artificial iris with embedded fiber meshwork was trephanized and then sutured in the ciliary sulcus. The ultrasound and clinical examination did not reveal any detectable bleeding source. The bleeding stopped spontaneously after 3 months with the need for topical and systemic antiglaucomatous medication and topical cycloplegics for this period of time.

Scanning electron microscopy of the leftover parts of the trephanized iris showed a variety regarding the smoothness and roughness of the edges and the protrusion of fibers in implants with fiber (Figure 8(a)) and without fiber meshwork (Figure 8(b)), eventually depending on the sharpness of the used trephines.

It seems that chronic movement of the trephined artificial iris edges on the ciliary body leading to defects on the

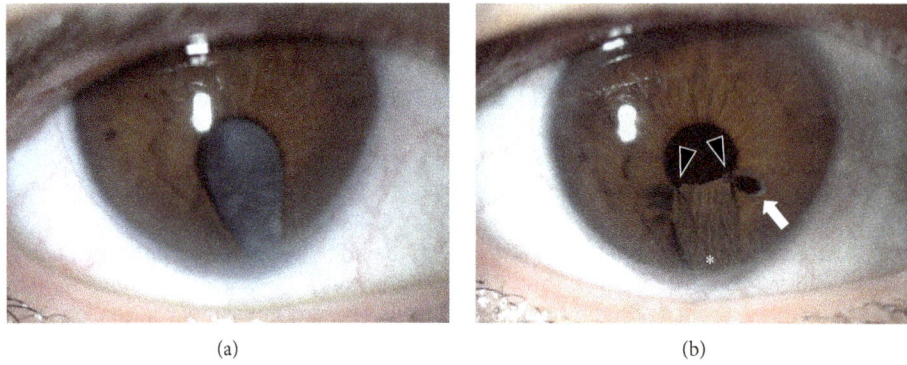

(a)   (b)

FIGURE 1: Congenital iris coloboma with cataract before (a) and after (b) implantation of a sector-shaped artificial iris (*) and intraocular lens in a combined surgery. Three months after surgery, the suture at the pupillary rim (arrowheads) cut through the remnant iris tissue and formed a new pupillary aperture (arrow). This patient did not suffer from visual impairment.

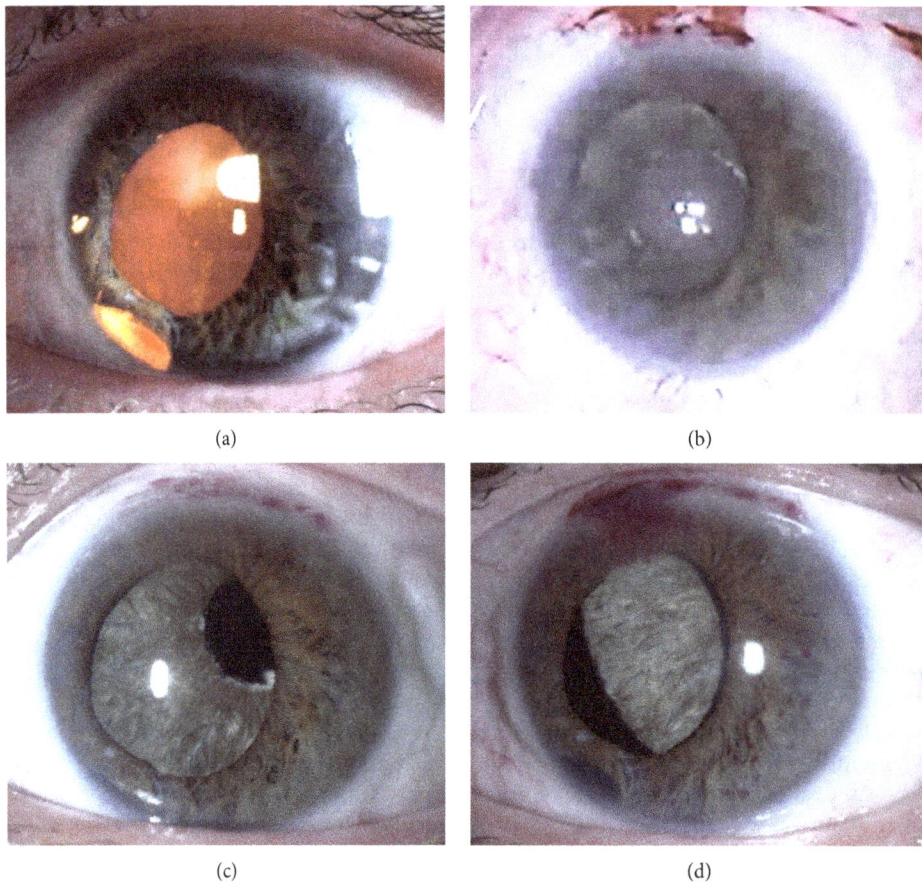

(a)   (b)

(c)   (d)

FIGURE 2: Continued.

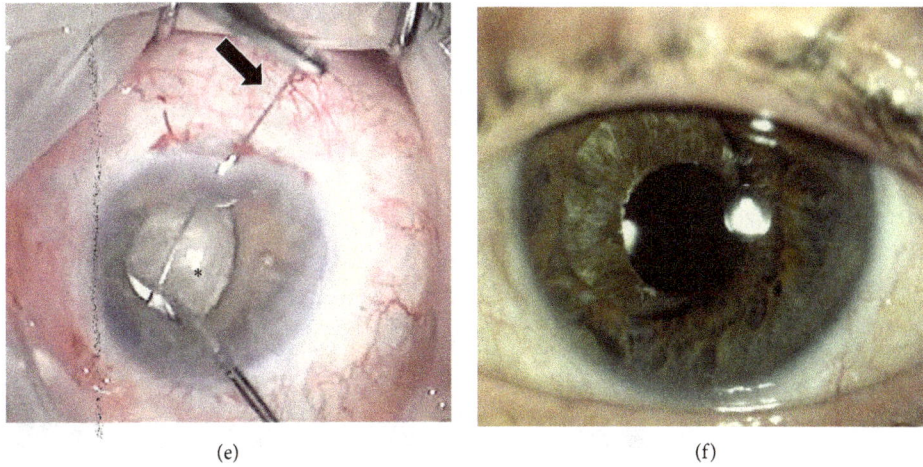

(e)

(f)

FIGURE 2: Patient (51 y, m) with an initially traumatic iris defect and a sclera-fixed intraocular lens (a). At the end of surgery, the artificial iris was located in the ciliary sulcus without sutures (b). (c) Slight decentralization of the pupillary aperture and subluxation of the artificial iris the first day after surgery. (d) Severe dislocation of the implant threatening to fall down into the vitreous the second day after surgery. Immediate operative intervention (e) with picking up the implant and fixing the device with a double-armed 10.0 polypropylene suture to the sclera (arrow). (f) Stable location of the implant and intraocular lens 1 year after surgery.

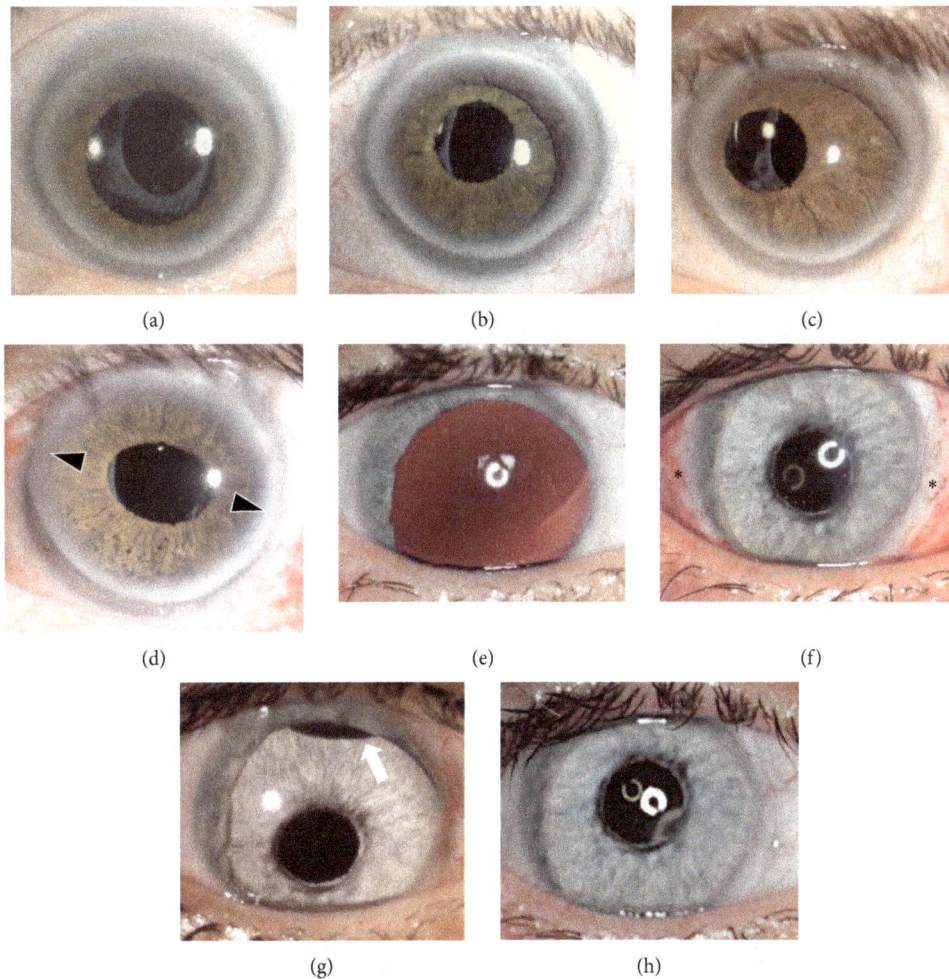

(a)

(b)

(c)

(d)

(e)

(f)

(g)

(h)

FIGURE 3: Two patients after artificial iris implantation with subluxation of the implant: Patient 1 (a–d) suffered from persistent traumatic mydriasis (a) and received a ciliary sulcus embedded fiber-free prosthesis without suture fixation (b). The prosthesis decentered after 2 years with visual disturbances (c) and had to be refixed with sutures (d). This led to slight oval pupil shape. Patient 2 (e–h) suffered from aphakic and subtotal aniridia. An intraocular lens was attached to the artificial iris by sutures. This "sandwich" was implanted and sutured to the sclera at the 3 and 9 o'clock position (f, **). After 4 weeks, the implant tilted with the upper rim into the anterior chamber (g, arrow). Refixation with a third suture at the 11 o'clock position resolved that problem (h).

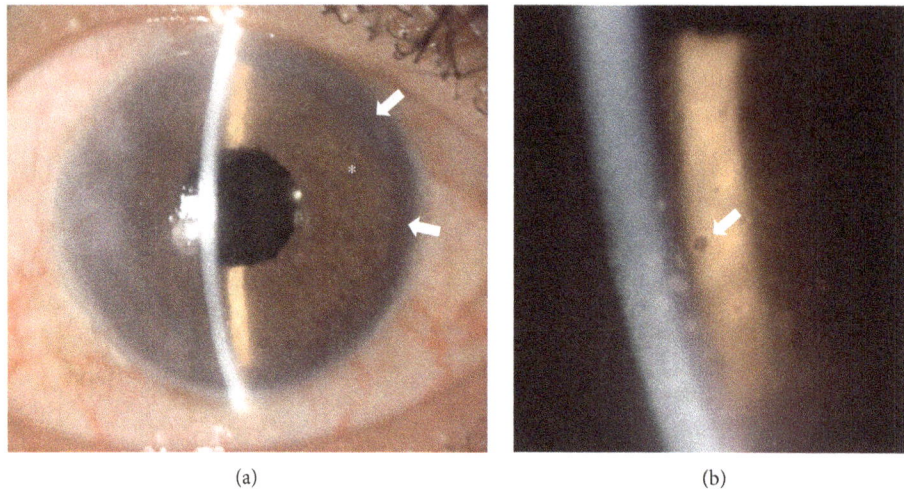

(a)   (b)

FIGURE 4: Anterior segment 2 years after artificial iris implantation with originally subtotal traumatic mydriasis (a) with intraocular pressure elevation (32 mm/Hg). Brown artificial iris (*) with fixed pupillary aperture. Residual iris rim is barely visible (arrows). Magnification of the cornea (b): pigment dispersion and clumps in Arlt's triangle on the endothelium (arrow).

ciliary body may have been the reason of the observed recurrent bleedings. As a consequence, from that incidence on, we have always used single-use sharp trephines to achieve clean cutting edges in view of eliminating this possible problem.

Early transient postoperative IOP rise is normally well controlled with antiglaucomatous eyedrops and systemic carboanhydrase inhibitors. The one case with prolonged and severe IOP rise due to pigment dispersion syndrome that was not sufficiently controlled with antiglaucomatous medication required glaucoma shunt surgery. This mentioned patient had a dark brown residual iris, implicating eventually a higher risk for pigmented dispersion in patients with dark irides. We were not able to differentiate the cause for IOP decompensation in the other patients (decompensated glaucoma versus artificial iris implantation).

On the other side of the spectrum, temporary bulbar hypotonia usually depended on the surgical technique especially in case of larger entries for specific lens diameters and sutureless pars plana vitrectomies. The expected hypotonia in those cases resolved within one week and was not a problem at any time [23].

A challenging situation may occur when a sector-shaped artificial iris is implanted, for example, in cases with partial aniridia or coloboma (Figure 1(a)): Constant movement of the residual iris can result in cutting sutures especially at the rim of the pupillary sphincter (Figure 1(b), arrow) with a secondary pupil and disturbed vision. This happened to both sector-shaped implants in our study. Because of that and the fact that the implantation procedure is more complex because of time-consuming iris sutures, we, since then, avoided this implantation technique with sector-shaped artificial iris implants [24]. The advantage to use a complete artificial iris over a sector-shaped one is the easier implantation procedure, better predictable centration of a perfectly round pupil, avoiding of sharp implant edges and prevention of cutting sutures. Primary sutures for the artificial iris fixation are

recommended and necessary in cases with missing anterior and/or posterior device support, for example, in aphakic eyes or absent of the lens capsules [24].

Suture-fixed implants last as long as the material of the sutures endures. In this series, we used durable polypropylene 10-0 sutures (Ethicon®). This UV-stable material should last at least for several years [25]. The postoperative follow-up time for our first operated patients is 5 years. Future follow-up examinations will show whether this fixation will last in younger patients with a life expectancy longer than the life span of the suture material. Supposedly, similar to suture-fixed ciliary sulcus IOLs, the sutured iris implants should hold less potential for complications.

Subluxations occurred either within the first two days or only after months after the implantation procedure (Figures 2 and 3). Decentration of the new pupil may result in difficulties to choose the correct diameter of the implant as well as presumed mechanical manipulation by the patient. Furthermore, loosening of the sutures (e.g., caused by aging) can cause a dislocation. The reasons for the early subluxations were preexisting scars, synechiae, adhesions at the implantation site, or loose structures resulting from the former trauma. This may lead to unstable artificial iris fixation. Exemplary, postoperative eye movement or gravity can force the artificial iris to leave its intended position, forming a "slide-off phenomenon" (Figure 3): The artificial iris tilts to one side of the suture axis heading towards the vitreous with the risk of causing severe mechanical retinal damage. In artificial irides without embedded meshwork, sutures could cut through the silicone tissue more easily. Those sutures prevent the refixated artificial iris from swinging on the suture-fixed intraocular lens and hold it in place (Figure 3(f)). Removing the artificial iris out of the posterior segment would need a removal of both, the artificial iris and the intraocular lens, to be removed and then refixated. Until now, we could not observe a suture cut through in fiber-free implants.

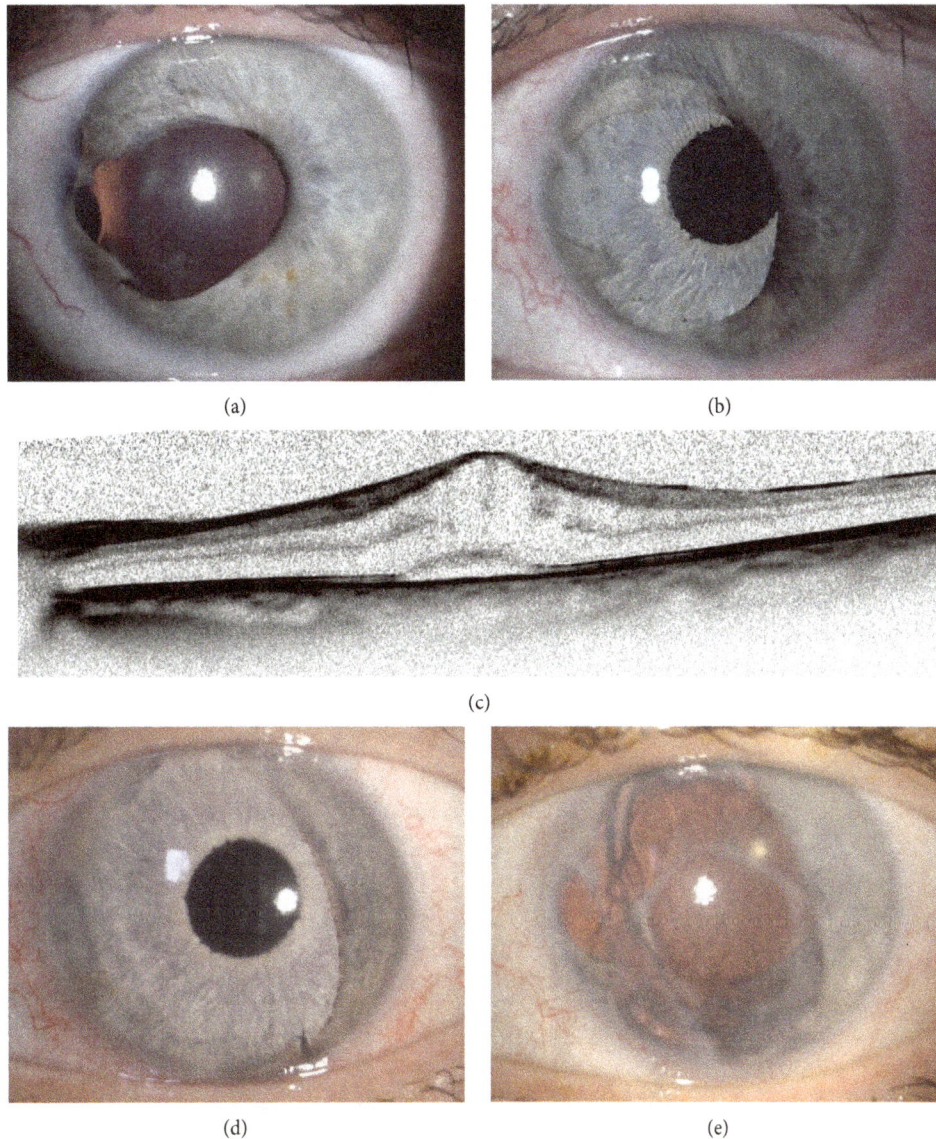

Figure 5: A 47-year-old woman with a 34-year iris defect and cataract after trauma (a). Results one year after artificial iris implantation: BCVA 20/20, clear media and stable situation (b). Two months later, the patient complained of a decreased BCVA of 20/200 and elevated IOP. Optical coherence tomography showed a cystoid macular edema (c), and slit lamp examination revealed descemet folds and corneal haze (d). Topical, intravitreal, and systemic medication did not improve BCVA. Explantation of the artificial iris (e) followed by perforating keratoplasty due to chronic inflammation and corneal decompensation. BCVA was 40/200 one year later.

In our group, we had one case with retinal detachment that had to undergo vitreoretinal surgery 4 weeks after implantation of the artificial iris. Vitreoretinal surgery in general is feasible because of the fixed pupil size of the implanted artificial iris. The fundus of the affected eyes can be examined up to the periphery despite the lack of pupil dilation. This can be seen during implantation surgery of an artificial iris. The visualization extends up to the peripheral retina, even the ora could be visualized using indentation.

As described in a previously published work, the corneal endothelium cell loss is about 11.3% and comparable to a standard cataract surgery [23]. The amount of endothelial cell loss caused by the implantation of an artificial iris itself is not significantly higher than after standard cataract surgery, but the preoperative circumstances after severe ocular trauma often result in a reduced endothelial cell count before surgery. Increased loss of endothelial cells is an additional risk factor of the patients' traumatized eyes and remains the difficulty in the reconstruction surgery. In anticipation of that, three patients needed keratoplasty after artificial iris implantation. Therefore, the risk for corneal decompensation is more likely to be attributed to the primary ocular circumstances than the surgical trauma. Regarding the patient with corneal decompensation after artificial iris implantation and macular edema, we successfully removed the artificial iris implant and performed a keratoplasty that had no complications during and after surgery.

TABLE 2: Graduation of complications related to the artificial iris (AI) implantation.

Grade	Description	Event	n	% of total n = 51
0 (none)	Postoperative uneventful course of disease		38	74.5
1 (mild)	Unexpected events needed for noninvasive intervention *with* full recovery	Recurrent bleedings with IOP raise	1	2.0
		Minor but stable deviation of the iris	1	2.0
		Need for laser-assisted capsulotomy	2	3.9
		Suture cut through residual iris	1	2.0
2 (moderate)	Unexpected events needed for noninvasive intervention *without* full recovery	New onset of glaucoma with need for local therapy	3	5.9
		New onset of clinically corneal decompensation	3	5.9
		Suture loosening of AI/lens	2	3.9
		Artificial iris sub-/dislocation	3	5.9
		New vitreous strands or synechiae in the anterior chamber	2	3.9
3 (severe)	Unexpected or expected events leading to any surgical intervention	New onset or aggravation of glaucoma with need for surgical intervention (valve drainage device)	2	3.9
		New onset or aggravation of clinically corneal decompensation with a need for amniotic membrane transplantation	2	3.9
		New onset or aggravation of clinically corneal decompensation with a need for keratoplasty	5	9.8
		CME	3	5.9
		Retinal detachment	1	2.0

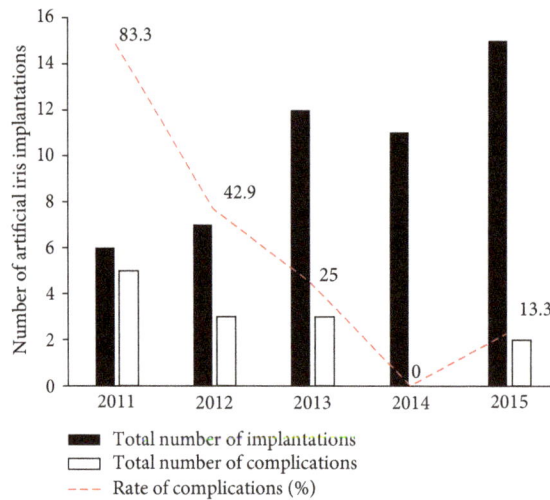

FIGURE 6: Incidence of complications after artificial iris implantation and complication rate. The surgeon's learning curve can be seen in the decreasing rate of complications with increasing numbers of implantations over the time. After 2 years—or 13 artificial iris implantations—the complication rate is below 25% and the surgical learning curve is significantly flattened.

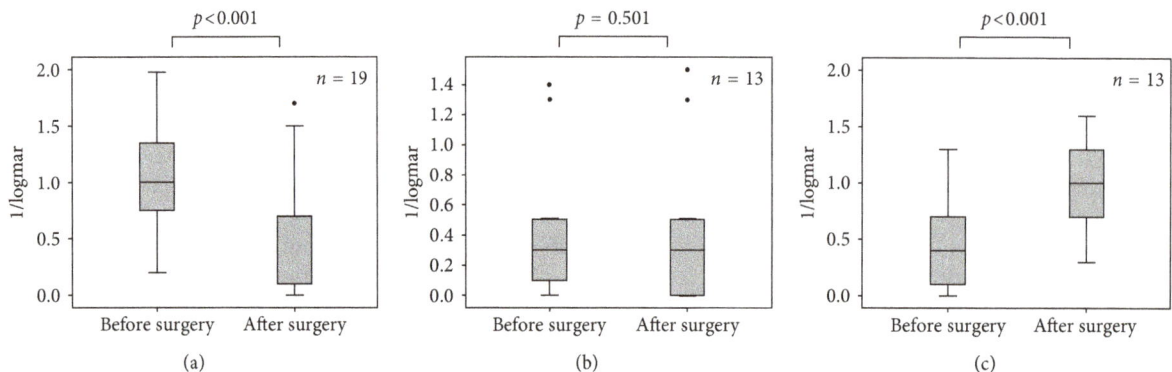

FIGURE 7: Development of visual acuity (logMAR) in 45 eyes after artificial iris implantation. Nineteen patients had a significant BCVA increase (>2 lines of a Snellen projection chart, $p < 0.001$) (a); 13 patients remained unchanged (±2 lines of a Snellen projection chart, $p = 0.501$) (b); 13 patients (37.8%) suffered from a significant BCVA decrease (>2 lines of a Snellen projection chart, $p < 0.001$) (c).

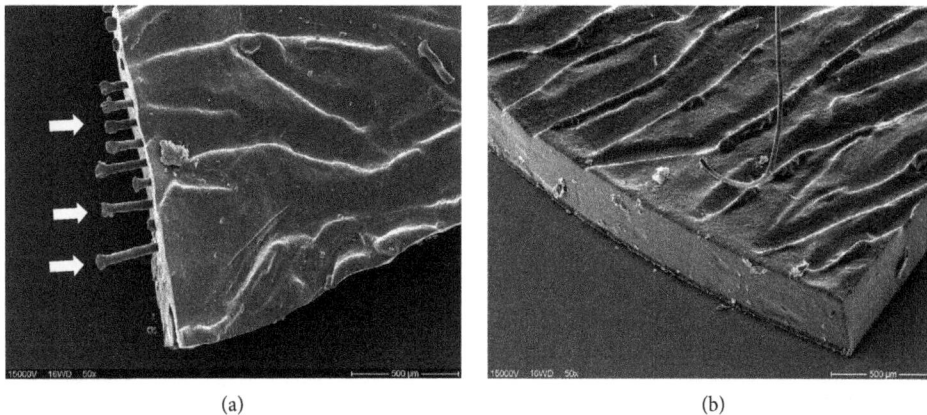

(a) (b)

FIGURE 8: Electron microscopic images of the edge of an artificial iris with embedded fiber meshwork (a). Outstanding sharp-edged fibers of the smooth silicon tissue are shown (arrows) caused eventually by use of a reusable trephine in this case. These could cause chronic bleeding in contact areas between the artificial iris and adjacent intraocular surfaces. (b) Smoothly trephined edge of an implant without embedded fiber meshwork with a single-use trephine.

5. Conclusion

In conclusion, iris reconstruction with ArtificialIris® implantation is an outstanding and rare ophthalmic surgery with potential unexpected events and a profoundly improving learning curve after a dozen implantations. After artificial iris implantation, the postoperative development can reveal unexpected adverse events of various quality and quantity. In summary, pupillary reconstruction with the used artificial iris implant should not be underestimated regarding its follow-up management and therefore requires significant surgical experience to avoid unnecessary pitfalls. Consequently, we would advise the use of artificial iris implants in specialized centers and focus on few surgeons.

Conflicts of Interest

The authors do not have any commercial interest in any of the materials and methods used in this study.

References

[1] J. McKelvie, B. McArdle, and C. McGhee, "The influence of tilt, decentration, and pupil size on the higher-order aberration profile of aspheric intraocular lenses," *Ophthalmology*, vol. 118, no. 9, pp. 1724–1731, 2011.

[2] J. Li, G. Yuan, L. Ying, B. Yu, and X. Dong, "Modified implantation of black diaphragm intraocular lens in traumatic aniridia," *Journal of Cataract and Refractive Surgery*, vol. 39, no. 6, pp. 822–825, 2013.

[3] T. Reinhard, S. Engelhardt, and R. Sundmacher, "Black diaphragm aniridia intraocular lens for congenital aniridia: long-term follow-up," *Journal of Cataract and Refractive Surgery*, vol. 26, no. 3, pp. 375–381, 2000.

[4] S. Srinivasan, D. S. Ting, M. E. Snyder, S. Prasad, and H. R. Koch, "Prosthetic iris devices," *Canadian Journal of Ophthalmology/Journal Canadien d'Ophtalmologie*, vol. 49, no. 1, pp. 6–17, 2014.

[5] R. Sundmacher, T. Reinhard, and C. Althaus, "Black-diaphragm intraocular lens for correction of aniridia," *Ophthalmic Surgery*, vol. 25, no. 3, pp. 180–185, 1994.

[6] J. Wolff, "Prosthetic iris devices," *Der Ophthalmologe: Zeitschrift der Deutschen Ophthalmologischen Gesellschaft*, vol. 108, no. 8, pp. 714–719, 2011.

[7] Y. S. Mostafa, A. A. Osman, D. H. Hassanein, A. M. Zeid, and A. M. Sherif, "Iris reconstruction using artificial iris prosthesis for management of aniridia," *European Journal of Ophthalmology*, vol. 28, no. 1, pp. 103–107, 2018.

[8] M. Rana, V. Savant, and J. I. Prydal, "A new customized artificial iris diaphragm for treatment of traumatic aniridia," *Contact Lens & Anterior Eye*, vol. 36, no. 2, pp. 93–94, 2013.

[9] M. S. Spitzer, E. Yoeruek, M. A. Leitritz, P. Szurman, and K. U. Bartz-Schmidt, "A new technique for treating post-traumatic aniridia with aphakia: first results of haptic fixation of a foldable intraocular lens on a foldable and custom-tailored iris prosthesis," *Archives of Ophthalmology*, vol. 130, no. 6, pp. 771–775, 2012.

[10] P. Szurman and G. Jaissle, "Artificial iris," *Der Ophthalmologe: Zeitschrift der Deutschen Ophthalmologischen Gesellschaft*, vol. 108, no. 8, pp. 720–727, 2011.

[11] C. Haritoglou, "Artificial iris after severe trauma of the orbit," *Der Ophthalmologe: Zeitschrift der Deutschen Ophthalmologischen Gesellschaft*, vol. 112, no. 7, pp. 599–601, 2015.

[12] C. Kniestedt, R. Eberhard, and J. Fleischhauer, "Implantation of an artificial iris in 11 patients," *Klinische Monatsblatter fur Augenheilkunde*, vol. 233, no. 4, pp. 365–368, 2016.

[13] K. R. Koch, L. M. Heindl, C. Cursiefen, and H. R. Koch, "Artificial iris devices: benefits, limitations, and management of complications," *Journal of Cataract and Refractive Surgery*, vol. 40, no. 3, pp. 376–382, 2014.

[14] J. Magnus, R. Trau, D. G. Mathysen, and M. J. Tassignon, "Safety of an artificial iris in a phakic eye," *Journal of Cataract and Refractive Surgery*, vol. 38, no. 6, pp. 1097–1100, 2012.

[15] S. Roman, H. Cherrate, J. P. Trouvet, M. Ullern, and C. Baudouin, "Artificial iris intraocular lenses in aniridia or iris deficiencies," *Journal Français d'Ophtalmologie*, vol. 32, no. 5, pp. 320–325, 2009.

[16] B. C. Thomas, T. M. Rabsilber, and G. U. Auffarth, "Aniridia-IOL and artificial iris reconstruction," *Klinische Monatsblatter fur Augenheilkunde*, vol. 230, no. 8, pp. 786–790, 2013.

[17] C. S. Mayer, L. Reznicek, and A. E. Hoffmann, "Pupillary reconstruction and outcome after artificial iris implantation," *Ophthalmology*, vol. 123, no. 5, pp. 1011–1018, 2016.

[18] B. Le Du, M. Boukhrissa, and J. P. Nordmann, "Acute angle-closure attack secondary to BrightOcular((c)) cosmetic iris implant and subsequent subluxation of contralateral iris implant," *Journal Francais d'Ophtalmologie*, vol. 39, no. 6, pp. e141–e144, 2016.

[19] A. M. Mansour, I. I. K. Ahmed, B. Eadie et al., "Iritis, glaucoma and corneal decompensation associated with BrightOcular cosmetic iris implant," *British Journal of Ophthalmology*, vol. 100, no. 8, pp. 1098–1101, 2016.

[20] A. Rickmann, P. Szurman, K. Januschowski et al., "Long-term results after artificial iris implantation in patients with aniridia," *Graefe's Archive for Clinical and Experimental Ophthalmology = Albrecht von Graefes Archiv fur klinische und experimentelle Ophthalmologie*, vol. 254, no. 7, pp. 1419–1424, 2016.

[21] M. S. Spitzer, A. Nessmann, J. Wagner et al., "Customized humanoptics silicone iris prosthesis in eyes with post-traumatic iris loss: outcomes and complications," *Acta Ophthalmologica*, vol. 94, no. 3, pp. 301–306, 2016.

[22] C. Forlini, M. Forlini, R. Rejdak et al., "Simultaneous correction of post-traumatic aphakia and aniridia with the use of artificial iris and IOL implantation," *Graefe's Archive for Clinical and Experimental Ophthalmology = Albrecht von Graefes Archiv fur klinische und experimentelle Ophthalmologie*, vol. 251, no. 3, pp. 667–675, 2013.

[23] C. S. Mayer and A. E. Hoffmann, "Surgical treatment with an artificial iris," *Der Ophthalmologe: Zeitschrift der Deutschen Ophthalmologischen Gesellschaft*, vol. 112, no. 10, pp. 865–868, 2015.

[24] C. Mayer, T. Tandogan, A. E. Hoffmann, and R. Khoramnia, "Artificial iris implantation in various iris defects and lens conditions," *Journal of Cataract and Refractive Surgery*, vol. 43, no. 6, pp. 724–731, 2017.

[25] W. S. Van Meter, "Long-term safety of polypropylene knots under scleral flaps for transsclerally sutured posterior chamber lenses," *Transactions of the American Ophthalmological Society*, vol. 95, no. 2, pp. 307–321, 1997.

5

Verisyse versus Veriflex Phakic Intraocular Lenses: Refractive Outcomes and Endothelial Cell Density 5 Years after Surgery

Dilek Yaşa ⓘ **and Alper Ağca** ⓘ

Beyoğlu Eye Research and Training Hospital, Bereketzade Mah, No. 2, Beyoglu, Istanbul, Turkey

Correspondence should be addressed to Dilek Yaşa; dilekyasa2@gmail.com

Academic Editor: Naoki Okumura

Purpose. To compare refractive stability, central endothelial cell density (ECD), and complications between Verisyse (Abbott Medical Optics, Netherlands) and Veriflex (Abbott Medical Optics, Netherlands) phakic intraocular lenses (pIOL) over five years. *Methods.* We retrospectively reviewed the medical records of patients who underwent Verisyse or Veriflex pIOL implantation for surgical correction of myopia. Patients with a 5-year follow-up period were included in the study. Uncorrected distance visual acuity (UDVA), corrected distance visual acuity (CDVA), spherical equivalent of manifest refraction (SE), and ECD were compared between the groups preoperatively and 1, 3, and 5 years postoperatively. *Results.* The study included 47 eyes in the Verisyse group and 50 eyes in the Veriflex group. There was no significant difference in mean SE, UDVA, CDVA, and ECD preoperatively or postoperatively. In both groups, there was a statistically significant myopic shift between 1-year and 5-year visits (-0.25 ± 0.30 D and -0.23 ± 0.48 D in the Verisyse and Veriflex groups, respectively). There was no significant difference between the groups in terms of efficacy and safety indexes at 5 years. ECD loss was highest during the first year (3.9% loss in the Verisyse group and 3.9% loss in the Veriflex group, $p = 0.670$). At 5 years, the mean cumulative ECD losses in the Verisyse and Veriflex groups were 7.42% and 7.64%, respectively ($p = 0.709$). Cataracts developed in 2.1% of the eyes in the Verisyse group and in 2.0% of those in the Veriflex group. No sight-threatening complications were observed. *Conclusion.* Verisyse and Veriflex pIOLs are highly effective for treating high myopia up to 5 years after surgery. Longitudinal studies with longer follow-up periods are necessary to determine the endothelial safety profile.

1. Introduction

Phakic intraocular lens (pIOL) implantation is a surgical method for treatment of high myopia [1]. Other options are corneal refractive surgery and clear lens extraction [2, 3]. pIOL implantation offers some advantages in highly myopic individuals. It allows maintenance of accommodation and results in better quality of vision when compared with corneal refractive surgery [4].

However, most early designs have been abandoned because of high rates of complications such as cataracts, glaucoma, and excessive endothelial cell loss in the long term [5, 6]. Verisyse (Abbott Medical Optics, Netherlands) and Veriflex (Abbott Medical Optics, Netherlands) are pIOLs that are considered to have good safety and efficacy [7–10]. Both of them are implanted in the same location with the same mechanism of fixation, but they have different material properties and require different incision sizes. Thus, they may have different efficacy and safety profiles.

There are only a limited number of studies comparing the long-term clinical outcomes following implantation of these lenses [11]. As a result, there is still a need for data on long-term follow-up and comparison of these lenses to establish their long-term efficacy and safety profiles. The aim of this study was to compare Verisyse and Veriflex in terms of the refractive results, central endothelial cell density (ECD), and complications over the long term.

2. Materials and Methods

This study was approved by the Institutional Review Board. Tenets of Declaration of Helsinki were followed. Medical records of patients who underwent an iris-claw pIOL implantation were evaluated retrospectively. The operative records of a single surgeon (senior author, AA) were queried, and patients with a 5-year follow-up period were included in the study. Uncorrected distance visual acuity (UDVA), corrected distance visual acuity (CDVA), spherical equivalent of manifest refraction (SE), and ECD were compared between the groups preoperatively and 1, 3, and 5 years postoperatively.

All patients received a full ophthalmological examination including refraction, UDVA and CDVA measurement, slit-lamp evaluation, Goldman applanation tonometry, fundoscopy, anterior-chamber depth measurement (from endothelium) using IOL Master (Carl Zeiss Meditec, Germany), and ECD measurement using a specular microscope (CEM 530, NIDEK, Japan). The patients were scheduled for yearly follow-up after the first year of surgery, which is routine in our clinic. A lens opacity that results in the loss of ≥ 2 lines of CDVA during follow-up was defined as cataract.

2.1. Verisyse Phakic Intraocular Lens Implantation.
Myopic model 206 was used for myopia less than -15.5 D, and model 204 was used for higher myopia. The target was emmetropia in all cases. Power calculation was performed using the modified vergence formula provided by the manufacturer. A surgical caliper was used to mark the planned borders of a 6 mm main incision centered at 12 o'clock. Two paracenteses were performed on two sides of the planned main incision. Acetylcholine 0.01% (Miochol-EO, Novartis) was injected into the anterior chamber from one of the paracenteses to constrict the papilla. The anterior chamber was filled with a cohesive viscoelastic material (Provisc, Alcon), and then the main incision was performed. The Artisan IOL was introduced from the main incision and rotated inside the eye until it was horizontal. The IOL optic was grasped with specially designed forceps, and the iris was enclaved in the claws of the pIOL using a special needle introduced from the paracentesis. Iridotomy was performed, and two interrupted nylon sutures were used to close the main incision.

2.2. Veriflex Phakic Intraocular Lens Implantation.
The target was emmetropia in all cases. Power calculation was performed using the modified vergence formula provided by the manufacturer. Two paracenteses were performed on two sides of the planned main incision. Next, 0.01% acetylcholine (Miochol-EO, Novartis) was injected into the anterior chamber from one of the paracentheses to constrict the pupilla. A 2.75 mm main incision centered at 12 o'clock was performed with a slit knife. The anterior chamber was filled with a cohesive viscoelastic material (Provisc, Alcon), and the Veriflex IOL was introduced from the main incision and rotated inside the eye until it was horizontal. The IOL optic was grasped with specially designed forceps, and the iris was enclaved in the claws of the pIOL using a special needle introduced from the paracentesis. Iridotomy was performed, and the incisions were hydrated with BSS.

2.3. Statistical Methods.
Statistical analysis was performed using SPSS for Windows (version 21.0; IBM, Armonk, NY), and the associated graphics were generated with Microsoft Excel 2013 (Microsoft Corporation, Seattle, WA, USA). The mean, standard deviation, and frequency were used in the statistical analysis. The variable distribution was determined using the Shapiro–Wilk test. A paired t-test was used to analyze parametric data, and a Wilcoxon signed-rank test was used to analyze nonparametric data. Chi-square and Fisher's exact tests were used to compare categorical variable. One-way repeated measures analysis of variance (ANOVA) was used to evaluate ECD during follow-up. The annual ECD loss was calculated according to the following formula:

$$\text{ECD loss/year} = \frac{\text{ECDf} - \text{ECDi}}{\text{ECDi} \times t}, \quad (1)$$

where ECDf is the endothelial cell count at the last visit, ECDi is the preoperative cell count, and t is the time in years between the two endothelial cell count measurements.

3. Results

The study included 97 eyes from 63 subjects. There were 40 (63%) male subjects and 23 (37%) female subjects. There were 47 eyes in the Verisyse group and 50 eyes in the Veriflex group. The preoperative patient characteristics are shown in Table 1. There were no statistically significant differences between the preoperative characteristics of the groups.

Figures 1(a) and 1(b) show the postoperative cumulative Snellen visual acuities (UDVA and CDVA) of the Verisyse and Veriflex groups, respectively. The efficacy indices (preoperative CDVA and postoperative UDVA) at 5 years were 1.14 ± 0.60 and 1.04 ± 0.47 in the Verisyse and Veriflex groups, respectively ($p > 0.05$).

Table 2 shows the SE of manifest refraction preoperatively and at postoperative visits. In both groups, SE was similar between the groups preoperatively and at the postoperative visits at 1, 3, and 5 years. However, postoperative SE increased significantly during the five-year follow-up in both groups. In both groups, there was a statistically significant myopic shift (-0.25 ± 0.30 D and -0.23 ± 0.48 D in Veriflex and Verisyse groups, respectively) between 1-year and 5-year visits. At the end of the follow-up (5-years), the mean SE was -0.68 ± 0.44 and -0.72 ± 0.40 in the Veriflex and Verisyse groups, respectively. Tables 3 and 4 list refractive sphere and refractive cylinder during follow-up. The refractive sphere increased significantly during the five-year follow-up in both groups. In Veriflex group, there was no significant change in the refractive cylinder during follow-up. In Verisyse group, the refractive cylinder was not significantly different at the end of follow-up when compared with preoperative cylinder.

At the 1-year postoperative visit, 74% of the eyes in both groups were within ± 0.5 D of emmetropia. However, at the 5-year postoperative visit, only 40% and 56% of the eyes were within ± 0.5 D of emmetropia in the Verisyse and Veriflex groups, respectively (Figures 2(a) and 2(b)). The difference

Table 1: Preoperative characteristics.

Parameter	Verisyse group Mean ± SD (range)	Veriflex group Mean ± SD (range)	p
Age (years)	31 ± 5 (20 to 42)	30 ± 5 (20 to 41)	0.247
SE (D)	−12.50 ± 3.51 (−6.25 to −20.00)	−11.50 ± 3.46 (−4.75 to −20.75)	0.207
Cylinder (D)	0.75 ± 0.53 (0 to 2.00)	0.59 ± 0.56 (0 to 2.00)	0.176
CDVA (logMAR)	0.34 ± 0.22 (0 to 1.00)	0.26 ± 0.16 (0 to 0.70)	0.095
ECD (cells/mm^2)	2681 ± 275 (2278 to 3220)	2656 ± 270 (2258 to 3205)	0.692
ACD (mm)	3.27 ± 0.21 (3.03 to 3.69)	3,32 ± 0.26 (3.02 to 3.82)	0.316
AL (mm)	28.44 ± 1.58 (24.45 to 31.62)	28.11 ± 1.49 (23.70 to 30.08)	0.342

SD: standard deviation; D: diopters; SE: spherical equivalent; CDVA: corrected distance visual acuity; WTW: white-to-white; ECD: endothelial cell density; Sim K: simulated keratometry; IOP: intraocular pressure; AL: axial length.

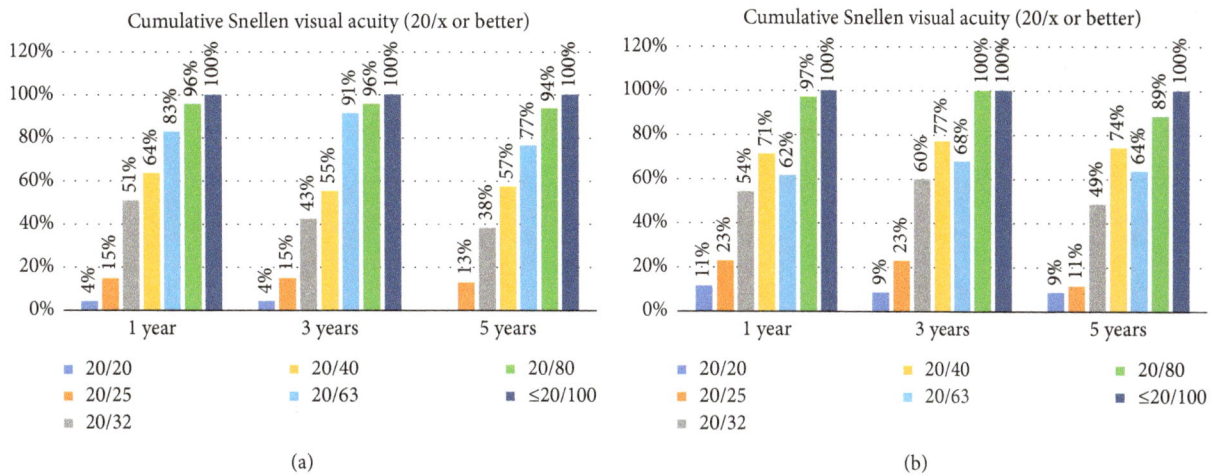

Figure 1: Cumulative uncorrected distance visual acuity in Verisyse (a) and Veriflex (b) groups.

Table 2: Spherical equivalent (SE) of subjective manifest refraction during follow-up.

	Preoperative (mean ± SD)	1 year (mean ± SD)	3 years (mean ± SD)	5 years (mean ± SD)	p
Veriflex	−11.50 ± 3.46	−0.36 ± 0.43	−0.49 ± 35	−0.68 ± 0.44	$p < 0.001^*$
Verisyse	−12.50 ± 3.51	−0.43 ± 0.34	−0.54 ± 0.39	−0.72 ± 0.40	$p < 0.001^{**}$
$p^\dagger$	0.207	0.398	0.554	0.595	

*Repeated measures ANOVA, p value for all visits. Post hoc analysis: statistically significant difference was observed from the preoperative visit to the 1-year visit ($p < 0.001$), from the 1-year visit to 3-year visit ($p = 0.036$), and from 3-year visit to 5-year visit ($p = 001$). **Repeated measures ANOVA, p value for all visits. Post hoc analysis: statistically significant difference was observed from the preoperative visit to the 1-year visit ($p < 0.001$), from the 1-year visit to 3-year visit ($p = 0.003$), and from 3-year visit to 5-year visit ($p < 0.001$). †Independent samples t-test.

Table 3: Refractive Sphere during follow-up.

	Preoperative (mean ± SD)	1 year (mean ± SD)	3 years (mean ± SD)	5 years (mean ± SD)	p
Veriflex	−11.21 ± 3.28	−0.10 ± 0.46	−0.24 ± 0.40	−0.41 ± 0.47	$p < 0.001^*$
Verisyse	−12.13 ± 3.34	−0.11 ± 0.39	−0.20 ± 0.43	−0.38 ± 0.46	$p < 0.001^{**}$
$p^\dagger$	0.223	0.909	0.740	0.752	

*Repeated measures ANOVA, p value for all visits. Post hoc analysis: statistically significant difference was observed from the preoperative visit to the 1-year visit ($p < 0.001$), from the 1-year visit to 3-year visit ($p = 0.026$), and from 3-year visit to 5-year visit ($p < 0.001$). **Repeated measures ANOVA, p value for all visits. Post hoc analysis: statistically significant difference was observed from the preoperative visit to the 1-year visit ($p < 0.001$), from the 1-year visit to 3-year visit ($p = 0.010$), and from 3-year visit to 5-year visit ($p < 0.001$). †Independent samples t-test.

between the groups was statistically insignificant (Chi-square test, $p = 0.156$).

None of the patients lost ≥2 lines of CDVA (Figure 3). The safety indices (preoperative CDVA and postoperative CDVA) at 5 years were $1.39 ± 0.63$ and $1.31 ± 0.50$ in the Verisyse and Veriflex groups, respectively ($p > 0.05$).

In one patient in the Veriflex group, one of the haptics of the iris-claw lens was refixated at the 1-year visit because it was loosely fixated to the iris. It was mobile and slightly decentered. This patient did not report a history of trauma, allergy, or eye-rubbing behavior, and the pIOL was stable and centralized at the last follow-up. The decentration was

TABLE 4: Refractive cylinder during follow-up.

	Preoperative (mean ± SD)	1 year (mean ± SD)	3 years (mean ± SD)	5 years (mean ± SD)	p^*
Veriflex	−0.59 ± 0.56	−0.52 ± 0.56	−0.51 ± 0.52	−0.54 ± 0.53	$p = 0.069$
Verisyse	−0.75 ± 0.53	−0.64 ± 0.46	−0.68 ± 0.49	−0.70 ± 0.48	$p = 0.036^\dagger$
p^{**}	0.207	0.398	0.554	0.595	

*Repeated measures ANOVA, p value for all visits. **Independent samples t-test. †Post hoc analysis: statistically significant difference was observed from the preoperative visit to the 1-year visit ($p = 0.006$) and from the preoperative visit to the 3-year visit ($p = 0.018$). There was no statistically significant difference from the preoperative visit to the 5-year visit ($p = 0.162$).

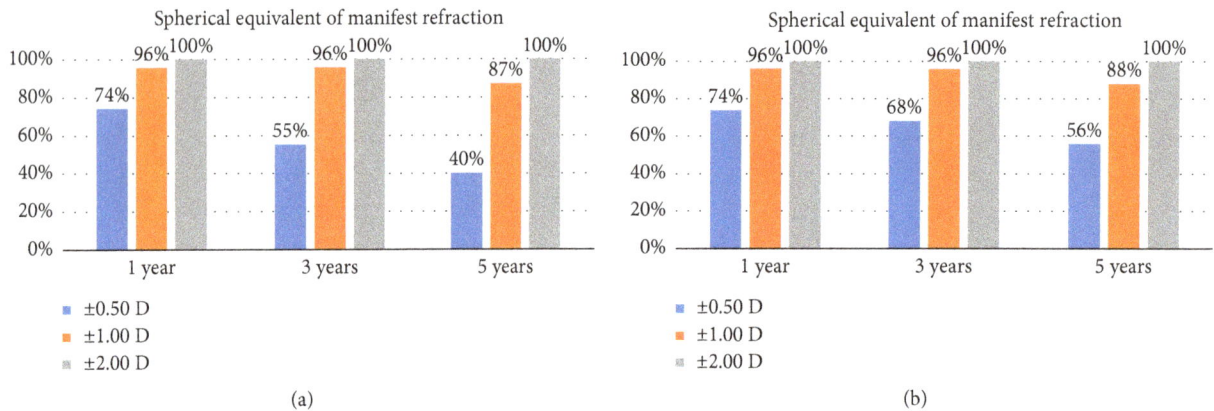

FIGURE 2: Spherical equivalent of mean manifest refraction in Verisyse (a) and Veriflex (b) groups.

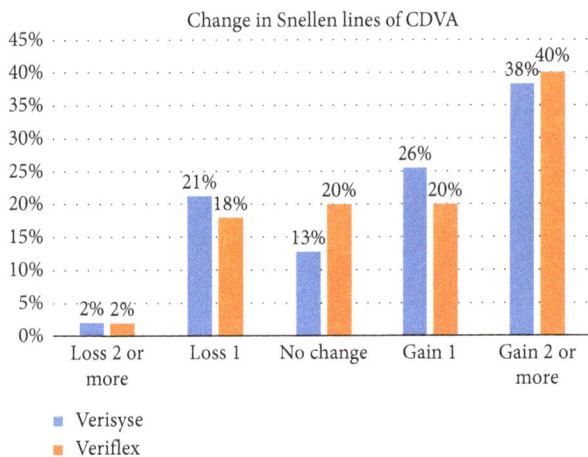

FIGURE 3: Change in corrected distance visual acuity (CDVA).

probably due to inappropriate enclavation during the surgery. The haptic was re-enclaved with a second operation just after the 1-year visit, and the patient experienced no further complications. Intraocular pressures (IOP) during follow-up are listed in Table 5. In all patients, IOP was ≤21 mmHg at all postoperative visits.

Table 6 shows the endothelial changes over the course of the study. ECD was similar between the groups preoperatively and postoperatively at all visits. At 5 years, the mean cumulative ECD losses in the Verisyse and Veriflex groups were 7.42% and 7.64%, respectively ($p = 0.709$). None of the patients lost ≥25% of their baseline ECD during the 5-year follow-up. Annual ECD loss for Verisyse was 3.05% in the first year, 1.23% between 1 and 3 years, and

1.02% between 3 and 5 years. The annual ECD loss for Veriflex was 3.05% in the first year, 1.24% between 1 and 3 years, and 1.05% between 3 and 5 years.

4. Discussion

In this study, we evaluated and compared the long-term results after implantation of two different types of iris-claw pIOLs. In line with previous studies, the refractive and visual results were satisfactory in both groups. There were no significant differences between the groups in terms of MRSE, UDVA, and CDVA during the follow-up period.

There are only a few studies comparing these two pIOLs in the long term. Bohac et al. [11] compared the refractive outcomes of Verisyse and Veriflex pIOLs for 36 months after surgery and found that SE was similar at the 36-month visit. However, CDVA was significantly better in the Veriflex group, in contrast to our study. An improvement in CDVA has been reported in the literature, and results from the magnification effect of pIOLs were compared with spectacles. A difference between the CDVA of the groups is difficult to reveal before the operation, and the difference probably results from preoperative patient characteristics in the study reported by Bohac et al. [11].

High refractive predictability after phakic iris-claw has been reported [7–9,11,12]. In a clinical trial study from the United States Food and Drug Administration (FDA), Stulting et al. reported that 71.7% of eyes were within 0.5 D of the target refraction and 94.7% were within 1.0 D postoperatively. In line with the FDA study, we found that 74% and 96% of the eyes in the Verisyse group were within ±0.5 D and ±1.00 D, respectively [7]. The percentages of the eyes that were in ±0.5 D and ±1.00 D were equal in the Veriflex

TABLE 5: Intraocular pressure during follow-up.

	Preoperative Mean ± SD (range)	1 year Mean ± SD (range)	3 years Mean ± SD (range)	5 years Mean ± SD (range)	p^*
Veriflex	13.6 ± 1.7 (10 to 16)	13.9 ± 2.6 (10 to 21)	13.9 ± 2.1 (10 to 18)	13.5 ± 2.1 (10 to 21)	$p = 0.792$
Verisyse	13.9 ± 2.0 (10 to 17)	13.9 ± 2.6 (9 to 20)	14.0 ± 1.5 (11 to 18)	14.3 ± 2.2 (10 to 20)	$p = 0.703$
p^{**}	0.561	0.950	0.825	0.088	

*Repeated measures ANOVA, p value for all visits. **Independent samples t-test.

TABLE 6: Endothelial changes over the course of the study.

	Preoperative	1 year	3 years	5 years	p^*
	Central ECD (cells/mm^2) (mean ± SD (% of cumulative ECD loss))				
Verisyse	2681 ± 275 (N/A)	2599 ± 242 (3.05)	2534 ± 238 (5.48)	2482 ± 242 (7.42)	$p < 0.001^{\dagger}$
Veriflex	2656 ± 270 (N/A)	2575 ± 253 (3.04)	2512 ± 251 (5.42)	2460 ± 282 (7.64)	$p < 0.001^{\dagger\dagger}$
p^{**}	0.692	0.670	0.678	0.709	
	Coefficient of variation of cell area (%)				
Verisyse	30.8 ± 5.5	29.0 ± 5.7	29.4 ± 4.3	29.1 ± 5.8	0.083
Veriflex	30.0 ± 5.2	30.6 ± 5.2	30.5 ± 5.4	31.2 ± 6.0	0.233
$p^{\dagger}$	0.515	0.185	0.699	0.117	
	Hexagonal cells (%)				
Verisyse	65.4 ± 7.5	66.1 ± 7.3	64.8 ± 6.9	66.0 ± 8.2	0.114
Veriflex	62.7 ± 7.7	64.7 ± 8.4	63.9 ± 8.2	64.4 ± 8.8	0.142
$p^{\dagger}$	0.130	0.422	0.601	0.396	

*Repeated measures ANOVA, p value for all visits. **Independent samples t-test. †Post hoc analysis: statistically significant difference was observed from the preoperative visit to the 1-year visit ($p < 0.001$), from the 1-year visit to 3-year visit ($p < 0.001$), and from 3-year visit to 5-year visit ($p < 0.001$). ††Post hoc analysis: statistically significant difference was observed from the preoperative visit to the 1-year visit ($p < 0.001$), from the 1-year visit to 3-year visit ($p < 0.001$), and from 3-year visit to 5-year visit ($p < 0.001$).

group. However, we found that the refractive results were not stable in the long term. There was a small but statistically significant regression at the 1-year and 5-year visits in both groups (-0.25 ± 0.30 D and -0.23 ± 0.48 D in the Verisyse and Veriflex groups, respectively). The amount of regression was not statistically different in both groups, and it is probably related to an increase in axial length. Several studies report that the refractive results are stable after pIOL implantation, while others report that regression of the refractive effect occurs, and it is probably related to a progressive increase in the axial length in at least some patients. Guell et al. [13] reported a 5-year follow-up study of 399 phakic Artisan-Verisyse IOLs. Among the patients with myopia, only 10% of the eyes in the 5 mm optic Verisyse PIOL group and 38% of the eyes in the 6 mm optic Verisyse PIOL group were within 0.5 D of the target refraction. Additional refractive surgery was performed in 60% and 20% of the 5 and 6 mm optics groups, respectively. The stability in the refractive results in several studies probably results from the amount of initial myopia, relatively short follow-up, low number of patients, or lack of sufficient statistical power to find a difference, or a combination of these factors.

Despite a regression during follow-up, we found the efficacy index to be 1.14 and 1.04 in the Verisyse and Veriflex groups ($p > 0.05$), respectively. It is also our clinical experience that most patients still have a UDVA equal to or better than the preoperative CDVA, even in the presence of a residual refractive error. The increase in CDVA is probably the reason for the high efficacy index, despite the residual

refractive errors and a small but statistically significant regression over time.

Approximately 20% of the eyes gained ≥1 line, and one-third of the eyes gained ≥2 lines. The exact mechanism of the increase in CDVA is unclear, but the reason for the improvement may be the relative magnification of the image after an anterior chamber pIOL implantation when compared with spectacle lenses [14]. There is agreement in the literature that improvement occurs in CDVA after corneal refractive surgery or pIOL implantation [15–17].

A prospective, multicenter U.S. FDA trial reported the most detailed data with the highest level of evidence on the ECD loss after a similar rigid iris-claw pIOL (Artisan). The ECD loss was $-4.8\% \pm 7.8\%$ from baseline to 3 years, with a 2.4% loss between 2 and 3 years [7]. Benedetti et al. [18] reported an ECD loss of 4.7% at two years and 9% at five years after Artisan pIOL implantation. A European prospective multicenter study evaluated the surgical results of Artiflex, and the mean endothelial cell changes were -0.05%, 1.79%, and -1.07% at 6 months, 1 year, and 2 years, respectively [10]. All of these values are higher than the normal ECD loss in a nonoperated eye. The ECD loss after implantation of iris-claw and posterior chamber phakic IOLs are comparable. Thus, it is not clear if one design has an advantage over the other in terms of ECD [7,18–20]. The most detailed data with the highest level of evidence on the ECD loss after a posterior chamber pIOL implantation was reported during the U.S. FDA trial (526 eyes, 4 years). In that study, ECD loss was $3.3 \pm 7.6\%$ at one year (90% confidence limits: 2.4% to 4.3%) and 9.7 ± 9.3 at 4 years [19, 20].

Recently, Yasa et al. [21] reported a mean ECD loss of 3.9% at one year after implantation of a new posterior chamber phakic IOL.

Several studies report that endothelial damage occurs primarily during the surgical procedure, and the decrease stabilizes after a certain time [22–24]. However, there are reports of late endothelial decompensation, which indicate progressive cell loss in at least some patients. Saxena et al. [25] found a significant negative correlation between ACD and endothelium cell loss. Doors et al. [26] found that a shallow ACD and smaller distance between the pIOL edge and the endothelium were risk factors for ECD loss. In a recent study, Jonker et al. [27] reported that in a group of 507 eyes, ECD had decreased by ≥25% in 7.9% of them, and ECD was <1500 cells/mm^2 in 3.9% at 10 years after implantation. Risk factors for increased ECD loss were a shallow ACD and a smaller distance between the central and peripheral pIOL edge to the endothelium. However, it is still not clear if ECD loss in eyes that do not have these risk factors is still higher than normal ECD loss in a nonoperated eye.

Verisyse and Veriflex have similar designs and fixation mechanisms but different material properties. Hedayatfar et al. [28] compared chronic subclinical inflammation induced after implantation of Artisan versus Artiflex phakic intraocular lenses (pIOLs). Anterior chamber flare was assessed quantitatively using laser flare photometry (LFP). They concluded that the inflammatory response induced by implantation of either type of pIOLs is short-lived without statistically significant difference between the two models. However, there are reports showing that the silicon optic material that is used in Veriflex may cause inflammation and might be increasing the incidence of pigment deposits postoperatively [10, 29, 30]. No chronic inflammation was seen in our patients. However, inflammation was not assessed quantitatively, and we highlight the possibility that mild inflammation in the early postoperative period could have gone unnoticed. This weakness of the study should be considered when interpreting the results.

Although there are several studies reporting long-term ECD loss for both phakic IOLs, it is difficult to compare the effect of lenses on ECD. It is difficult to draw a conclusion by comparing different studies because surgeries are performed by different surgeons and preoperative patient characteristics are different in these studies. For example, in the prospective multicenter U.S. FDA trial, one site had a mean cell loss of 5.0%, and the others combined had a mean cell loss of 1.7% [13].

In this study, we evaluated two different iris-claw lenses with different material properties. All the surgeries were performed by a single surgeon, all the patients had ACD ≥ 3.00 mm from the endothelium, and preoperative patient characteristics were similar between the groups. In addition, the follow-up duration was reasonably long. We found that the central ECD loss was similar in both groups at all follow-up points. ECD loss was highest during the first year (3.05% and 3.04% in the Verisyse and Veriflex groups, respectively), and at five years, the cumulative loss was 7.42% and 7.64% in the Verisyse and Veriflex groups, respectively. The results

correspond to an annual ECD loss of 1.02 and 1.05% in Verisyse and Veriflex pIOLs between 3-year and 5-year visits.

ECD loss was highest during the first year and diminished thereafter. However, it is still not possible to conclude that the ECD loss is similar to a normal non-operated eye. In early cross-sectional studies, the average annual endothelial cell loss rate in normal eyes was found to be approximately 0.3 to 0.5% [31, 32]. In a longitudinal study, in which the same subjects were examined again at a later date, Bourne et al. reported an annual loss of 0.6 ± 0.5% over 10 years [33]. In a recent longitudinal study, the annual rate of cell loss after refractive surgery was found to be 0.6% ± 0.8 % over 9 years [34]. Thus, we believe that lifelong ECD follow-up is needed in patients who have undergone pIOL implantation.

In both groups, there were no serious intraoperative complications, and the safety index was not statistically significantly different between the groups. None of the patients lost more than 2 lines, and 1 patient in both groups lost 2 lines at 5 years (2.1% and 2.0% in the Verisyse and Veriflex groups, respectively). In both patients, the reason for CDVA loss was cataracts. Most of the patients undergoing pIOL implantation are young adults. Thus, cataract formation is a major concern when implanting a pIOL. In a meta-analysis of 6,338 eyes, Chen et al. [35] reported that the incidence of cataract formation was 1.29%, 1.11%, and 9.60% with anterior-chamber, iris-fixated, and posterior-chamber pIOLs. However, the rate of cataract formation may be higher in longer follow-up. Moshirfar et al. [36] evaluated the incidence rate and indications to investigate Verisyse pIOLs implanted over a 13.6-year period by one surgeon at one institution with a mean follow-up of 5.6 years per eye. Similar to our study, they reported that the occurrence of cataract formation in this patient population was 2.3%.

In our patient group, the only other complication was a slight decentration of the pIOL due to improper enclavation of one of the haptics in the iris. This patient did not report a history of trauma, allergy, or eye rubbing, and the decentration was probably due to inappropriate enclavation during the surgery. The haptic was re-enclaved with a second operation just after the 1-year visit, and the patient did not have any additional complications in the remaining follow-up period. No pigment dispersion, glaucoma, or pupillary block was observed in this patient group.

The most important weakness of this study is its retrospective nature. For example, there were no cases of pigment dispersion in our patients. Although intraocular pressure measurement is routine at every visit in our clinic, gonioscopy was not performed. Thus, very mild clinical pigment dispersion in some patients could have gone unnoticed.

We found a myopic shift during 5 years in our patient group. This was an expected finding as most of our patients had high axial myopia. Thus, a correlation could have been found between the axial length (AL) change and the change in SE if we had performed an analysis. However, it is unusual to measure AL routinely in postoperative visits. Thus, AL measurement was not part of our routine postoperative examinations. Accordingly, neither this study nor the other retrospective studies in the literature report an analysis of correlation between the change in SE and the change in AL [18, 22, 25]. This is a weakness of this study that results from its retrospective nature and can be addressed in prospective studies.

Postoperative examinations were performed by different residents during the 5-year follow-up, and mild anterior subcapsular cataracts that do not affect visual acuity or slight pupil ovalization in a patient may have gone unnoticed. In addition, it was not possible to measure the distance between the pIOL edge and the endothelium postoperatively to evaluate its long-term effect on ECD because of the retrospective nature of the study. However, the advantages of this study are the longitudinal follow-up of ECD measurements for 5-years in 97 patients for two different pIOLs implanted by the same surgeon in patients with similar preoperative characteristics and a minimum ACD of 3.02 mm.

In conclusion, we have found that refractive results and visual acuities were clinically similar after implantation of both designs of iris-claw pIOLs in patients with high myopia. Both pIOLs were highly effective for the surgical treatment of high myopia, and the incidence of perioperative and postoperative complications is rare when patients are selected carefully. Central ECD loss was similar in both the Verisyse and Veriflex groups and slowed down dramatically after the first year. However, we believe that ECD and intraocular lens position should continue to be monitored as these patients are usually young and will continue to live with the implanted lens for many decades. Prospective studies with larger patient groups and longer follow-up periods are needed to reveal long-term ECD loss profiles.

Conflicts of Interest

The authors declare that there are no conflicts of interest regarding the publication of this article.

References

[1] M. Lundstrom, S. Manning, P. Barry, U. Stenevi, Y. Henry, and P. Rosen, "The European registry of quality outcomes for cataract and refractive surgery (EUREQUO): a database study of trends in volumes, surgical techniques and outcomes of refractive surgery," *Eye and Vision*, vol. 2, no. 1, p. 8, 2015.

[2] J. Burazovitch, D. Naguzeswski, T. Beuste, and M. Guillard, "Predictability of SMILE over four years in high myopes," *Journal Français d'Ophtalmologie*, vol. 40, no. 6, pp. e201–e209, 2017.

[3] J. L. Arne, "Phakic intraocular lens implantation versus clear lens extraction in highly myopic eyes of 30- to 50-year-old patients," *Journal of Cataract & Refractive Surgery*, vol. 30, no. 10, pp. 2092–2096, 2004.

[4] H. Kobashi, K. Kamiya, A. Igarashi, K. Matsumura, M. Komatsu, and K. Shimizu, "Long-term quality of life after posterior chamber phakic intraocular lens implantation and after wavefront-guided laser in situ keratomileusis for myopia," *Journal of Cataract & Refractive Surgery*, vol. 40, no. 12, pp. 2019–2024, 2014.

[5] J. L. Guell, M. Morral, D. Kook, and T. Kohnen, "Phakic intraocular lenses part 1: historical overview, current models, selection criteria, and surgical techniques," *Journal of Cataract & Refractive Surgery*, vol. 36, no. 11, pp. 1976–1993, 2010.

[6] T. Kohnen, D. Kook, M. Morral, and J. L. Guell, "Phakic intraocular lenses: part 2: results and complications," *Journal of Cataract & Refractive Surgery*, vol. 36, no. 12, pp. 2168–2194, 2010.

[7] R. D. Stulting, M. E. John, R. K. Maloney et al., "Three-year results of Artisan/Verisyse phakic intraocular lens implantation. Results of the United States Food And Drug Administration clinical trial," *Ophthalmology*, vol. 115, no. 3, pp. 464–472, 2008.

[8] N. Nassiri, S. Ghorbanhosseini, E. Jafarzadehpur, S. Kavousnezhad, N. Nassiri, and K. Sheibani, "Visual acuity, endothelial cell density and polymegathism after iris-fixated lens implantation," *Clinical Ophthalmology*, vol. 12, pp. 601–605, 2018.

[9] C. Albarran-Diego, G. Munoz, T. Ferrer-Blasco, S. Garcia-Lazaro, and L. Belda-Salmeron, "Foldable iris-fixated phakic intraocular lens vs femtosecond laser-assisted LASIK for myopia between -6.00 and -9.00 diopters," *Journal of Refractive Surgery*, vol. 28, no. 6, pp. 380–386, 2012.

[10] H. B. Dick, C. Budo, F. Malecaze et al., "Foldable artiflex phakic intraocular lens for the correction of myopia: two-year follow-up results of a prospective European multicenter study," *Ophthalmology*, vol. 116, no. 4, pp. 671–677, 2009.

[11] M. Bohac, M. Anticic, N. Draca et al., "Comparison of verisyse and veriflex phakic intraocular lenses for treatment of moderate to high myopia 36 months after surgery," *Seminars in Ophthalmology*, vol. 32, no. 6, pp. 725–733, 2017.

[12] Q. Qasem, C. Kirwan, and M. O'Keefe, "5-year prospective follow-up of Artisan phakic intraocular lenses for the correction of myopia, hyperopia and astigmatism," *Ophthalmologica*, vol. 224, no. 5, pp. 283–290, 2010.

[13] J. L. Guell, M. Morral, O. Gris, J. Gaytan, M. Sisquella, and F. Manero, "Five-year follow-up of 399 phakic Artisan-Verisyse implantation for myopia, hyperopia, and/or astigmatism," *Ophthalmology*, vol. 115, no. 6, pp. 1002–1012, 2008.

[14] I. S. Barequet, T. Wygnanski-Jaffe, and A. Hirsh, "Laser in situ keratomileusis improves visual acuity in some adult eyes with amblyopia," *Journal of Refractive Surgery*, vol. 20, no. 1, pp. 25–28, 2004.

[15] S. W. Kwon, H. S. Moon, and K. H. Shyn, "Visual improvement in high myopic amblyopic adult eyes following phakic anterior chamber intraocular lens implantation," *Korean Journal of Ophthalmology*, vol. 20, no. 2, pp. 87–92, 2006.

[16] A. Agca, E. B. Ozgurhan, O. Baz et al., "Laser in situ keratomileusis in adult patients with anisometropic amblyopia," *International Journal of Ophthalmology*, vol. 6, no. 3, pp. 362–369, 2013.

[17] N. Cagil, N. Ugurlu, H. B. Cakmak, S. I. Kocamis, D. Turak, and S. Simsek, "Photorefractive keratectomy in treatment of refractive amblyopia in the adult population," *Journal of Cataract & Refractive Surgery*, vol. 37, no. 12, pp. 2167–2174, 2011.

[18] S. Benedetti, V. Casamenti, and M. Benedetti, "Long-term endothelial changes in phakic eyes after Artisan intraocular lens implantation to correct myopia: five-year study," *Journal*

of Cataract & Refractive Surgery, vol. 33, no. 5, pp. 784–790, 2007.

[19] H. F. Edelhauser, D. R. Sanders, R. Azar, H. Lamielle, and ICLiToMS Group, "Corneal endothelial assessment after ICL implantation," *Journal of Cataract & Refractive Surgery*, vol. 30, no. 3, pp. 576–583, 2004.

[20] D. R. Sanders, K. Doney, M. Poco, and ICLiToMS Group, "United States Food and Drug Administration clinical trial of the implantable collamer lens (ICL) for moderate to high myopia: three-year follow-up," *Ophthalmology*, vol. 111, no. 9, pp. 1683–1692, 2004.

[21] D. Yasa, U. Urdem, A. Agca et al., "Early results with a new posterior chamber phakic intraocular lens in patients with high myopia," *Journal of Ophthalmology*, vol. 2018, Article ID 1329874, 8 pages, 2018.

[22] D. Yasa, A. Agca, Z. Alkin et al., "Two-year follow-up of Artisan Iris-supported phakic anterior chamber intraocular lens for correction of high myopia," *Seminars in Ophthalmology*, vol. 31, no. 3, pp. 280–284, 2016.

[23] C. Budo, J. C. Hessloehl, M. Izak et al., "Multicenter study of the Artisan phakic intraocular lens," *Journal of Cataract & Refractive Surgery*, vol. 26, no. 8, pp. 1163–1171, 2000.

[24] Y. Chen, Q. Liu, C. Xue, Z. Huang, and Y. Chen, "Three-year follow-up of secondary anterior iris fixation of an aphakic intraocular lens to correct aphakia," *Journal of Cataract & Refractive Surgery*, vol. 38, no. 9, pp. 1595–1601, 2012.

[25] R. Saxena, S. S. Boekhoorn, P. G. Mulder, B. Noordzij, G. van Rij, and G. P. Luyten, "Long-term follow-up of endothelial cell change after Artisan phakic intraocular lens implantation," *Ophthalmology*, vol. 115, no. 4, pp. 608–613, 2008.

[26] M. Doors, D. W. Cals, T. T. Berendschot et al., "Influence of anterior chamber morphometrics on endothelial cell changes after phakic intraocular lens implantation," *Journal of Cataract & Refractive Surgery*, vol. 34, no. 12, pp. 2110–2118, 2008.

[27] S. M. R. Jonker, T. Berendschot, A. E. Ronden, I. E. Y. Saelens, N. J. C. Bauer, and R. Nuijts, "Long-term endothelial cell loss in patients with artisan myopia and Artisan toric phakic intraocular lenses: 5- and 10-year results," *Ophthalmology*, vol. 125, no. 4, pp. 486–494, 2018.

[28] A. Hedayatfar, H. Hashemi, S. Asghari, N. Badie, and M. Miraftab, "Chronic subclinical inflammation after phakic intraocular lenses implantation: comparison between Artisan and Artiflex models," *Journal of Current Ophthalmology*, vol. 29, no. 4, pp. 300–304, 2017.

[29] M. L. Passos, R. C. Ghanem, and V. C. Ghanem, "Removal of persistent cellular deposits after foldable iris-fixated phakic IOL implantation," *Journal of Refractive Surgery*, vol. 33, no. 6, pp. 426–428, 2017.

[30] M. J. Koss, M. Cichocki, and T. Kohnen, "Posterior synechias following implantation of a foldable silicone iris-fixated phakic intraocular lens for the correction of myopia," *Journal of Cataract & Refractive Surgery*, vol. 33, no. 5, pp. 905–909, 2007.

[31] R. W. Yee, M. Matsuda, R. O. Schultz, and H. F. Edelhauser, "Changes in the normal corneal endothelial cellular pattern as a function of age," *Current Eye Research*, vol. 4, no. 6, pp. 671–678, 1985.

[32] K. H. Carlson, W. M. Bourne, J. W. McLaren, and R. F. Brubaker, "Variations in human corneal endothelial cell morphology and permeability to fluorescein with age," *Experimental Eye Research*, vol. 47, no. 1, pp. 27–41, 1988.

[33] W. M. Bourne, L. R. Nelson, and D. O. Hodge, "Central corneal endothelial cell changes over a ten-year period,"

Investigative Ophthalmology & Visual Science, vol. 38, no. 3, pp. 779–782, 1997.

[34] S. V. Patel and W. M. Bourne, "Corneal endothelial cell loss 9 years after excimer laser keratorefractive surgery," *Archives of Ophthalmology*, vol. 127, no. 11, pp. 1423–1427, 2009.

[35] L. J. Chen, Y. J. Chang, J. C. Kuo, R. Rajagopal, and D. T. Azar, "Metaanalysis of cataract development after phakic intraocular lens surgery," *Journal of Cataract & Refractive Surgery*, vol. 34, no. 7, pp. 1181–1200, 2008.

[36] M. Moshirfar, L. M. Imbornoni, E. M. Ostler, and V. Muthappan, "Incidence rate and occurrence of visually significant cataract formation and corneal decompensation after implantation of Verisyse/Artisan phakic intraocular lens," *Clinical Ophthalmology*, vol. 8, pp. 711–716, 2014.

6

Comparison of Individual Retinal Layer Thicknesses after Epiretinal Membrane Surgery with or without Internal Limiting Membrane Peeling

Chul Hee Lee ⑩,[1] Min Woo Lee,[1] Eun Young Choi,[1] Suk Ho Byeon,[2] Sung Soo Kim,[2] Hyoung Jun Koh,[2] Sung Chul Lee,[2] and Min Kim ⑩[1]

[1]Department of Ophthalmology, Institute of Vision Research, Gangnam Severance Hospital, Yonsei University College of Medicine, Seoul, Republic of Korea
[2]Department of Ophthalmology, Institute of Vision Research, Severance Hospital, Yonsei University College of Medicine, Seoul, Republic of Korea

Correspondence should be addressed to Min Kim; minkim76@gmail.com

Academic Editor: Glenn Yiu

Purpose. To compare changes in the retinal layer thickness and visual outcomes in patients undergoing epiretinal membrane (ERM) surgery with or without internal limiting membrane (ILM) peeling. *Methods*. Seventy-six eyes of 76 patients who underwent ERM surgery from January 2013 to March 2015 at the Department of Ophthalmology, Yonsei University College of Medicine, Seoul, South Korea, were analyzed. While ERM removal with ILM peeling was performed in ILM peeling (P) group ($n = 39$), ILM peeling was not performed in non-ILM peeling (NP) group ($n = 37$). Retinal layer segmentation was performed using optical coherence tomography images. Individual retinal layer thicknesses before and at 6 months after ERM surgery were compared. The postoperative best-corrected visual acuity (BCVA) was also compared. *Results*. In the P group, the thicknesses of retinal nerve fiber layer (RNFL), ganglion cell layer (GCL), and inner plexiform layer (IPL) were significantly reduced. In the NP group, significant decreases in the RNFL, GCL, IPL, inner nuclear layer, and outer plexiform layer were observed. The P group manifested a greater mean postoperative GCL ($35.56 \pm 1.53 \mu$m vs $29.86 \pm 2.16 \mu$m; $p = 0.033$) and less loss of GCL ($-10.26 \pm 1.91 \mu$m vs $-19.86 \pm 2.74 \mu$m; $p = 0.004$) compared to the NP group. No statistically significant differences were observed when comparing the changes in BCVA. *Conclusions*. This study demonstrates that ILM peeling for ERM surgery may result in better preservation of GCL compared to no ILM peeling.

1. Introduction

The epiretinal membrane (ERM) is an avascular proliferative fibrous tissue composed of extracellular matrix and a polymorphous population of cells, which develops between the vitreous and the internal limiting membrane (ILM). Tangential tractional force on the retina asserted by an ERM leads to distortion of normal retinal structure and layers, causing symptoms such as impairment of central vision, metamorphopsia, macropsia, and monocular diplopia [1, 2]. For many years, the treatment of choice for symptomatic ERMs had been pars plana vitrectomy (PPV) with membranectomy [3]. As ILM peeling has greatly improved the

anatomical success rate of macular hole surgery in randomized controlled trials [4, 5], ILM removal has been favored in the treatment of ERM. Although previous studies have described some advantages of ILM peeling for ERM surgery [6, 7], there is still debate over the visual outcomes, safety, and indications for ILM peeling in patients with ERM.

The advantages of ILM removal during ERM surgery include better anatomical outcomes, lower recurrence rates, and better final visual acuity [6–9]. ILM is a transparent structure that defines the boundary between the retina and the vitreous body. It serves as the footplate of Müller cells, astrocytes, and fibroblasts, permitting adhesion and gliosis

[10, 11]. ILM removal, therefore, inhibits fibrous membrane formation by removing the scaffold for astrocyte and fibroblast proliferation, which explains its association with lower recurrence and better anatomical success rates. However, ILM peeling during ERM removal may be traumatic to retinal layers resulting in irregularities and indentations on the inner surface of the retina and thinning of the temporal retina [12]. Additionally, some comparative studies have shown that ILM peeling during ERM operations provides no definite functional benefit with respect to improving visual acuity [3, 13].

With the development of automated segmentation of retinal layers using optical coherence tomography (OCT), analysis of changes in individual retinal layers has become possible. A recent study has validated the accuracy of automated segmentation analysis [14, 15]; therefore, segmentation of retinal layers using OCT can be a useful tool for evaluating changes in retinal layers before and after vitreoretinal surgery. Previous studies indicated that preoperative integrity of the inner segment and outer segment line (IS/OS line) [16], preoperative photoreceptor outer segment length [17], and postoperative ganglion cell layer (GCL) thickness [18] are significantly correlated with postoperative best-corrected visual acuity (BCVA). However, there has been no prior comparative analysis of the changes in individual retinal layers by automated segmentation between patients who have undergone ERM surgery with ILM peeling versus without ILM peeling.

The purpose of this study is to analyze the changes in individual retinal layer thickness by automated segmentation in patients who have undergone ERM surgery with or without ILM peeling.

2. Methods

2.1. Enrollment of Study Population. This was a single-center retrospective study. We analyzed patient records, operative reports, and operation videos of 103 patients (103 eyes) who underwent ERM surgery by two surgeons (MK and SSK) at the Department of Ophthalmology, Yonsei University College of Medicine, Seoul, South Korea, between January 2013 and March 2015. The patients were classified into two groups depending on whether they underwent ILM peeling: ILM peeling (P) group with PPV plus epiretinal membranectomy plus ILM peeling and non-ILM peeling (NP) group with PPV plus epiretinal membranectomy. Only patients diagnosed with idiopathic ERM were included. Patients with other combined forms of maculopathy, such as macular hole, lamellar macular hole, diabetic macular edema, or retinal vein occlusion were excluded. Patients were also excluded from the analysis if they required reoperation or intravitreal injections within the 1-year follow-up period to treat postoperative complications such as retinal detachment, dislocation of intraocular lens, pseudophakic cystoid macular edema, and choroidal neovascularization. Only those patients who did not show significant posterior capsular opacity after the ERM surgery were included in the study. This study was approved by the institutional review board of Yonsei University College of Medicine (IRB approval number: 3-2016-0278) and was conducted in accordance with the tenets of the Declaration of Helsinki.

2.2. Preoperative Examination and Automated Segmentation. All past medical history and preoperative ophthalmologic data for each patient were reviewed. Results of the following preoperative evaluations were recorded: BCVA obtained by the Snellen visual acuity chart, which was converted to a logarithm of the minimum angle of resolution (logMAR) value for statistical analysis; slit-lamp biomicroscopy; intraocular pressure, as determined using a noncontact tonometer; color fundus photography; biometry measurements, obtained by the ZEISS IOLMaster® 500 (Carl Zeiss AG; Heidenheim, Germany); and OCT images, taken by the spectral domain OCT (SD-OCT; Spectralis®; Heidelberg Engineering, Heidelberg, Germany).

Automated segmentation of retinal layers was performed by the built-in software, which automatically calculated the average retinal thickness in each of the individual retinal layers: retinal nerve fiber layer (RNFL), GCL, inner plexiform layer (IPL), inner nuclear layer (INL), outer plexiform layer (OPL), outer nuclear layer (ONL), photoreceptor layer (PRL), and retinal pigment epithelium (RPE). The segmentation analysis was performed by two independent observers (CHL and EYC). Analysis was performed within a 6-mm diameter circle centered on the fovea, as defined in the Early Treatment of Diabetic Retinopathy Study (ETDRS) [19]. The diameters of the central circle, inner ring, and outer ring were 1 mm, 3 mm, and 6 mm, respectively (Figure 1).

2.3. Surgical Technique. For all patients, a 25-gauge PPV was performed (CONSTELLATION® Vision System, Alcon, Fort Worth, TX, USA). After performing core vitrectomy, triamcinolone was injected intravitreally to better visualize the vitreous gel and ERM. After removing the detached vitreous gel and the posterior hyaloid membrane, removal of the ERM was performed using intraocular forceps.

In the P group, the ILM was stained with 0.2 mL of 1 mg/mL indocyanine green (ICG) solution (DID-Indocyanine Green inj, Dongindang Pharmaceutical, Siheung, Republic of Korea). Both surgeons used the same concentration of ICG dye. After injecting the 1 mg/mL ICG solution at the macula area, the infusion was turned on immediately followed by aspiration of ICG dye with the vitrectomy cutter for minimal ICG dye circulation within the vitreous cavity. The ILM was peeled of an area of approximately 2 to 3 disc diameters centered on the macula using a 25-gauge ILM forceps. After the initial ILM peeling, ICG dye solution was reinjected to visualize residual ILM. Residual ILM was peeled until there was no ILM visible by ICG dye staining within 2 to 3 disc diameters of the macular center (Figure 2(a)).

In the NP group, ICG dye solution was injected over the macula region after epiretinal membranectomy to ensure that ILM remained intact. Patients with ILM unstained after simple membranectomy were excluded from the NP group (Figure 2(b)).

(a)

(b)

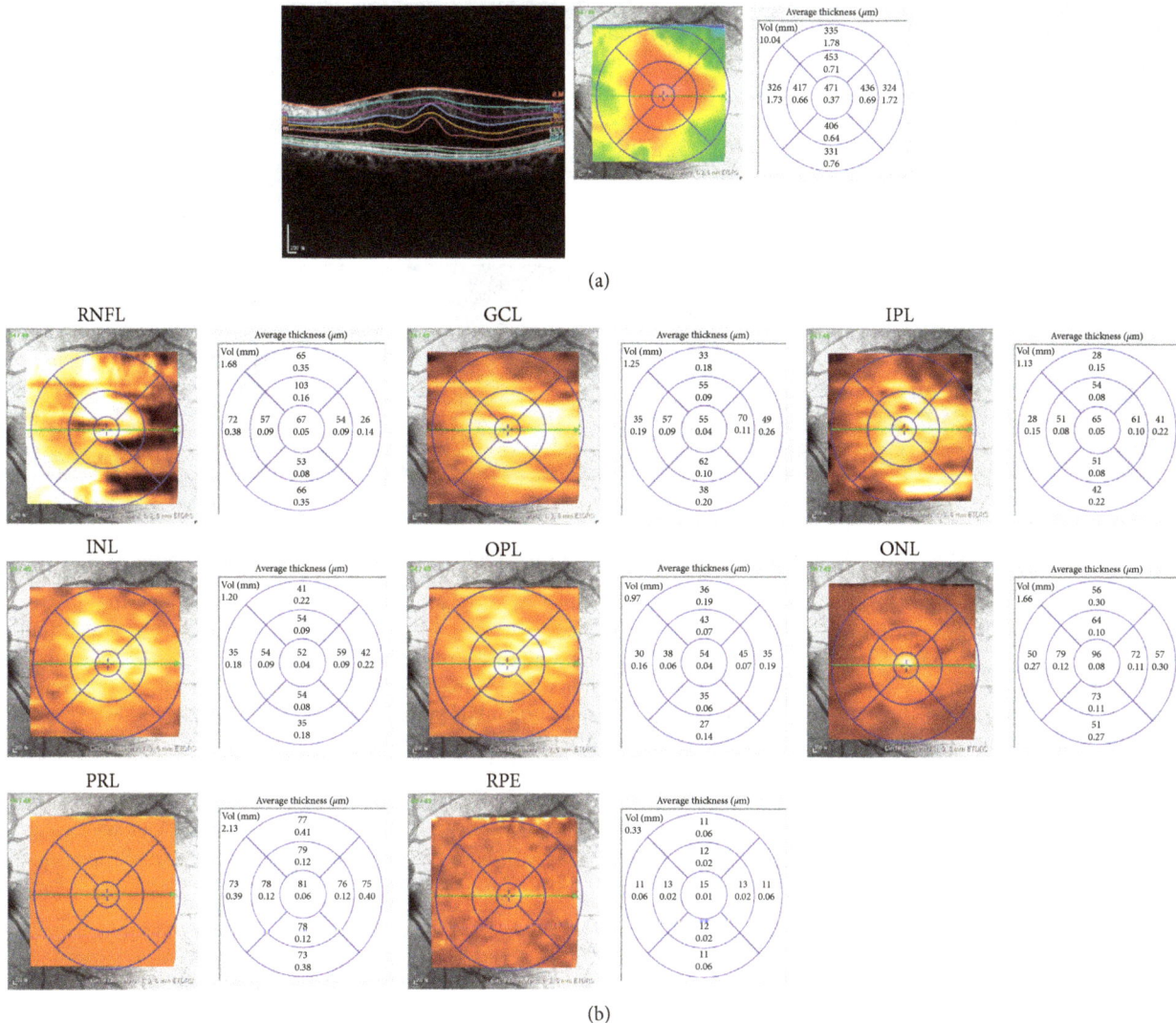

FIGURE 1: An example of automated retinal layer segmentation performed preoperatively on a patient with an epiretinal membrane. (a) Automated segmentation of retinal layers was performed by the built-in software of spectral domain OCT (SD-OCT; Spectralis®; Heidelberg Engineering, Heidelberg, Germany). (b) The segmentation analysis was performed within a 6-mm diameter circle centered on the fovea, as defined in the Early Treatment of Diabetic Retinopathy Study (ETDRS). The average retinal thickness in each of the 8 macular sectors was automatically calculated: retinal nerve fiber layer (RNFL), ganglion cell layer (GCL), inner plexiform layer (IPL), inner nuclear layer (INL), outer plexiform layer (OPL), outer nuclear layer (ONL), photoreceptor layer (PRL), and retinal pigment epithelium (RPE). The average retinal layer thickness at each macular sector was calculated at the 1-mm center circle, 3-mm inner ring, and 6-mm outer ring of the ETDRS.

2.4. Postoperative Examination. To determine the effects of ILM peeling on BCVA and anatomical structure of the retinal layers, the BCVA and automated segmentation analysis of SD-OCT at 6 months after the operation were analyzed. The change in retinal layer thickness was determined by subtracting the preoperative retinal layer thickness from the postoperative retinal layer thickness at the 1 mm central circle. The change in BCVA was calculated by subtracting the preoperative BCVA from the postoperative BCVA at 6 months follow-up.

2.5. Statistical Analyses. For all segmentation data, only the retinal layer thicknesses in the central circle at 1 mm were compared. The mean age and preoperative BCVA, biometry data, and segmentation data of the two groups (P group and NP group) were compared using independent Student's t-tests. The mean postoperative BCVA and segmentation data of the two groups were also compared using independent Student's t-tests. Within each group, the significance of the change in thickness of each retinal layer from before surgery to 6 months after surgery was determined by paired sample t-tests. The correlation between the thickness of each layer and postoperative BCVA was calculated by Pearson's correlation coefficient. A value of $p < 0.05$ was accepted as statistically significant.

Interrater agreement between the two observers was analyzed for all segmentation data by calculating intraclass correlation coefficients (ICCs). All statistical analyses of the data were performed using IBM SPSS 23.0 software for

(a)

(b)

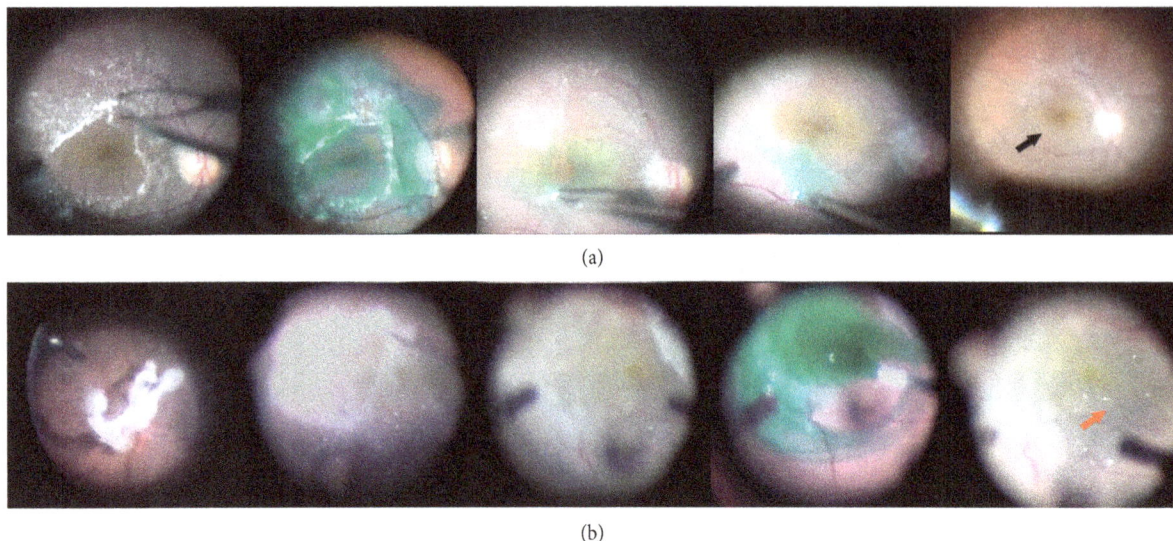

Figure 2: Examples of epiretinal membrane surgery with and without internal limiting membrane peeling. (a) For the ILM peeling (P) group, initial removal of posterior hyaloid membrane and ERM was performed using intraocular forceps with assistance of triamcinolone injection for better visualization. The ILM was double stained with 0.2 mL of 1 mg/mL indocyanine green (ICG) solution (DID-Indocyanine Green inj, Dongindang Pharmaceutical, Siheung, Republic of Korea). The ILM, which was stained light-green, was peeled using a 25-gauge ILM forceps. An area of approximately 2 to 3 disc diameters centered on the macula of the ILM was peeled. After the initial ILM peeling, ICG dye solution was reinjected to visualize residual ILM. There was no residual ILM visible by ICG dye staining within 2 to 3 disc diameters of the macular center (black arrow). (b) For the non-ILM peeling (NP) group, after initial posterior hyaloid membrane and ERM removal, ICG dye solution was injected over the macula region to ensure that ILM remained intact (red arrow).

Windows (SPSS/IBM Corporation, Chicago, IL, USA). Data are presented as mean ± standard deviation, except where indicated otherwise.

3. Results

3.1. Baseline Characteristics. Out of the 103 patients who underwent ERM surgery, 76 patients (76 eyes) with clinically confirmed idiopathic ERM satisfied the inclusion criteria and were included in the final analysis (P group $n = 39$, NP group $n = 37$). Sample size calculation was done by using the modified Cochran's formula. By using this formula, the sample size of 76 eyes met 95% confidence level with 6% margin of error about the population of 103 cases that underwent ERM surgery by two surgeons (MK and SSK) at the Department of Ophthalmology, Yonsei University College of Medicine between January 2013 and March 2015. There were no significant differences in patient age, BCVA, axial length, and spherical equivalent diopter between the two groups (Table 1). In addition, the mean preoperative segmented retinal layer thicknesses at each macular sector did not exhibit any significant differences (Table 1). Simultaneous cataract surgery was performed for all phakic eyes (P group: 61.5%; NP group: 62.2%; independent Student's t-tests, $p = 0.999$), and posterior capsular opacities were removed in all pseudophakic patients (P group: 38.5%; NP group: 37.8%; $p = 0.999$). In the P group, the average ILM removal time was 2.4 ± 0.5 minutes for surgeon 1 (MK) and 2.3 ± 0.7 for surgeon 2 (SSK) ($p = 0.999$). In the NP group, the average ERM removal time was 2.2 ± 0.2 minutes

for surgeon 1 (MK) and 2.2 ± 0.4 minutes for surgeon 2 (SSK) ($p = 0.999$).

3.2. Individual Retinal Layer Segmentation and BCVA at 6 Months Postoperatively. At 6 months postoperatively, the mean GCL thickness was significantly higher in the P group than in the NP group (P group: 35.56 ± 1.53 μm; NP group: 29.86 ± 2.16 μm; $p = 0.033$; Table 2). There was no significant difference in BCVA between the two groups (P group: 0.11 ± 0.02; NP group: 0.16 ± 0.02; $p = 0.099$; Table 2). No significant correlation between postoperative GCL and postoperative BCVA was observed in both groups (P group: Pearson $r = 0.218$, $p = 0.182$; NP group: Pearson $r = 0.049$, $p = 0.775$).

In the analysis of mean differences in retinal layer thickness before and after 6 months operation, the P group exhibited less loss of GCL thickness when compared to the NP group (P group: −10.26 ± 1.91 μm; NP group: −19.86 ± 2.74 μm; $p = 0.004$; Table 3). The mean change in thickness in all other segmented layers showed no significant differences (Table 3).

In paired t-test analysis, the P group showed significant reduction in the RNFL, GCL, and IPL thicknesses at 6 months after surgery. On the other hand, significant decreases in thickness that extended into the deeper layers, including the RNFL, GCL, IPL, INL, and OPL, were observed in the NP group (Table 3). The BCVA of both groups improved significantly after surgery (P group: $p < 0.0001$; NP group: $p = 0.006$; paired t-tests).

TABLE 1: Baseline characteristics and preoperative automated retinal layer segmentation.

	P group (ILM peeling) (n = 39) Mean ± SD	NP group (non-ILM peeling) (n = 37) Mean ± SD	p value
Age (years)	66.59 ± 1.41	68.73 ± 1.14	0.245
Preoperative BCVA (logMAR)	0.23 ± 0.03	0.27 ± 0.03	0.255
Spherical equivalent (D)	0.41 ± 0.36	0.43 ± 0.31	0.958
Axial length (mm)	23.72 ± 0.20	23.31 ± 0.18	0.135
Total retinal thickness (μm)	466.4 ± 11.31	458.7 ± 10.25	0.616
RNFL thickness (μm)	84.46 ± 11.79	70.78 ± 9.81	0.378
GCL thickness (μm)	45.82 ± 1.39	49.73 ± 1.97	0.106
IPL thickness (μm)	45.97 ± 1.76	46.43 ± 1.86	0.858
INL thickness (μm)	50.49 ± 1.70	52.38 ± 1.71	0.435
OPL thickness (μm)	37.82 ± 1.32	40.46 ± 1.68	0.217
ONL thickness (μm)	114.2 ± 4.60	111.4 ± 4.35	0.660
PRL thickness (μm)	71.56 ± 0.69	70.84 ± 0.64	0.444
RPE thickness (μm)	16.21 ± 0.47	16.84 ± 0.52	0.369

BCVA = best-corrected visual acuity; SD = standard deviation; ILM = internal limiting membrane; RNFL = retinal nerve fiber layer; GCL = ganglion cell layer; IPL = inner plexiform layer; INL = inner nuclear layer; OPL = outer plexiform layer; ONL = outer nuclear layer; PRL = photoreceptor layer; RPE = retinal pigment epithelium. Independent Student's t-test for statistical analysis between Group 1 and Group 2 for retinal layers, BCVA, age, spherical equivalent, and axial length.

TABLE 2: Automated retinal layer segmentation and best-corrected visual acuity at 6 months after epiretinal membrane surgery.

	P group (ILM peeling) (n = 39) Mean ± SD	NP group (non-ILM peeling) (n = 37) Mean ± SD	p value
Total retinal thickness (μm)	378.9 ± 5.89	360.8 ± 8.94	0.091
RNFL thickness (μm)	21.67 ± 1.47	23.95 ± 1.80	0.327
GCL thickness (μm)	35.56 ± 1.53	29.86 ± 2.16	0.033*
IPL thickness (μm)	34.05 ± 1.17	31.41 ± 1.81	0.219
INL thickness (μm)	45.46 ± 1.55	44.49 ± 2.45	0.735
OPL thickness (μm)	35.05 + 1.16	33.30 ± 1.49	0.353
ONL thickness (μm)	117.5 ± 3.90	109.5 ± 2.98	0.112
PRL thickness (μm)	72.77 ± 0.72	72.05 ± 0.67	0.470
RPE thickness (μm)	17.13 ± 0.93	17.24 ± 0.80	0.926
BCVA (logMAR)	0.11 ± 0.02	0.16 ± 0.02	0.099

BCVA = best-corrected visual acuity; SD = standard deviation; ILM = internal limiting membrane; RNFL = retinal nerve fiber layer; GCL = ganglion cell layer; IPL = inner plexiform layer; INL = inner nuclear layer; OPL = outer plexiform layer; ONL = outer nuclear layer; PRL = photoreceptor layer; RPE = retinal pigment epithelium. Independent Student's t-test for statistical analysis between Group 1 and Group 2 for retinal layers and BCVA.

The ICCs for the preoperative and postoperative segmentation data indicated excellent interrater agreement in all layers.

4. Discussion

ILM peeling for ERM surgery resulted in less loss of GCL thickness compared to no ILM peeling.

A novel finding of this study is that the P group exhibited significantly lower reduction of GCL thickness compared to the NP group. This contradicts many previous concerns regarding iatrogenic trauma and retinal toxicity produced by ICG dye guided ILM peeling.

In previous studies using electron microscopy, findings indicated possible Müller cell damage caused by the ILM peeling procedure [20, 21]. However, these peeled ILM samples only contained Müller cells and myofibroblasts and were void of ganglion cells, photoreceptors, or RPE cells [20]. Another recent study showed that specimens acquired from ILM abrasion using a tano diamond-dusted membrane scraper did not contain RNFL or neuronal cells that lay beneath the ILM [22]. In accordance with our results, these studies suggest that iatrogenic trauma may be confined to Müller cells, and other neuronal cells are minimally affected by the procedure.

Unfortunately, we could not perform auto fluorescence, microperimetry, or visual field testing for evaluating ICG dye toxicity in terms of RPE cell function. However, our study shows that the use of ICG dye with 1 mg/mL concentration during ERM surgery does not induce significant retinal toxicity, in terms of preserving retinal thickness, including the RPE layer. In agreement with our results, Kwok et al. have demonstrated that there was no clinically significant ICG toxicity after ILM peeling angiographically [23]. There have been some case reports of poor visual outcomes due to ICG dye toxicity after successful macular

TABLE 3: Difference in segmented retinal layer thicknesses and best-corrected visual acuity before and at 6 months after epiretinal membrane surgery.

Difference	P group (ILM peeling)	p value (preop vs POD 6 month)	NP group (non-ILM peeling)	p value (preop vs POD 6 month)	p value (P group vs NP group)
Total retinal thickness (μm)	-87.51 ± 9.87	$<0.0001^{\dagger}$	-97.95 ± 8.35	$<0.0001^{\dagger}$	0.425
RNFL thickness (μm)	-62.79 ± 11.43	$<0.0001^{\dagger}$	-46.84 ± 9.21	$<0.0001^{\dagger}$	0.283
GCL thickness (μm)	-10.26 ± 1.91	$<0.0001^{\dagger}$	-19.86 ± 2.74	$<0.0001^{\dagger}$	0.004**
IPL thickness (μm)	-11.92 ± 1.89	$<0.0001^{\dagger}$	-15.03 ± 2.37	$<0.0001^{\dagger}$	0.306
INL thickness (μm)	-5.03 ± 2.49	0.050	-7.89 ± 3.29	0.022*	0.486
OPL thickness (μm)	-2.77 ± 1.71	0.114	-7.16 ± 1.58	0.002**	0.064
ONL thickness (μm)	3.26 ± 5.29	0.542	-1.89 ± 4.88	0.721	0.478
PRL thickness (μm)	1.21 ± 0.77	0.126	1.22 ± 0.82	0.194	0.992
RPE thickness (μm)	0.92 ± 0.93	0.326	0.41 ± 0.78	0.672	0.672
BCVA (logMAR)	-0.11 ± 0.02	$<0.0001^{\dagger}$	-0.11 ± 0.03	0.006**	0.950

BCVA = best-corrected visual acuity; POD = postoperative day; SD = standard deviation; ILM = internal limiting membrane; RNFL = retinal nerve fiber layer; GCL = ganglion cell layer; IPL = inner plexiform layer; INL = inner nuclear layer; OPL = outer plexiform layer; ONL = outer nuclear layer; PRL = photoreceptor layer; RPE = retinal pigment epithelium. Independent Student's t-test for statistical analysis between Group 1 and Group 2 for difference of retinal layers and BCVA: $^{*}p < 0.05$, $^{**}p < 0.01$, $^{\dagger}p < 0.001$. Paired sample t-test within Group 1 and Group 2 for statistical analysis: $^{*}p < 0.05$, $^{**}p < 0.01$, $^{\dagger}p < 0.001$.

hole closure [24]. However, with a macular hole, the RPE and other retinal layers at the fovea are directly exposed to the vitreous cavity, whereas in the presence of an ERM, these layers are enclosed by the fibrotic membrane and ILM. We speculate that the risk of foveal exposure to ICG dye would be lower in patients with an ERM.

The reason for the relative preservation of postoperative GCL in the P group is unclear. However, we hypothesize that induction of Müller cell injury during ILM peeling may have triggered reactive gliosis, resulting in subsequent thickening of GCL compared to the NP group. On the retinal side of the ILM obtained after ERM surgery, electron micrographs revealed segments of Müller cell footplates in ILM specimens, which shows that ILM peeling generates Müller cell injury [21]. In addition, injured Müller cells have a role in retinal neural regeneration and repair as described in previous studies performed on rodent and human retinal tissues [25–28]. Hypothetically, ILM peeling, having induced Müller cell injury, may have activated reactive gliosis at the GCL level with the RNFL serving as Müller cell footplate.

However, it is unclear whether greater GCL thickness as shown by our study necessarily means a recovery of healthy neuronal cells. Previous studies have shown decreased retinal function on multifocal electroretinogram and visual field sensitivity after ILM peeling [21, 29]. Our study showed that there was no correlation between postoperative GCL thickness and postoperative BCVA in the P group (Pearson $r = 0.218$, $p = 0.182$). The relative preservation of GCL after ILM peeling may be a result of a reactive gliosis after initial injury on Müller cells, rather than a healthy regeneration of ganglion cells. Further study about the changes that occur at cellular level after ILM peeling is required to clarify these results.

There is no significant difference in postoperative BCVA between ILM peeling and no ILM peeling for ERM surgery. Both groups exhibited significant improvements in BCVA after ERM surgery. However, ILM peeling did not

result in superior visual outcomes regarding central visual acuity. Our results agree with a recent randomized controlled study that compared the BCVA of ILM peeling and no ILM peeling [30]. In other studies, some have reported superior outcomes in ILM peeling group, while some have reported opposing results [6, 7, 31]. However, the advantage of our study over these previous studies is that the proportion of eyes with and without ILM peeling was similar (P group: 51.3% versus NP group: 48.7%), which adds representativeness and objectivity to our data.

Our study has a few limitations. First, although the surgical protocols in the two groups were identical except for ILM peeling, two surgeons performed operations. However, there was no significant difference between the two surgeons in operation time, ERM removal time, or ILM removal time. Also, since there were a sufficient and approximately equal number of each surgeon's patients in both groups, the surgeon factors may have been minimized. Second, epiretinal membranectomy without ILM peeling does not necessarily result in complete preservation of the ILM, as ILM could be removed along with the ERM during the membrane removal procedure. Unfortunately, we could not perform a histological study proving that the ILM was completely preserved after ERM removal in the NP Group. As an alternative to a histological study, we have done the best we could clinically by thoroughly reviewing our surgical videos to include only those eyes that showed complete peeling of ILM in the P group and cases with ILM as completely preserved as possible in the NP Group grossly (Figure 2). Third, there are insufficient data about the changes that occur at cellular levels after surgical manipulation of the ILM, a key finding to explain our data.

In conclusion, this study demonstrates a novel finding that ILM peeling during ERM surgery may result in better preservation of GCL compared to ERM surgery without ILM peeling. We cautiously speculate that the removal of ILM and subsequent Müller cell injury may have induced reactive gliosis. Future studies regarding the changes inflicted on Müller cells after ILM removal in the human retina are required to support our results and confirm our findings.

Conflicts of Interest

The authors declare that they have no conflicts of interest.

Acknowledgments

This study was supported by a faculty research grant of Yonsei University College of Medicine, 2017-32-0037.

References

[1] H. Liu, S. Zuo, C. Ding, X. Dai, and X. Zhu, "Comparison of the effectiveness of pars plana vitrectomy with and without internal limiting membrane peeling for idiopathic retinal membrane removal: a meta-analysis," *Journal of Ophthalmology*, vol. 2015, Article ID 974568, 10 pages, 2015.

[2] F. S. Ting and A. K. Kwok, "Treatment of epiretinal membrane: an update," *Hong Kong Medical Journal*, vol. 11, no. 6, pp. 496–502, 2005.

[3] H. Shimada, H. Nakashizuka, T. Hattori, R. Mori, Y. Mizutani, and M. Yuzawa, "Double staining with brilliant blue G and double peeling for epiretinal membranes," *Ophthalmology*, vol. 116, no. 7, pp. 1370–1376, 2009.

[4] N. Lois, J. Burr, J. Norrie et al., "Full-thickness Macular H et al: internal limiting membrane peeling versus no peeling for idiopathic full-thickness macular hole: a pragmatic randomized controlled trial," *Investigative Opthalmology & Visual Science*, vol. 52, no. 3, pp. 1586–1592, 2011.

[5] L. Ternent, L. Vale, C. Boachie, J. M. Burr, and N. Lois, "Full-Thickness Macular H, Internal Limiting Membrane Peeling Study G: cost-effectiveness of internal limiting membrane peeling versus no peeling for patients with an idiopathic full-thickness macular hole: results from a randomised controlled trial," *British Journal of Ophthalmology*, vol. 96, no. 3, pp. 438–443, 2012.

[6] D. W. Park, P. U. Dugel, J. Garda et al., "Macular pucker removal with and without internal limiting membrane peeling: pilot study," *Ophthalmology*, vol. 110, no. 1, pp. 62–64, 2003.

[7] E. H. Bovey, S. Uffer, and F. Achache, "Surgery for epimacular membrane: impact of retinal internal limiting membrane removal on functional outcome," *Retina*, vol. 24, no. 5, pp. 728–735, 2004.

[8] R. Sorcinelli, "Surgical management of epiretinal membrane with indocyanine-green-assisted peeling," *Ophthalmologica*, vol. 217, no. 2, pp. 107–110, 2003.

[9] A. M. Maguire, W. E. Smiddy, S. K. Nanda, R. G. Michels, Z. de la Cruz, and W. R. Green, "Clinicopathologic correlation of recurrent epiretinal membranes after previous surgical removal," *Retina*, vol. 10, no. 3, pp. 213–222, 1990.

[10] C. Guidry, "The role of Muller cells in fibrocontractive retinal disorders," *Progress in Retinal and Eye Research*, vol. 24, no. 1, pp. 75–86, 2005.

[11] I. Iandiev, O. Uckermann, T. Pannicke et al., "Glial cell reactivity in a porcine model of retinal detachment," *Investigative Opthalmology & Visual Science*, vol. 47, no. 5, pp. 2161–2171, 2006.

[12] K. Kumagai, M. Hangai, and N. Ogino, "Progressive thinning of regional macular thickness after epiretinal membrane surgery," *Investigative Opthalmology & Visual Science*, vol. 56, no. 12, pp. 7236–7242, 2015.

[13] H. N. Oh, J. E. Lee, H. W. Kim, and I. H. Yun, "Clinical outcomes of double staining and additional ILM peeling during ERM surgery," *Korean Journal of Ophthalmology*, vol. 27, no. 4, pp. 256–260, 2013.

[14] J. Tian, B. Varga, G. M. Somfai, W. H. Lee, W. E. Smiddy, and D. C. DeBuc, "Real-time automatic segmentation of optical coherence tomography volume data of the macular region," *PLoS One*, vol. 10, no. 8, Article ID e0133908, 2015.

[15] D. Y. Kim, H. S. Yang, Y. J. Kook, and J. Y. Lee, "Association between microperimetric parameters and optical coherent tomographic findings in various macular diseases," *Korean Journal of Ophthalmology*, vol. 29, no. 2, pp. 92–101, 2015.

[16] C. I. Falkner-Radler, C. Glittenberg, S. Hagen, T. Benesch, and S. Binder, "Spectral-domain optical coherence tomography for monitoring epiretinal membrane surgery," *Ophthalmology*, vol. 117, no. 4, pp. 798–805, 2010.

[17] A. Shiono, J. Kogo, G. Klose et al., "Photoreceptor outer segment length: a prognostic factor for idiopathic epiretinal membrane surgery," *Ophthalmology*, vol. 120, no. 4, pp. 788–794, 2013.

[18] S. W. Park, I. S. Byon, H. Y. Kim, J. E. Lee, and B. S. Oum, "Analysis of the ganglion cell layer and photoreceptor layer using optical coherence tomography after idiopathic epiretinal membrane surgery," *Graefe's Archive for Clinical and Experimental Ophthalmology*, vol. 253, no. 2, pp. 207–214, 2015.

[19] Early Treatment Diabetic Retinopathy Study Research Group, "Early Treatment Diabetic Retinopathy Study design and baseline patient characteristics: ETDRS report number 7," *Ophthalmology*, vol. 98, no. 5, pp. 741–756, 1991.

[20] R. G. Schumann, M. Remy, M. Grueterich, A. Gandorfer, and C. Haritoglou, "How it appears: electron microscopic evaluation of internal limiting membrane specimens obtained during brilliant blue G assisted macular hole surgery," *British Journal of Ophthalmology*, vol. 92, no. 3, pp. 330–331, 2008.

[21] S. R. Tari, O. Vidne-Hay, V. C. Greenstein, G. R. Barile, D. C. Hood, and S. Chang, "Functional and structural measurements for the assessment of internal limiting membrane peeling in idiopathic macular pucker," *Retina*, vol. 27, no. 5, pp. 567–572, 2007.

[22] D. R. Almeida, E. K. Chin, R. M. Tarantola et al., "Effect of internal limiting membrane abrasion on retinal tissues in macular holes," *Investigative Opthalmology & Visual Science*, vol. 56, no. 5, pp. 2783–2789, 2015.

[23] A. K. Kwok, T. Y. Lai, D. T. Yew, and W. W. Li, "Internal limiting membrane staining with various concentrations of indocyanine green dye under air in macular surgeries," *American Journal of Ophthalmology*, vol. 136, no. 2, pp. 223–230, 2003.

[24] D. Stanescu-Segall and T. L. Jackson, "Vital staining with indocyanine green: a review of the clinical and experimental studies relating to safety," *Eye*, vol. 23, no. 3, pp. 504–518, 2009.

[25] A. V. Das, K. B. Mallya, X. Zhao et al., "Neural stem cell properties of Muller glia in the mammalian retina: regulation

by Notch and Wnt signaling," *Developmental Biology*, vol. 299, no. 1, pp. 283–302, 2006.

[26] J. M. Lawrence, S. Singhal, B. Bhatia et al., "MIO-M1 cells and similar muller glial cell lines derived from adult human retina exhibit neural stem cell characteristics," *Stem Cells*, vol. 25, no. 8, pp. 2033–2043, 2007.

[27] S. Ooto, T. Akagi, R. Kageyama et al., "Potential for neural regeneration after neurotoxic injury in the adult mammalian retina," *Proceedings of the National Academy of Sciences*, vol. 101, no. 37, pp. 13654–13659, 2004.

[28] J. Wan, H. Zheng, Z. L. Chen, H. L. Xiao, Z. J. Shen, and G. M. Zhou, "Preferential regeneration of photoreceptor from Muller glia after retinal degeneration in adult rat," *Vision Research*, vol. 48, no. 2, pp. 223–234, 2008.

[29] J. W. Lim, J. H. Cho, and H. K. Kim, "Assessment of macular function by multifocal electroretinography following epi-retinal membrane surgery with internal limiting membrane peeling," *Clinical Ophthalmology*, vol. 4, pp. 689–694, 2010.

[30] P. Tranos, S. Koukoula, D. G. Charteris et al., "The role of internal limiting membrane peeling in epiretinal membrane surgery: a randomised controlled trial," *British Journal of Ophthalmology*, vol. 101, no. 6, pp. 719–724, 2017.

[31] A. Sivalingam, R. C. Eagle Jr., J. S. Duker et al., "Visual prognosis correlated with the presence of internal-limiting membrane in histopathologic specimens obtained from epi-retinal membrane surgery," *Ophthalmology*, vol. 97, no. 11, pp. 1549–1552, 1990.

7

Epi-Off versus Epi-On Corneal Collagen Cross-Linking in Keratoconus Patients

F. Cifariello,[1,2] **M. Minicucci,**[3] **F. Di Renzo** (ORCID),[1] **D. Di Taranto,**[1] **G. Coclite,**[1] **S. Zaccaria,**[1] **S. De Turris,**[1] **and C. Costagliola** (ORCID)[1,2,3]

[1]*Department of Medicine and Health Science, University of Molise, Campobasso, Italy*
[2]*Casa di Cura "Villa Maria", Campobasso, Italy*
[3]*I.R.C.S.S. Neuromed, Pozzilli, Isernia, Italy*

Correspondence should be addressed to C. Costagliola; ciro.costagliola@unimol.it

Academic Editor: Antonio Queiros

Aim. To evaluate two different techniques of cross-linking: standard epithelium-off (CXL epi-off) versus transepithelial (CXL epi-on) cross-linking in patient with progressive keratoconus. *Methods.* Forty eyes from 32 patients with progressive keratoconus were prospectively enrolled from June 2014 to June 2015 in this nonblinded, randomized comparative study. Twenty eyes were treated by CXL epi-off and 20 by CLX epi-on, randomly assigned, and followed for 2 years. All patients underwent a complete ophthalmologic testing that included uncorrected and best corrected visual acuity, central and peripheral corneal thickness, corneal astigmatism, simulated maximum, minimum, and average keratometry, corneal confocal microscopy, Schirmer I and break-up time (BUT) tests, and the Ocular Surface Disease Index. Intra- and postoperative complications were recorded. The solution used for CXL epi-off comprised riboflavin 0.1% and dextran 20.0% (Ricrolin), whereas the solution for CXL epi-on (Ricrolin TE) comprised riboflavin 0.1%, dextran 15.0%, trometamol (Tris), and ethylenediaminetetraacetic acid. Ultraviolet-A treatment was performed with a UV-X system at 3 mW/cm^2. *Results.* In both groups, a significant improvement in visual function (Group 1: baseline 0.36 ± 0.16 logMAR, two-year follow-up 0.22 ± 0.17 logMAR, $p = 0.01$; Group 2: baseline 0.32 ± 0.18 logMAR, 2-year follow-up 0.27 ± 0.19 logMAR, $p = 0.01$) was recorded. Keratometry remained unchanged in both groups. The mean corneal thickness showed a significant reduction (mean difference of corneal thickness: -55 micron and -71 micron, resp.). One-month after treatment, OSDI© reached 13.56 ± 2.15 in Group 1 ($p = 0.03$) and 11.26 ± 2.12 in Group 2 ($p = 0.04$). At confocal microscopy, abnormal corneal nerve alterations were found in both groups. Fibrotic reaction (43.75%) and activated keratocyte (62.6%) were more commonly recorded in Group 1 than in Group 2 (25.0% and 18.75%), with $p = 0.668$ and 0.356, respectively. *Conclusion.* Our findings demonstrate that both procedures are able to slow keratoconus progression. Both treatment modalities are equivalent in terms of results and related complications. CXL epi-on technique is preferable to CXL epi-off since it preserves the corneal thickness and improves visual acuity, also reducing the postoperative ocular discomfort during the study period.

1. Introduction

Corneal collagen cross-linking (CXL) has acquired nowadays popularity for the treatment of progressive corneal ectasia. This technique, stabilizing the progression of keratoconus, delays the need for keratoplasty and, thus, decreases the chance of corneal transplantation [1], through an increase of the corneal biomechanical strength [2]. The method was developed in 1997 at the Dresden University and was carried out in Italy for the first time in 2005 [3]. It involves the photoactivation of riboflavin with ultraviolet-A (UVA) radiation, that unfolds a series of photochemical reactions inducing inter- and intrafibrillary cross links in the corneal stromal lamellae [4]. In this way, the tensile strength of the cornea prevent further thinning and deformation of the corneal profile [5] and deterioration of vision and offers some degree of functional improvement [6]. The original protocol was an epithelium-off (epi-off) procedure: the central corneal epithelium (about 8 mm) is removed, and riboflavin solution (0.1% riboflavin-5-phosphate and 20% dextran T-500) is applied to the exposed corneal stroma. CXL epi-off has been modified over time in favor of a method that does not involve the epithelium debridement [7, 8], that is, the technique called epithelium-on CXL [9]. This new approach was introduced to reduce the postoperative side effects of conventional epi-off CXL, as corneal infections, subepithelial haze, sterile infiltrates, reactivation of herpetic keratitis, and endothelial damage [10]. Transepithelial technique combines some advantages of the conventional technique, maintaining a higher safety profile, but it increases the risk of failure with a possible need of further treatment [11]. In fact, the diffusion process of riboflavin in the stroma is limited by corneal epithelial tight junctions [12–14]. Riboflavin penetration through the epithelium can be increased by different strategies, such as changing the physicochemical properties of the riboflavin molecule by adding chemical enhancers in the riboflavin formulation [15] besides the mechanical disruption of corneal epithelium [16].

Iontophoresis is a novel noninvasive system aimed at enhancing the delivery of charged molecules into tissues using small electric current [17]. Riboflavin, in the formulation used for iontophoresis, is negatively charged [18]. This last technique seems to be the best option to lock the progression of keratoconus [19, 20]. Moreover, the UV penetration in this procedure is limited by the riboflavin impregnated intact corneal epithelium, making it safer compared to the epi-off.

The aim of this study has been to compare these two techniques and to evaluate the efficacy and safety of the two treatments.

2. Materials and Methods

Forty eyes from 32 patients with progressive keratoconus, followed at the University of Molise, Italy, from June 2014 to June 2015, were included in this nonblinded, randomized comparative study. The patients were randomly assigned to one of the two treatment groups (20 eyes were treated with CLX epi-off, and the other 20 eyes were treated with CLX epi-on). Progression of keratoconus was documented through a clinical and instrumental (topographic, pachymetric, or aberrometric) worsening in the previous 6 months of observation. Inclusion criteria were patients with evolving keratoconus, aged between 18 and 40 years, and with no evidence of corneal scarring. Exclusion criteria were patients with central and paracentral corneal opacities, Vogt's striae, previous intraocular surgery, history of herpetic keratitis, severe dry eye, and concomitant autoimmune diseases.

All patients underwent a complete ophthalmologic testing that included uncorrected and best corrected visual acuity (BCVA), central and peripheral corneal thickness, corneal astigmatism, simulated maximum, minimum, and average keratometry, corneal confocal microscopy, Schirmer I and break-up time (BUT) tests, and the Ocular Surface Disease Index. All intra and postoperative adverse events were recorded.

BCVA was determined using Snellen's chart and was converted to logarithm of the minimum angle of resolution (logMAR). Central and peripheral corneal thickness, K flat, K steep, and mean K were evaluated with Sirius (CSO spa, Firenze, Italy) and Pentacam® (OCULUS, Germany) topographs. Fibrotic reaction, corneal alteration of nerves, activated keratocytes, and corneal opacities were evaluated through confocal microscopy HRT III (Heidelberg Engineering, with Rostock Cornea Module, Heidelberg, Germany).

Cornea was examined for anterior thinning, the presence of inflammatory cells associated with the lenticule, and activation of corneal keratocytes, which may indicate the development of fibrosis [21, 22]. Images of corneal alteration nerves were acquired using the same illumination intensity and by focusing the microscope beneath the basal epithelium. Approximately five images were randomly selected for qualitative analysis from the basal epithelium. The subbasal nerve fibre was assessed. The confocal images were selected and analyzed by two clinicians (F.C. and M.M.). Activation of stromal keratocytes was assessed considering the degree of keratocyte activation by comparing the data obtained with a grading scale. The grading scale consisted of a series of images derived from concurrent studies of stromal keratocyte activation using confocal microscopy [23]. The examinations for corneal opacities were performed by two clinicans (F.C. and M.M.), and manual quantitative analysis of keratocytes was attempted twice: first by the examiner and then by an expert observer (C.C.). Two consecutive section images were taken at a depth of $150\,\mu m$ (measured from the epithelial surface) to subjectively estimate the pre- and postoperative anterior stromal cell density [24]. Lastly, eye discomfort was evaluated before treatment and one-month later in all subjects using the Ocular Surface Disease Index (OSDI) questionnaire. The unit of measurement was expressed in OSDI© (Allergan, USA).

Epi-off CXL technique was performed after instilling 4% lidocaine for topical anesthesia and 1.0% pilocarpine to reduce the risk for ultraviolet light exposure. A 9.0 mm of corneal epithelium was mechanically removed. Riboflavin (0.1% in 20% dextran solution; Ricrolin; Sooft, Montegiorgio, Italy) was administered topically every 2 minutes for 30 minutes. The administration was continued every 2 minutes during UVA exposure. The cornea was exposed to UVA 370 nm light (UV-X System; Peschke Meditrade GmbH, Hünenberg, Switzerland) for 30 minutes at an irradiance of $3.0\,mW/cm^2$. At the end of the procedure, ofloxacin and cyclopentolate eye drops were administered, and therapeutic contact lens (LAC ACUVUE-etafilcon A) was then applied and was removed 3 days after surgery. Topical tobramycin (four times daily for 1 week) and dexamethasone phosphate 0.1% (four times daily for 2 weeks) were prescribed. The therapeutic contact lens was removed three days later. Lubricating eye drops were prescribed for the following three months.

In the epi-on CXL group, corneal epithelial was not removed. Corneal imbibition was obtained with 0.1% riboflavin–15% dextran solution supplemented with Trishydroxymethylaminomethane and sodium ethylenediaminetetraacetic acid (Ricrolin TE; Sooft, Montegiorgio, Italy) applied every 5 minutes for 30 minutes. One drop of 1% pilocarpine was administered 30 minutes before treatment to reduce the risk for UVA exposure. Ten minutes later, a single dose of 4% lidocaine eye drops was administered to anaesthetize the cornea. Postoperatively, topical tobramycin (four times daily for 1 week) was prescribed. All patients were operated by the same surgeons (F.C. and M.M.). The patients were checked at day 1, 3, 7, and 15 and then after 1, 6, 12, and 24 months.

The study was approved by the Institutional Review Board (CTS, Department of Medicine and Health Sciences, University of Molise, Ref. no. 0001-05-2018; ClinicalTrials. gov Identifier: NCT01350323), and each patient gave their written informed consent after a detailed description of the procedure used and of the aim of the work.

3. Data Analysis

The significance between parameters was assessed by Student's t-test for paired values and chi-square test for non-parametric variables. The differences between the values of the two groups at the baseline and after therapy were evaluated with two sample t-test. Significance was set at $p < 0.05$.

4. Results

The mean age of patients in Group 1 was 24 ± 7 years (ranging from 15 to 31 years; 13 male/7 female). In Group 2, the mean age was 31 ± 10 years (ranging from 19 to 44 years; 16 male/4 female).

In Group I, BCVA at the baseline was 0.36 ± 0.16 logMAR and improved to 0.22 ± 0.17 logMAR in postoperative 2 years ($p = 0.01$), whereas in Group 2, the values progressed from 0.32 ± 0.18 logMAR to 0.27 ± 0.19 logMAR ($p = 0.01$). At the end of the follow-up, the difference between the two groups was also significant ($p = 0.01$).

Mean K at the baseline was 46.19 ± 2.82 D and 47.00 ± 2.79 D, respectively (Group 1 and Group 2); these two values in the postoperative period of 2 years remained unchanged: 46.16 ± 3.15 D ($p = 0.57$) (Group 1) and 47.82 ± 4.06 D (Group 2) ($p = 0.10$). In addition, the differences between the two values were not significant ($p = 0.08$).

K steep and K flat at the baseline in Group 1 were, respectively, 47.75 ± 3.20 D and 44.62 ± 2.63 D and in Group 2 were 48.86 ± 3.27 D and 45.84 ± 2.53 D. Two years after treatment, K steep and K flat of Group 1 reached 47.76 ± 3.47 D ($p = 0.10$) and 44.71 ± 3.03 D ($p = 0.33$), whereas in Group 2, they were 49.75 ± 3.47 D ($p = 0.60$) and 46.44 ± 3.67 D ($p = 0.25$). On the contrary, at the end of the follow-up, the difference between the two groups was significant for both parameters ($p = 0.01$).

Mean corneal thickness after 2 years significantly change in both groups (from $556.45 \pm 23.56\,\mu$m to $501.41 \pm 21.91\,\mu$m ($p = 0.01$) and from $565.41 \pm 31.91\,\mu$m to $495.45 \pm 43.16\,\mu$m ($p = 0.01$), resp.), but the difference between groups was not significant ($p = 0.10$).

At the baseline, the OSDI© score was 4.85 ± 1.18 and 4.98 ± 1.32, respectively (p not significant). After one month, the score increased to 13.56 ± 2.15 in Group 1 ($p = 0.01$) and 11.26 ± 2.12 in Group 2 ($p = 0.04$). The difference between the two groups was also significant ($p = 0.02$).

Confocal microscopy data in both groups revealed corneal nerve alterations: 93.8% in the epi-off group (Group 1) and 87.5% in the epi-on group (Group 2). Activated keratocyte and fibrotic reaction in Group 1 represented 62.5% and 43.75%, respectively, whereas in Group 2, they were recorded in a significantly lowest percentage (25% and 18.75%; $p = 0.001$ in both).

The main complications were observed in 3 patients: two in Group 1 (Vogt's striae in a patient; in another patient corneal haze type II) and one in Group 2 (Vogt's striae and in the same eye follicular conjunctivitis). Schirmer and BUT tests did not reveal lacrimation defects in both groups.

5. Discussion

Our findings report for the first time OSDI© (Ocular Surface Disease Index) difference in patients who underwent CXL. Through the OSDI©, we evaluated the degree of ocular discomfort in the patient treated with the two different methods. The results show that the score was lower in patients of Group 2 ($p < 0.05$). At the baseline, the score was 4.85 ± 1.18 and 4.98 ± 1.32 OSDI©, respectively. After treatment, the score increased to 13.56 ± 2.15 OSDI© in Group 1 and 11.26 ± 2.12 OSDI© in Group 2. Despite the use of topical anesthetics, the greater mean postoperative pain in the epi-off CXL group compared to the epi-on CXL group probably depends on the exposure of the corneal nerves and the release of inflammatory mediators, especially prostaglandins and neuropeptides after epithelium removal and related healing processes [25] (Tables 1 and 2).

Statistical analyses show that the mean corneal thickness, two years later, change significantly in both groups (from $556.45 \pm 23.56\,\mu$m to $501.41 \pm 21.91\,\mu$m ($p = 0.01$) and from $565.41 \pm 31.91\,\mu$m to $495.45 \pm 43.16\,\mu$m ($p = 0.01$), resp.), as already reported [20, 26, 27]. Although epithelial remodeling and stroma edema disappear few days after treatment, it has been reported to be responsible of corneal thickness changes also over a longer time [28]. This could justify the rethickening to preoperative levels 12 months after surgery reported in the previous studies, especially in the epi-on procedure [9, 18, 25, 27]. On the contrary, our findings demonstrate that corneal thickness decreases two-year postoperatively. This suggests the involvement of different factors, that is, compression of collagen fibrils, changes in both corneal hydration and glycosaminoglycans synthesis, and keratinocyte apoptosis, that alone or in combination may play a detrimental role in the corneal rethickening [28].

A significant increase in BCVA compared to the baseline was recorded in both groups ($p = 0.01$). However, the epi-on group exhibits a better improvement compared to the epi-off group at the end of the follow-up ($p = 001$) (Table 3). Our results are consistent with those achieved by three previous randomized clinical trials [18, 27, 29], which demonstrated a more important recovery of BCVA in the epi-on group versus the epi-off. However, it has been shown that, for progressive keratoconus patients, the standard cross-linking

TABLE 1: Group 1 (epi-off): comparison of analyzed parameters (mean ± SD) before and after treatment at the end of the follow-up (2 years).

	Preoperative	Postoperative	p value
Mean corneal thickness (μm)	556.45 ± 23.56	501.41 ± 21.91	0.01*
K flat (D)	44.62 ± 2.63	44.71 ± 3.03	0.33
K steep (D)	47.75 ± 3.20	47.76 ± 3.47	0.10
Mean K (D)	46.19 ± 2.82	46.16 ± 3.15	0.57
BCVA (logMAR)	0.36 ± 0.14	0.22 ± 0.12	0.01*
OSDI© (before and one-month later)	4.85 ± 1.18	13.56 ± 2.15	0.01*

BCVA: best corrected visual acuity; OSDI: Ocular Surface Disease Index; *Student's t-test for paired values.

TABLE 2: Group 2 (epi-on): comparison of analyzed parameters (mean ± SD) before and after treatment at the end of the follow-up (2 years).

	Preoperative	Postoperative	p value
Mean corneal thickness (μm)	565.41 ± 31.91	495.45 ± 43.16	0.01*
K flat (D)	45.84 ± 2.53	46.44 ± 3.67	0.25
K steep (D)	48.86 ± 3.27	49.75 ± 3.47	0.60
Mean K (D)	47.00 ± 2.79	47.82 ± 4.06	0.10
BCVA (logMAR)	0.32 ± 0.16	0.27 ± 0.13	0.01*
OSDI© (before and one-month later)	4.98 ± 1.32	11.26 ± 2.12	0.04*

BCVA: best corrected visual acuity; OSDI: Ocular Surface Disease Index; *Student's t-test for paired values.

TABLE 3: Epi-off versus epi-on after 2-year follow-up (mean ± SD).

	Epi-off	Epi-on	p value
Mean corneal thickness (μm)	501.41 ± 21.91	495.45 ± 43.16	0.10
K flat (D)	44.71 ± 3.03	46.44 ± 3.67	0.01*
K steep (D)	47.76 ± 3.47	49.75 ± 3.47	0.01*
Mean K (D)	46.16 ± 3.15	47.82 ± 4.06	0.08
BCVA (logMAR)	0.22 ± 0.12	0.27 ± 0.13	0.01*
OSDI© (before and one-month later)	13.56 ± 2.15	11.26 ± 2.12	0.02

BCVA: best corrected visual acuity; OSDI: Ocular Surface Disease Index; *Student's t-test for paired values.

TABLE 4: Ocular Surface Disease Index (OSDI©).

	All of the time	Most of the time	Half of the time	Some of the time	None of the time
Have you experienced any of the following during the last week:					
(1) Eyes that are sensitive to light?	4	3	2	1	0
(2) Eyes that feel gritty?	4	3	2	1	0
(3) Painful or sore eyes?	4	3	2	1	0
(4) Blurred vision?	4	3	2	1	0
(5) Poor vision?	4	3	2	1	0
	Subtotal	Score			A
Have problems with your eyes limited you in performing any of the following during the last week:					
(6) Reading	4	3	2	1	0
(7) Driving at night?	4	3	2	1	0
(8) Working with a computer or bank machine (ATM)?	4	3	2	1	0
(9) Watching TV?	4	3	2	1	0
	Subtotal	Score			B
Have your eyes felt uncomfortable in any of the following situations during the last week:					
(10) Windy conditions?	4	3	2	1	0
(11) Places or areas with low humidity (very dry)?	4	3	2	1	0
(12) Areas that are air conditioned?	4	3	2	1	0
	Subtotal	Score			C

Add subtotals A, B, and C to obtain the result.

procedure yields better results and increases the chances of stopping the disease's progression in the long term [30]. This discrepancy could be explained assuming that the effects of cross-linking mainly reflects the biomechanical impact on stiffening the thinning cornea rather than the reforming cornea shape [31]. Therefore, the significant difference in BCVA after two years between the two study groups is more easily understood (Tables 4 and 5).

TABLE 5: Postoperative confocal microscopy in epi-off versus epi-on patients after 2-year follow-up.

	Epi-off (%)	Epi-on (%)	p value
Corneal nerve alteration	93.80	87.50	Not significant
Fibrotic reaction	43.75	25.00	<0.01*
Alterated keratocyte	62.50	18.75	<0.001*

*Chi-square test for nonparametric variables.

The activated keratocyte and fibrotic reaction are more frequent in Group 1 patients. This might be due to a rearrangement of the corneal epithelium secondary to the treatment or more likely to the much deeper cross-linking activity in the epi-off group [14, 32].

Few side effects occurred in our study: in Group 1, two patients had complications (Vogt's striae and type II corneal hazes) and in Group 2, only one eye developed Vogt's striae at the apex of keratoconus. On the contrary, several complications have been reported in other previous series, especially after epi-off CXL, such as clinically significant corneal haze, endothelial damage, and sterile infiltrate infections [33, 34]. Lastly, the most significant complications after epi-off CXL are pain and photophobia, which required placement of bandage contact lens, sunglasses, and analgesia. Our study showed that these two important postoperative complications were minimal in the epi-on CXL patients, as assessed by the OSDI© questionnaire.

The limit of this study is the small number of patients in each group; the strengths are the prospective design, the long term follow-up (two years), and the evaluation of OSDI©.

Despite the different penetration stroma demonstrated in other studies, the clinical outcomes after CLX epi-off and epi-on procedures show that keratoconus was relatively stable after 24 months, and no differences were observed comparing the two procedures. Moreover, our findings demonstrate that the CXL epi-on technique is preferable to CXL epi-off since it reduces postoperative ocular discomfort, maintaining the same profile of safety and efficacy.

Conflicts of Interest

The authors declare that they have no conflicts of interest.

References

[1] M. Hovakimyan, R. F. Guthoff, and O. Stachs, "Collagen cross-linking: current status and future directions," *Journal of Ophthalmology*, vol. 2012, Article ID 406850, 12 pages, 2012.

[2] T. T. Andreassen, A. H. Simonsen, and H. Oxlund, "Biomechanical properties of keratoconus and normal corneas," *Experimental Eye Research*, vol. 31, no. 4, pp. 435–441, 1980.

[3] C. Mazzotta, T. Caporossi, R. Denaro et al., "Morphological and functional correlations in riboflavin UV A corneal collagen cross-linking for keratoconus," *Acta Ophthalmologica*, vol. 90, no. 3, pp. 259–265, 2012.

[4] L. Mastropasqua, "Collagen cross-linking: when and how? A review of the state of the art of the technique and new perspectives," *Eye and Vision*, vol. 2, no. 1, p. 19, 2015.

[5] E. Spoerl, M. Huhle, and T. Seiler, "Induction of cross links in corneal tissue," *Experimental Eye Research*, vol. 66, no. 1, pp. 97–103, 1998.

[6] C. Wittig-Silva, M. Whiting, E. Lamoureux, R. G. Lindsay, L. J. Sullivan, and G. R. Snibson, "A randomized controlled trial of corneal collagen cross-linking in progressive keratoconus: preliminary results," *Journal of Refractive Surgery*, vol. 24, no. 7, pp. S720–S725, 2008.

[7] C. Caruso, C. Ostacolo, R. L. Epstein et al., "Transepithelial corneal cross- linking with vitamin E-enhanced riboflavin solution and abbreviated low-dose UV-A:24-month clinical outcomes," *Cornea*, vol. 35, no. 2, pp. 145–150, 2016.

[8] G. Wollensak, H. Aurich, C. Wirbelauer et al., "Significance of the riboflavin film in corneal collagen crosslinking," *Journal of Cataract and Refractive Surgery*, vol. 36, no. 1, pp. 114–120, 2010.

[9] S. Nawaz, S. Gupta, V. Gogia, N. K. Sasikala, and A. Panda, "Trans-epithelial versus conventional corneal collagen crosslinking: a randomized trial in keratoconus," *Oman Journal of Ophthalmology*, vol. 8, no. 1, pp. 9–13, 2015.

[10] A. Leccisotti and T. Islam, "Transepithelial corneal collagen cross-linking in keratoconus," *Journal of Refractive Surgery*, vol. 26, no. 12, pp. 942–948, 2010.

[11] S. Baiocchi, C. Mazzotta, D. Cerretani, T. Caporossi, and A. Caporossi, "Corneal crosslinking: riboflavin concentration in corneal stroma exposed with and without epithelium," *Journal of Cataract and Refractive Surgery*, vol. 35, no. 5, pp. 893–899, 2009.

[12] G. Wollensak and E. Iomdina, "Biomechanical and histological changes after corneal crosslinking with and without epithelial debridement," *Journal of Cataract and Refractive Surgery*, vol. 35, no. 5, pp. 540–546, 2009.

[13] F. Raiskup-Wolf, A. Hoyer, E. Spoerl, and L. E. Pillunat, "Collagen cross-linking with riboflavin and ultraviolet A light in keratoconus: long-term results," *Journal of Cataract and Refractive Surgery*, vol. 34, no. 5, pp. 796–801, 2008.

[14] M. Filippello, E. Stagni, D. Buccoliero, V. Bonfiglio, and T. Avitabile, "Transepithelial cross-linking in keratoconus patients: confocal analysis," *Optometry and Vision Science*, vol. 89, no. 10, pp. e1–e7, 2012.

[15] V. Agrawal, "Long-term results of cornea collagen cross-linking with riboflavin for keratoconus," *Indian Journal of Ophthalmology*, vol. 61, no. 8, pp. 433-434, 2013.

[16] Z. Dong and X. Zhou, "Collagen cross-linking with riboflavin in a femtosecond laser-created pocket in rabbit corneas: 6-month results," *American Journal of Ophthalmology*, vol. 152, no. 1, pp. 22.e1–27.e1, 2011.

[17] G. Bikbova and M. Bikbov, "Standard corneal collagen crosslinking versus transepithelial iontophoresis-assisted corneal crosslinking, 24 months follow-up: randomized control trial," *Acta Ophthalmologica*, vol. 94, no. 7, pp. e600–e606, 2016.

[18] Y. Goldich, Y. Barkana, O Wussuku Lior et al., "Corneal collagen cross-linking for the treatment of progressive keratoconus: 3-year prospective outcome," *Canadian Journal of Ophthalmology*, vol. 49, no. 1, pp. 54–59, 2014.

[19] P. Vinciguerra, V. Romano, P. Rosetta et al., "Transepithelial iontophoresis versus standard corneal collagen cross-linking: 1-year results of a prospective clinical study," *Journal of Refractive Surgery*, vol. 32, no. 10, pp. 672–678, 2016.

[20] S. C. Kaufman and H. E. Kaufman, "How has confocal microscopy helped us in refractive surgery?," *Current Opinion in Ophthalmology*, vol. 17, no. 4, pp. 380–388, 2006.

[21] M Ünlü, E. Yüksel, and K. Bilgihan, "Effect of corneal cross-linking on contact lens tolerance in keratoconus," *Clinical and Experimental Optometry*, vol. 100, no. 4, pp. 369–374, 2017.

[22] B. Iaccheri, G. Torroni, C. Cagini et al., "Corneal confocal scanning laser microscopy in patients with dry eye disease treated with topical cyclosporine," *Eye*, vol. 31, no. 5, pp. 788–794, 2017.

[23] C. Mazzotta, F. Hafezi, G. Kymionis et al., "In vivo confocal microscopy after corneal collagen crosslinking," *Ocular Surface*, vol. 13, no. 4, pp. 298–314, 2015.

[24] S. Rossi, A. Orrico, C Santamaria et al., "Standard versus trans-epithelial collagen cross-linking in keratoconus patients suitable for standard collagen cross-linking," *Clinical Ophthalmology*, vol. 9, pp. 503–509, 2015.

[25] M. F. Al Fayez, S Al Fayez, and Y. Alfayez, "Transepithelial versus epithelium-off corneal collagen cross-linking for progressive keratoconus: a prospective randomized controlled trial," *Cornea*, vol. 34, no. 10, pp. S53–S56, 2015.

[26] A. Stojanovic, X. Chen, N. Jin et al., "Safety and efficacy of epithelium-on corneal collagen cross-linking using a multifactorial approach to achieve proper stromal riboflavin saturation," *Journal of Ophthalmology*, vol. 2012, Article ID 498435, 8 pages, 2012.

[27] N. Soeters, R. P. Wisse, D. A. Godefrooij, S. M. Imhof, and N. G. Tahzib, "Transepithelial versus epithelium-off corneal cross-linking for the treatment of progressive keratoconus: a randomized controlled trial," *American Journal of Ophthalmology*, vol. 159, no. 5, pp. 821.e3–828.e3, 2015.

[28] S. A. Greenstein, V. P. Shah, K. L. Fry, and P. S. Hersh, "Corneal thickness changes after corneal collagen crosslinking for keratoconus and corneal ectasia: one-year results," *Journal of Cataract and Refractive Surgery*, vol. 37, no. 4, pp. 691–700, 2011.

[29] M. Lombardo, D. Giannini, G. Lombardo, and S. Serrao, "Randomized controlled trial comparing transepithelial corneal cross-linking using iontophoresis with the Dresden protocol in progressive keratoconus," *Ophthalmology*, vol. 124, no. 6, pp. 804–812, 2017.

[30] A. Cantemir, A. I. Alexa, N. Anton et al., "Evaluation of iontophoretic collagen cross-linking for early stage of progressive keratoconus compared to standard cross-linking: a non-inferiority study," *Ophthalmology and Therapy*, vol. 6, no. 1, pp. 147–160, 2017.

[31] Y. Liu, Y. Liu, Y. N. Zhang et al., "Systematic review and meta-analysis comparing modified cross-linking and standard cross-linking for progressive keratoconus," *International Journal of Ophthalmology*, vol. 10, no. 9, pp. 1419–1429, 2017.

[32] C. Mazzotta, A. Balestrazzi, C. Traversi et al., "Treatment of progressive keratoconus by riboflavin-UVA-induced cross-linking of corneal collagen: ultrastructural analysis by Heidelberg retinal tomograph II in vivo confocal microscopy in humans," *Cornea*, vol. 26, no. 4, pp. 390–397, 2007.

[33] P. Rama, F. M. Diatteo, S. Matuska, G. Paganoni, and A. Spinelli, "Acanthamoeba keratitis with perforation after corneal crosslinking and bandage contact lens use," *Journal of Cataract and Refractive Surgery*, vol. 35, no. 4, pp. 788–791, 2009.

[34] P. Rama, F. Di Matteo, S. Matuska, C. Insacco, and G. Paganoni, "Severe keratitis following corneal cross-linking for keratoconus," *Acta Ophthalmologica*, vol. 89, no. 8, pp. e658–e659, 2011.

8

Comparison of the Techniques of Secondary Intraocular Lens Implantation after Penetrating Keratoplasty

Katarzyna Krysik ⓘ,[1] **Dariusz Dobrowolski** ⓘ,[1,2,3] **Ewa Wroblewska-Czajka,**[3]
Anita Lyssek-Boron,[1] **and Edward Wylegala**[2,3,4]

[1]Department of Ophthalmology with Paediatric Unit, St. Barbara Hospital, Trauma Center, Medykow Square 1, 41-200 Sosnowiec, Poland
[2]Chair and Clinical Department of Ophthalmology, School of Medicine with the Division of Dentistry in Zabrze, Medical University of Silesia in Katowice, Panewnicka 65 St., 40-760 Katowice, Poland
[3]Department of Ophthalmology, District Railway Hospital, Panewnicka 65 St., 40-760 Katowice, Poland
[4]Hebei Provincial Eye Hospital, Xingtai, China

Correspondence should be addressed to Dariusz Dobrowolski; dardobmd@wp.pl

Academic Editor: Matteo Forlini

Aim. To conduct a retrospective analysis of secondary IOL implantation in patients who underwent PK with no simultaneous IOL implantation. *Materials and Methods.* The retrospective study of the secondary implantation of IOLs was conducted in 46 eyes that underwent a primary operation with PK and cataract/lens extraction with no IOL implantation due to capsule rupture or combining corneal or intraocular complications. The minimum period from PK was 12 months. All secondary IOL implantations were performed from January 2011 to August 2017. Aphakic postkeratoplasty patients were treated using one of the surgical techniques for secondary IOL implantation. In-the-bag IOL implantation was possible if the posterior capsule was complete. If the lens capsule remnants were sufficient to provide secure IOL support, an in-the-sulcus IOL implantation was performed. Scleral fixation was offered in eyes with extensive capsular deficiency or the presence of the vitreous body in anterior chamber. BCVA and expected and achieved refraction were evaluated; we included using two biometry devices, and results were compared. *Results.* The corrected distance visual acuity (CDVA) before surgery ranged from 0.1 to 0.8 (mean 0.54 ± 0.17). After secondary IOL implantation, CDVA ranged from 0.2 to 0.8 (mean 0.43 ± 0.14) at postoperative 1 month and from 0.3 to 0.9 (mean 0.55 ± 0.15) at postoperative 6 months ($p < 0.05$). Comparison of the final refraction using two methods of biometry showed no statistically significant difference in the group that underwent scleral fixation of the IOL, similar to the findings for the in-the-bag and in-the-sulcus IOL implantation groups. In the scleral-fixation group, $p = 0.55$ for the USG biometry technique and $p = 0.22$ for the OB technique. p values for the IOL-implantation group were $p = 0.49$ and $p = 0.44$, respectively. *Conclusion.* Both implantation methods are safe for the patients. Final refraction is depending on the technique and indication to keratoplasty. Both biometry techniques deliver precise data for IOL choice.

1. Introduction

Eyes undergoing penetrating keratoplasty (PK) often have coexisting ocular pathologies which impede simultaneous intraocular lens (IOL) implantation. Lens injury with cataract formation frequently occurs in ocular trauma, intraocular inflammations, and after previous complicated surgeries. A typical triple procedure, consisting of PK, cataract extraction, and IOL implantation, leads to faster visual acuity improvement when compared with staged surgery, and it avoids successive surgeries [1, 2]. Conversely, the large refractive errors associated with triple procedures also need to be taken into account [3]. In some patients—such as those with ocular infections, insufficient capsular bag support, traumatic eyes with moderate to severe posterior segment injury, iris laceration or aniridia, lens subluxation, or loss of zonular integrity—a one-time IOL placement may be difficult and may carry intra- and postoperative risks [4]. Other risk factors associated with the open-sky state and the patient's health status, such as previous ocular surgery, ocular trauma, internal diseases (arterial hypertension, coronary heart disease, diabetes, atherosclerosis, etc.), and the choice of general anaesthesia, may also constitute contraindications for IOL implantation during a single surgery [5–9]. However, secondary IOL implantation is a challenging surgical procedure and demands suitable ocular conditions. Although the methods and timing of the surgical approach have changed over years, the functional reconstruction of the eye is often more difficult than the original attempt at anatomic reconstruction [3, 10]. If there are local or general contraindications for surgery, appropriate contact lens correction can be offered to the patient.

Aphakic patients need successive visual rehabilitation after undergoing PK. In unilateral cases, these patients often present with high ametropia and high anisometropia, which may be very difficult or impossible to correct with other than surgical methods. Implantation of IOLs also helps to separate the anterior from the posterior chamber and to avoid further complications, such as vitreous contact with the endothelium which can lead to corneal decompensation or cystoid macular oedema (CME) [4, 11]. The choice of a secondary implanted IOL includes anterior chamber intraocular lenses (ACIOL), iris-claw or angle-supported lenses, and posterior chamber (retropupillary approach) lenses (PCIOL), such as in-the-bag and in-the-sulcus implanted or scleral- or iris-fixated lenses [3, 12–15]. The main advantage of the PCIOLs is their more physiological location, which is closer to the normal crystalline lens plane, and the greater distance to the cornea [11, 16]. The surgical risks of this method, associated mainly with elderly patients, include a higher frequency of uveal or choroidal bleeding, damage to the blood-aqueous barrier in the ciliary body due to mechanical pressure of the haptics, and endophthalmitis caused by erosion of the scleral sutures and CME [17–19]. This type of surgical approach, although more time-consuming than ACIOL implantation, might have a lower rate of IOL dislocations, glaucoma, or endothelial cell loss with consecutive corneal decompensation and uveitis [18, 20, 21].

The aim of the present study was to conduct a retrospective analysis of secondary IOL implantation in patients who underwent PK with no simultaneous IOL implantation. We report on the surgical technique, its anatomical and refractive outcomes, and complications arising from this kind of treatment.

2. Materials and Methods

This was a retrospective study of the secondary implantation of IOLs in 46 eyes that underwent a primary operation with PK and cataract/lens extraction with no IOL implantation. All secondary IOL implantations were performed from January 2011 to August 2017 at the Ophthalmology Department of Saint Barbara Hospital, Trauma Centre,

Sosnowiec, Poland. All parts of the data analysis were conducted under the tenets of the Declaration of Helsinki. The most common reason for secondary IOL implantation in our group, rather than simultaneous with keratoplasty, was a lack of the optimal surgical and ocular conditions for safe IOL placement during keratoplasty (Table 1). The minimum period from PK was 12 months. The analysed data from the medical records included demographics, medical history, corrected distance preoperative and postoperative Snellen visual acuity, details and technique of the IOL calculation and IOL calculation formula, and the outcome and complications of surgery. All patients underwent a complete ophthalmic examination, including corrected distance visual acuity, IOP measurement by Goldmann applanation tonometry, and slit-lamp biomicroscopy and fundus examination with a dilated pupil (if examination was possible). In all the eyes, all corneal sutures were removed at least a month prior to IOL power calculation to avoid changes in corneal curvature.

Exclusion criteria were keratoconus or other corneal ectatic disorders, postkeratoplasty ocular diseases (rejection episode, secondary glaucoma), ocular surgery or trauma, and high astigmatism (>6.0 D), which could affect the final refractive treatment.

All PKs and secondary IOL implantations were performed by two experienced surgeons. All patients signed an informed consent form before any surgical procedure. The donor corneas for the PKs originated from our or cooperative tissue banks. We used a Hanna vacuum trephine system (Moria Inc., Antony, France) or Barron radial vacuum trephines (Katena Products Inc. Denville, New Jersey, USA) for trephination.

Aphakic postkeratoplasty patients were treated using one of three surgical techniques for IOL implantation. In-the-bag IOL implantation was possible if the posterior capsule was present (6 cases). If the lens capsule remnants were sufficient to provide secure IOL support, an in-the-sulcus IOL implantation was performed (11 cases). An AcrySof Multipiece MA60AC (Alcon, USA) was implanted in both methods. Indications for scleral fixation were extensive capsular deficiency or the presence of the vitreous body in the anterior chamber with need of an anterior vitrectomy (29 cases). The surgical technique included conjunctival periotomy adjoining the 3 o'clock and 9 o'clock limbus and creation of half-thickness triangular scleral flaps 3 mm posterior to the surgical limbus, avoiding the long posterior ciliary arteries. The corneal incision for lens implantation was made in the superior quadrants of the peripheral cornea, in the 120° area, back from the Vogt's palisades. A transscleral suture passage was made with an ab interno technique, using 10-0 polypropylene suture material, 1.5 mm posterior to the limbus, through the ciliary sulcus. The haptics of the IOL were placed in the ciliary sulcus. The external knot was covered with a scleral flap. A single-piece CZ 70 BD (Alcon, Fort Worth, TX, USA) PMMA IOL with a 7 mm diameter optic was used in all patients. As most IOL power calculations are based on the endocapsular IOL localisation, power adjustment is necessary to account for a more anteriorly positioned lens in the ciliary sulcus.

TABLE 1: Surgical techniques used for secondary IOL implantation and the indications for prior keratoplasty with lens extraction.

Characteristics	Total ($n = 46$), N (%)	Female ($n = 19$), N (%)	Male ($n = 27$), N (%)
IOL in-the-bag implantation	6 (13)	2 (33.3)	4 (66.7)
Indication for PK			
Ocular trauma	4 (8.7)	1 (5.26)	3 (11.11)
Ocular inflammation	1 (2.17)	0	1 (3.7)
Previous ocular surgery	1 (2.17)	1 (5.26)	0
IOL in-the-sulcus implantation	11 (24)	7 (63.6)	4 (36.4)
Indication for PK			
Ocular trauma	6 (13.04)	4 (21.06)	2 (7.41)
Ocular inflammation	3 (6.52)	2 (10.52)	1 (3.7)
Previous ocular surgery	2 (4.35)	1 (5.26)	1 (3.7)
IOL scleral fixation	29 (63)	10 (34.5)	19 (65.5)
Indication for PK			
Ocular trauma	18 (39.1)	6 (31.6)	12 (44.45)
Ocular inflammation	9 (19.6)	3 (15.78)	6 (22.23)
Previous ocular surgery	2 (4.35)	1 (5.26)	1 (3.7)

The intraocular lens power was determined using standard and corneal topography-derived keratometry with the SRK/T formula. We used two independent methods for IOL calculation: ultrasonic biometry (UB) with an A-Scan ultrasonic biometer (Quantel Medical, US) with an applanation technique under topical anaesthesia and interferometry (optical biometry; OB) with an AL-Scan optical biometer (Nidek Co., Ltd., Japan). Keratometric measurements were obtained after removal of the corneal sutures, a minimum of one year after keratoplasty. Primary keratometry and refraction of the operated eyes were unknown.

Because of the potential intrasurgical risks and the duration of this procedure, the scleral fixation was performed under peribulbar or general anaesthesia. Both the in-the-bag and in-the-sulcus IOL implantations were performed under topical anaesthesia. Following surgery, all patients received an intracameral injection of cefuroxime (1 mg).

This retrospective, observational study, according to Polish law, does not require approval by a local bioethics committee.

The XLSTAT-Biomed (Addinsoft SARL, France) computer software was used for statistical analysis and to calculate means and standard deviations. The parameter values were compared using Student's t-test or the Mann–Whitney U test. For normal and near-normal distributions, a variance analysis was performed using ANOVA, and the homogeneity of variance was then determined using Bartlett's test. The difference between the measurements with different methods was plotted against their mean in a Bland–Altman plot. The 95% limits of agreement (mean difference ± 1.96 standard deviation) gave the distance between the measurements by the methods with 95% confidence. A p value of <0.05 was considered statistically significant.

3. Results

Between January 2011 and August 2017, 46 secondary IOL implantations were performed in 46 eyes of post-PK patients. The study group consisted of 19 females at the age of 59.95 ± 14.5 (mean ± SD) years (range was: 35–82 years) at the time of the IOL implantation procedure and 27 males at age of 58.19 ± 15.13 (mean ± SD) years (range was: 27–83 years) at the time of the IOL implantation procedure. No statistically significant differences were noted for the group size or age in the female and male groups ($p < 0.05$). There were 46 surgeries, comprising 6 (13%) in-the-bag IOL implantations, 11 (24%) in-the-sulcus IOL implantations, and 29 (63%) scleral fixations of the IOL. All PKs were performed from January 2010 and October 2016. The age at the time of PK was 58.16 ± 14.38 (mean ± SD) (range was: 34–80 years) years for the female group and 56.67 ± 15.37 (mean ± SD) (range was: 25–82 years) years for the male group. The mean interval between PK and secondary IOL implantation was 21 months in the female group and 19 months in the male group. Table 1 shows the surgical techniques used for IOL implantation and the indications for PK.

The indications for PK and cataract/lens extraction were ocular trauma, 28 eyes (61%); inflammation (bacterial origin: 11 eyes, fungal origin: 2 eyes) of the anterior segment of the eye, 13 eyes (28%); and corneal scars and decompensation after ocular surgeries (including refractive intraocular surgery, glaucoma surgery, and pars plana vitrectomy), 5 eyes (11%).

The corrected distance visual acuity (CDVA) before secondary IOL implantation ranged from 0.1 to 0.8 (mean 0.54 ± 0.17). After secondary IOL implantation, the corrected distance visual acuity ranged from 0.2 to 0.8 (mean 0.43 ± 0.14) at postoperative 1 month and from 0.3 to 0.9 (mean 0.55 ± 0.15) at postoperative 6 months ($p < 0.05$). Figure 1 shows the changes in corrected distance visual acuity from the preoperative period to 1 and 6 months from the secondary IOL implantation.

Figures 2 and 3 show the corrected distance visual acuity, including the IOL implantation method.

Table 2 shows the corrected distance visual acuity before and after the secondary IOL implantation.

Comparative analysis of the mean CDVA in the three periods of secondary IOL implantation showed statistically

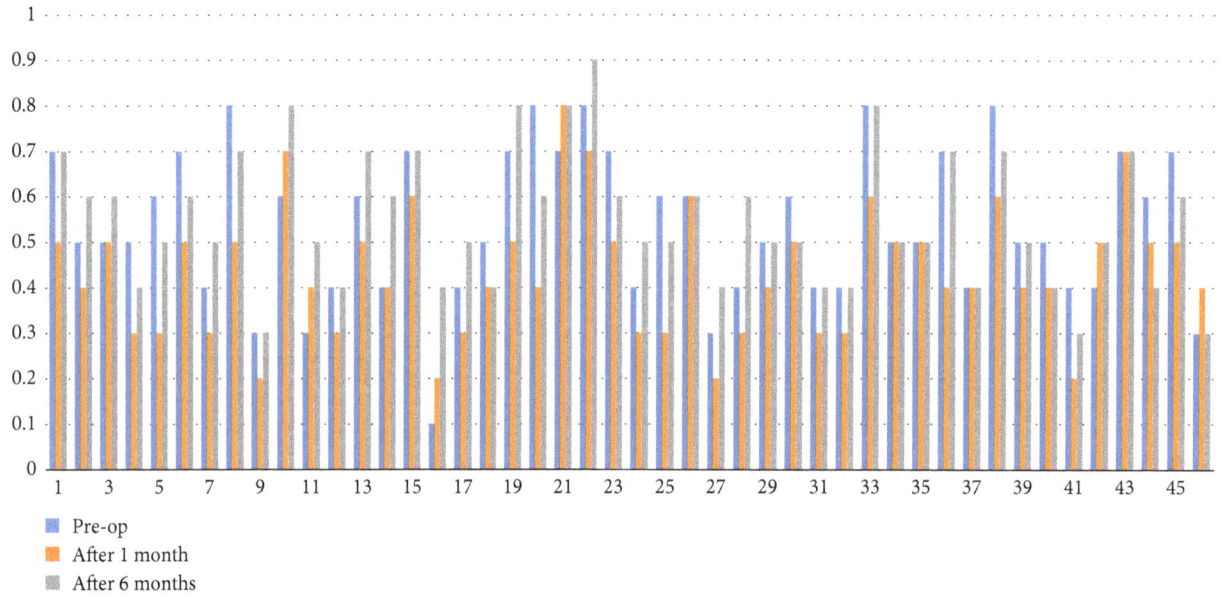

FIGURE 1: Corrected distance visual acuity at major points before IOL implantation, 1 month after surgery, and 6 months after surgery.

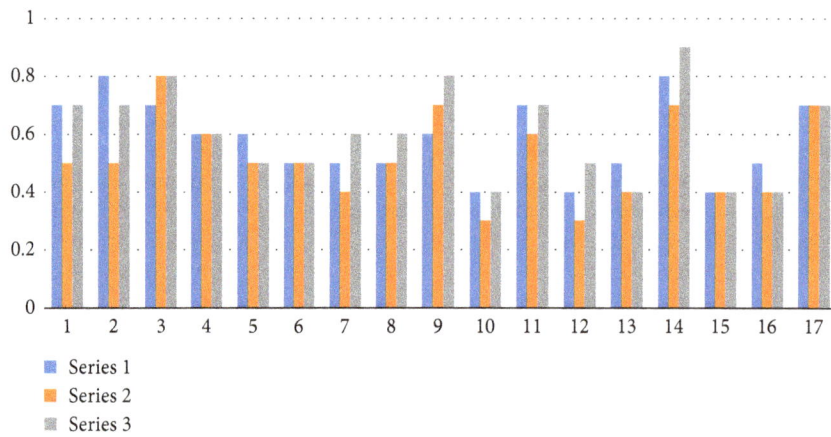

FIGURE 2: Corrected distance visual acuity. Series 1: before IOL implantation; series 2 : 1 month after surgery; series 3 : 3 months after in-the-bag and in-the-sulcus IOL implantation surgery.

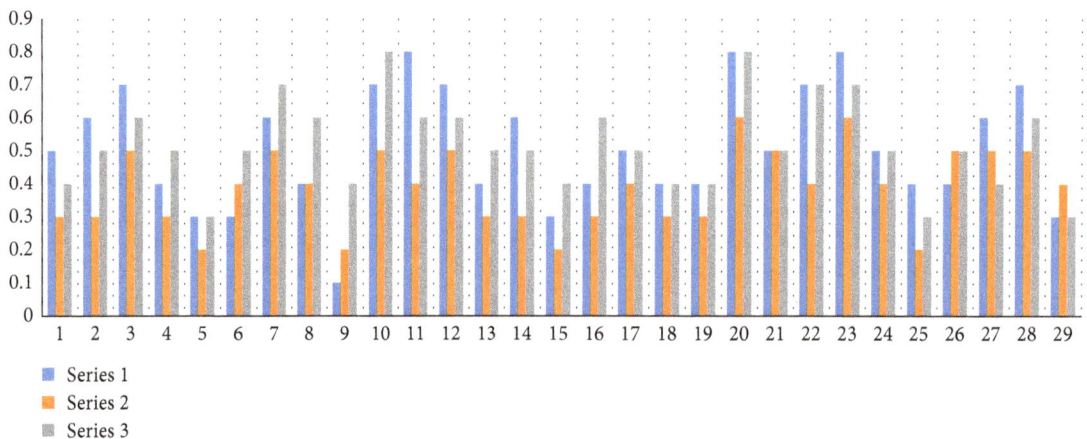

FIGURE 3: Corrected distance visual acuity. Series 1: before IOL implantation; series 2 : 1 month after surgery; series 3 : 3 months after scleral fixation surgery of the IOL.

TABLE 2: Corrected distance visual acuity before and after the secondary IOL implantation.

Characteristics	Total n (%) ($n = 46$)	Preoperative CDVA (range)	Postoperative CDVA (range) After one month	Postoperative CDVA (range) After 6 months
Procedure				
IOL in-the-bag implantation	6	0.5–0.8	0.5–0.8	0.5–0.8
IOL in-the-sulcus implantation	11	0.4–0.8	0.3–0.7	0.4–0.9
IOL scleral fixation	29	0.1–0.8	0.2–0.6	0.3–0.8

Preoperative uncorrected VA was below 0.1, and postoperative UCVA, if compared with corrected results was equal or lower; no more than 2 lines on Snellen charts were observed. Postoperative CDVA was better than or equal to preoperative CDVA in 83.3%, 72.2%, and 68.9% of cases, respectively; 2 cases of in-the-sulcus IOL lost more than 2 lines, and 3 cases of scleral-fixation IOL lost more than 2 lines at the end-point.

significant differences in the values between the preoperative period and 1 month after the secondary IOL implantation ($p = 0.002$) and between 1 month and 6 months after the surgery ($p < 0.001$). The preoperative and final mean CDVA in the study group showed no statistically significant difference ($p = 0.69$).

Figure 4 shows the Bland–Altman plots for the agreement between the two methods of refraction measurement. The dotted lines represent the mean refraction differences between the methods. The interline zones represent the area of 95% limits of agreement.

The differences between the expected and achieved final refraction with a myopic shift and a comparison of the expected and achieved refraction of the whole study group are presented in Figure 5.

The final corrected distance visual acuity and final refraction in the group of eyes operated with scleral fixation and secondary in-the-bag or in-the-sulcus techniques are shown in Figures 6 and 7.

Comparison of the final refraction using both methods of biometry showed no statistically significant difference in the group that underwent scleral fixation of the IOL, similar to the findings for the in-the-bag and in-the-sulcus IOL implantation groups. In the scleral-fixation group, $p = 0.55$ for the USG biometry technique and $p = 0.22$ for the OB technique. These values for the IOL-implantation group were $p = 0.49$ and $p = 0.44$, respectively.

Graft transparency was rated during each follow-up visit. Despite transient partial graft oedema in 6 eyes after scleral fixation (21%), a final full graft transparency was observed at the last control visit in all operated eyes. Other postoperative complications of secondary IOL implantation were glaucoma or ocular hypertension, observed in 7 eyes (24%) after scleral fixation and 2 eyes (18%) after in-the-sulcus IOL implantation. Most of these were treated with 1 or 2 topical agents (timolol 0.5%, brimonidine) with no need for consecutive glaucoma surgery. Moderate, transient irydocyclitis was reported in 4 eyes (14%) after scleral fixation and in 1 eye after in-the-sulcus IOL implantation (9%). Pseudophakic cystoid macular oedema appeared in 2 eyes after scleral fixation (7%), and topical and systemic anti-inflammatory medication was administered. A prolapsed vitreous, updrawn pupil, or anterior synechia was the condition that impeded the easy and safe secondary IOL implantation. In those 2 cases, the patient underwent anterior vitrectomy and anterior synechiolysis. No dislocation of the secondary implanted IOL or endophthalmitis was observed.

4. Discussion

The sequential procedure seems to be more accurate for the calculation of the IOL power when compared with the triple procedure (cataract surgery, IOL implantation, and PK). Conversely, the triple procedure allows a faster visual rehabilitation, although it might have a higher risk of intra- and postoperative intraocular infections and other complications [2, 19, 20, 22]. The longer duration of the open-sky state and a higher risk to the patient (including changes in intraocular pressure, posterior capsule rupture, prolapse of the vitreous body, and potential choroidal haemorrhage) frequently forces a need to divide the surgery into two separate approaches [2]. Numerous studies have reported the sequential surgical approach for combined corneal and lens diseases [3, 4, 15, 23].

The indication for secondary IOL implantation is to relieve discomfort or unsatisfactory correction with spectacles or contact lenses for medical, professional, or personal reasons [18]. Precise IOL power calculation is crucial to achieve the expected refraction after lens removal. Many studies have shown less postsurgical refractive error following a two-stage intervention [3, 23]. A very careful surgical approach should be established for globe reconstruction with secondary IOL implantation [10].

The current literature contains insufficient data regarding secondary PCIOL implantation in the eyes after PK and lens removal [3]. The patient profiles differ from those of patients who underwent only lens surgery with no corneal transplantation. The complication profile differed significantly for the patients who underwent scleral fixation versus the other two types of IOL implantation. Our results are compatible with those of Güell et al. [11] who emphasised that the main limitations of the study on secondary IOL implantation were the retrospective approach and the lack of a control group. In addition, a nonhomogeneous group of patients was analysed altogether.

The smaller frequency of intra- and postoperative complications in the groups that underwent the in-the-bag and in-the-sulcus IOL implantation results from an appropriate choice of IOL model, with a large optic and thin long-angulated haptics with more anatomical placement [24, 25]. Postoperative complications of scleral fixation in our study group were comparable to those following secondary scleral fixation in the eyes with no prior corneal surgery [14, 16]. However, we did not measure endothelial cell density, although another aspect of one-stage surgery is

(a)

(b)

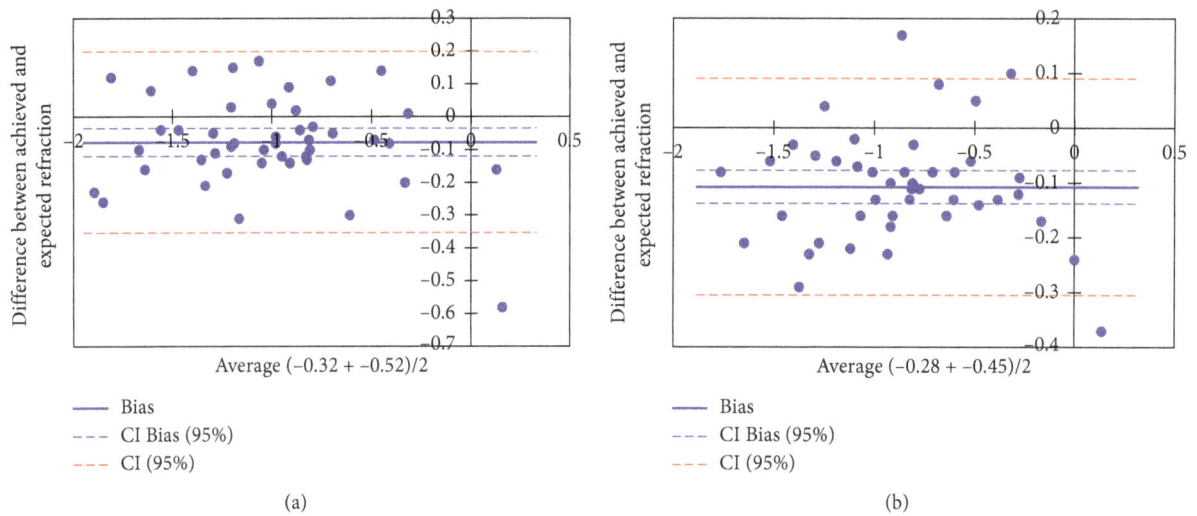

FIGURE 4: Bland–Altman tests showing the mean difference between the achieved and expected final refraction and the mean refraction in the ultrasound biometry measurement group (a) and the optical biometry measurement group (b).

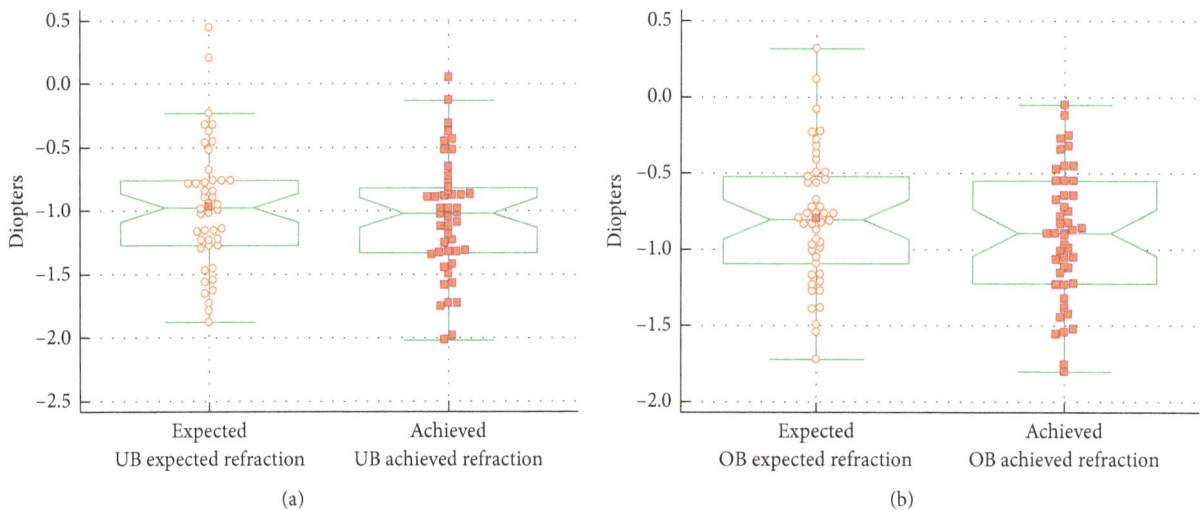

(a)

(b)

FIGURE 5: The difference between the expected and achieved refraction for both measurement methods with a myopic shift in the ultrasound biometry measurement group (a) and the optical biometry measurement group (b) ($p < 0.05$).

a lower risk of endothelial cell loss and stress to the corneal endothelium, due to the open anterior chamber and the lack of a corneal button during IOL implantation. When IOL implantation is performed in the two-stage approach, both the shape and the site of implantation should be taken into account [11, 13, 14, 17, 21, 25].

Ultrasound biometry is still in common use, but optical biometry is now considered the gold standard for IOL calculation. However, our comparison did not reveal any significant differences between these methods. Previous data are not applicable for IOL power evaluation in the eyes after PK. In our sample of patients, the final refraction using ultrasound and optical methods of biometry showed no statistically significantly different values. This demonstrates that even in the scleral-fixation group, despite the large corneal surgical cut, the impact on postoperative refraction

is not significant, and the achieved refraction is not statistically significant from that of patients undergoing surgery with small corneal cut. The visual outcomes are consistent with prognostic values: in our sample of patients with secondary IOL implantation, the final mean corrected distance visual acuity was comparable to the preoperative values.

Our findings are compatible with the results of authors who conducted secondary scleral fixation after complicated cataract surgery with no prior corneal surgery [14, 16, 21]. In our group of patients, we did not perform limbal wedge resection or relaxing incisions to improve the second surgery result, as suggested by Geggel [3].

Despite the delayed visual rehabilitation after the sequential surgical approach, the final refractive outcome is crucial [7]. In our opinion, the secondary implantation of the

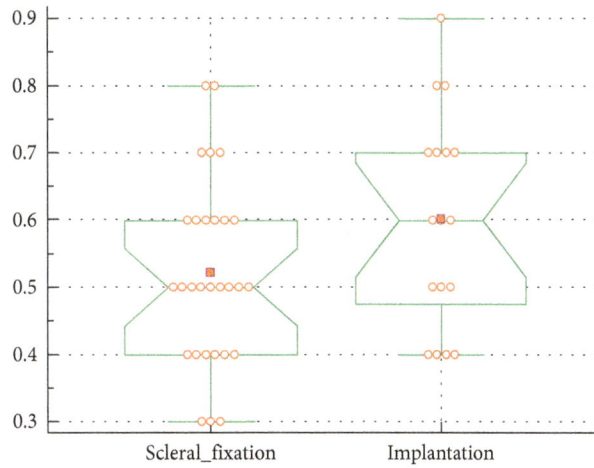

FIGURE 6: Final corrected distance visual acuity—surgical method comparison ($p = 0.12$).

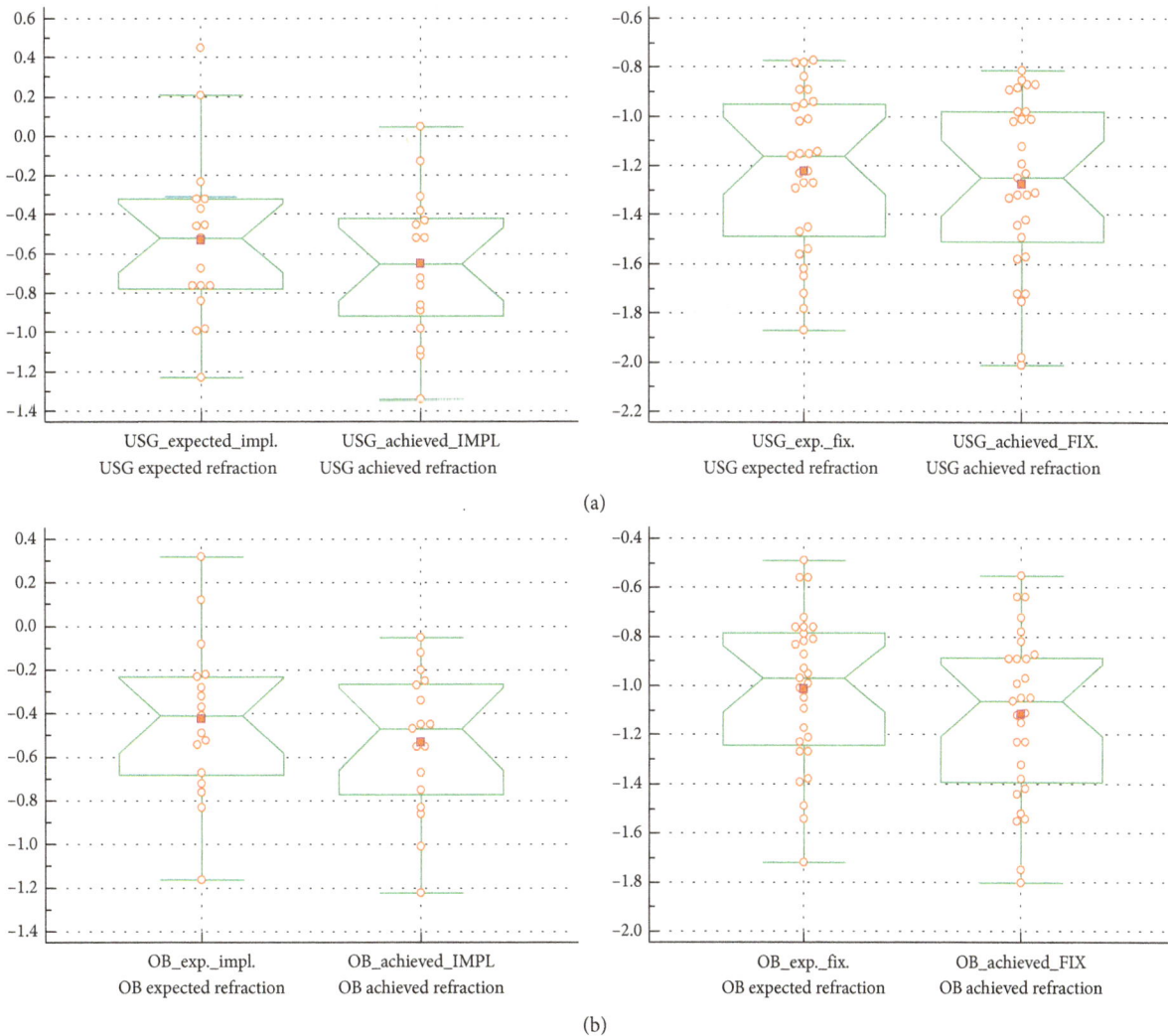

(a)

(b)

FIGURE 7: The difference between expected and achieved refraction in both measurement methods with myopic shift in the ultrasound biometry measurement group (a) and the optical biometry measurement group (b) ($p < 0.05$). USG_expected_impl: USB expected refraction; USG_achieved_IMPL: USG achieved refraction; USG_exp._fix.: USG expected refraction; USG_achieved_FIX.: USG achieved refraction; OB_exp._impl.: OB expected refraction; OB_achieved_IMPL: OB achieved refraction; OB_exp._fix.: OB expected refraction; OB_achieved_FIX: OB achieved refraction.

IOL after PK is a very challenging surgery. Because of the complex nature of the indications for surgery and their modalities, the choice of surgical technique and the results of surgical treatment depend on numerous factors. The surgeon has to consider many different factors, including the corneal shape, the anterior chamber depth and its configuration, and the state of the lens capsule and iris. An important consideration for safe lens implantation is accurate timing for the appropriate surgical technique [16, 21].

In summary, our results for the surgical treatment of aphakia after a one-time PK and lens removal show that there is no one-size-fits-all surgical approach. The surgeon's experience and a careful surgical strategy are crucial for the right choice of the IOL lens power and the method of its implantation.

Conflicts of Interest

The authors declare that there are no conflicts of interest regarding the publication of this paper.

References

[1] Y. Oie and K. Nishida, "Triple procedure: cataract extraction, intraocular lens implantation, and corneal graft," *Current Opinion in Ophthalmology*, vol. 28, no. 1, pp. 63–66, 2017.

[2] S. Yang, B. Wang, Y. Zhang et al., "Evaluation of an interlaced triple procedure: penetrating keratoplasty, extracapsular cataract extraction, and nonopen-sky intraocular lens implantation," *Medicine*, vol. 96, no. 35, p. e7656, 2017.

[3] H. S. Geggel, "Intraocular lens implantation after penetrating keratoplasty," *Ophthalmology*, vol. 97, no. 11, pp. 1460–1467, 1990.

[4] H. S. Sethi, M. P. Naik, and V. S. Gupta, "26-G needle-assisted sutureless glueless intrascleral haptic fixation for secondary ciliary sulcus implantation of three-piece polymethylmethacrylate intraocular lens during penetrating keratoplasty," *Taiwan Journal of Ophthalmology*, vol. 6, no. 3, pp. 141–144, 2016.

[5] A. Pillar, B. H. Jeng, and W. M. Munir, "Positive end-expiratory pressure as a risk factor for severe positive vitreous pressure during combined penetrating keratoplasty and cataract extraction," *Cornea*, vol. 35, no. 11, pp. 1491–1494, 2016.

[6] P. Bandivadekar, S. Gupta, and N. Sharma, "Intraoperative suprachoroidal hemorrhage after penetrating keratoplasty: case series and review of literature," *Eye & Contact Lens: Science & Clinical Practice*, vol. 42, no. 3, pp. 206–210, 2016.

[7] B. Seitz, A. Langenbucher, A. Viestenz, T. Dietrich, M. Küchle, and G. O. Naumann, "Cataract and keratoplasty-simultaneous or sequential surgery?," *Klinische Monatsblätter für Augenheilkunde*, vol. 220, no. 5, pp. 326–329, 2003.

[8] M. J. Groh, B. Seitz, A. Händel, and G. O. Naumann, "Expulsive hemorrhage in perforating keratoplasty-incidence and risk factors," *Klinische Monatsblatter für Augenheilkunde*, vol. 215, no. 9, pp. 152–157, 1999.

[9] F. W. Price Jr., W. E. Whitson, K. A. Ahad, and H. Tavakkoli, "Suprachoroidal hemorrhage in penetrating keratoplasty," *Ophthalmic Surgery*, vol. 25, no. 8, pp. 521–525, 1994.

[10] M. Fiorentzis, A. Viestenz, J. Heichel, B. Seitz, T. Hammer, and A. Viestenz, "Methods of fixation of intraocular lenses according to the anatomical structures in trauma eyes," *Clinical Anatomy*, vol. 31, no. 1, pp. 6–15, 2018.

[11] J. L. Güell, P. Verdaguer, D. Elies et al., "Secondary iris-claw anterior chamber lens implantation in patients with aphakia without capsular support," *British Journal of Ophthalmology*, vol. 98, no. 5, pp. 658–663, 2014.

[12] M. Forlini, W. Soliman, A. Bratu, P. Rossini, G. M. Cavallini, and C. Forlini, "Long-term follow-up of retropupillary iris-claw intraocular lens implantation: a retrospective analysis," *BMC Ophthalmology*, vol. 15, no. 1, p. 143, 2015.

[13] S. R. DeSilva, K. Arun, M. Anandan, N. Glover, C. K. Patel, and P. Rosen, "Iris-claw intraocular lenses to correct aphakia in the absence of capsule support," *Journal of Cataract and Refractive Surgery*, vol. 37, no. 9, pp. 1667–1672, 2011.

[14] T. C. Y. Chan, J. K. M. Lam, V. Jhanji, and E. Y. M. Li, "Comparison of outcomes of primary anterior chamber versus secondary scleral-fixated intraocular lens implantation in complicated cataract surgeries," *American Journal of Ophthalmology*, vol. 159, no. 2, pp. 221.e2–226.e2, 2015.

[15] C. H. Hsiao, J. J. Chen, P. Y. Chen, and H. S. Chen, "Intraocular lens implantation after penetrating keratoplasty," *Cornea*, vol. 20, no. 6, pp. 580–585, 2001.

[16] Z. Yalniz-Akkaya, A. Burcu, G. O. Uney et al., "Primary and secondary implantation of scleral-fixated posterior chamber intraocular lenses in adult patients," *Middle East African Journal of Ophthalmology*, vol. 21, no. 1, pp. 44–49, 2014.

[17] R. Bellucci, V. Pucci, S. Morselli, and L. Bonomi, "Secondary implantation of angle-supported anterior chamber and scleral-fixated posterior chamber intraocular lenses," *Journal of Cataract and Refractive Surgery*, vol. 22, no. 2, pp. 247–252, 1996.

[18] M. J. Koss and T. Kohnen, "Intraocular architecture of secondary implanted anterior chamber iris-claw lenses in aphakic eyes evaluated with anterior segment optical coherence tomography," *British Journal of Ophthalmology*, vol. 93, no. 10, pp. 1301–1306, 2009.

[19] E. C. Davies and R. Pineda II, "Complications of sleral-fixated intraocular lenses," *Seminars in Ophthalmology*, vol. 33, no. 1, pp. 23–28, 2018.

[20] J. B. Malta, M. Banitt, D. C. Musch, A. Sugar, S. I. Mian, and H. K. Soong, "Long-term outcome of combined penetrating keratoplasty with scleral-sutured posterior chamber intraocular lens implantation," *Cornea*, vol. 28, no. 7, pp. 741–746, 2009.

[21] M. D. Wagoner, M. D. Terry, A. Cox, R. G. Ariyasu, D. S. Jacobs, and C. L. Karp, "Intraocular lens implantation in the absence of capsular support," *Ophthalmology*, vol. 110, no. 4, pp. 840–859, 2003.

[22] M. Küchle, A. Händel, and G. O. Naumann, "Results of implantation of transsclerally sutured posterior chamber lenses in combination with penetrating keratoplasty," *Der Ophthalmologe*, vol. 95, no. 10, pp. 671–676, 1998.

[23] S. Shimmura, Y. Ohashi, H. Shiroma, J. Shimazaki, and K. Tsubota, "Corneal opacity and cataract: triple procedure versus secondary approach," *Cornea*, vol. 22, no. 3, pp. 234–238, 2003.

[24] P. S. Kemp and T. A. Oetting, "Stability and safety of MA50 intraocular lens placed in the sulcus," *Eye*, vol. 29, no. 11, pp. 1438–1441, 2015.

[25] H. V. Gimbel, R. Sun, M. Ferensowicz, E. Anderson-Penno, and A. Kamal, "Intraoperative management of posterior capsule tears in phacoemulsification and intraocular lens implantation," *Ophthalmology*, vol. 108, pp. 2186–2192, 2001.

9

Role of the Epipapillary Membrane in Maculopathy Associated with Cavitary Optic Disc Anomalies: Morphology, Surgical Outcomes, and Histopathology

Atsushi Tanaka,[1,2] Wataru Saito [iD],[1,3] Satoru Kase,[1] Kan Ishijima,[1] Kousuke Noda,[1] and Susumu Ishida[1]

[1]*Department of Ophthalmology, Faculty of Medicine and Graduate School of Medicine, Hokkaido University, Sapporo, Japan*
[2]*Enoki Eye Clinic, Sayama, Japan*
[3]*Kaimeido Eye and Dental Clinic, Sapporo, Japan*

Correspondence should be addressed to Wataru Saito; wsaito@med.hokudai.ac.jp

Academic Editor: Vlassis Grigoropoulos

Purpose. To evaluate the surgical outcomes of pars plana vitrectomy (PPV) with epipapillary membrane removal in patients with maculopathy associated with cavitary optic disc anomalies. *Methods*. Eight patients (8 eyes) with cavitary optic disc anomaly-associated maculopathy who underwent PPV with epipapillary membrane removal were retrospectively reviewed. The best-corrected visual acuity (BCVA) and macular and papillary morphologies using enhanced depth imaging optical coherence tomography (EDI-OCT) were evaluated before and after treatment. Immunohistochemistry for an intraoperatively excised epipapillary membrane tissue was also performed. *Results*. Before surgery, EDI-OCT revealed that epipapillary membrane was observed in all patients. Retinoschisis was resolved with no recurrence in all patients following vitrectomy regardless of a disease type or the presence or absence of preoperative posterior vitreous detachment. The mean final BCVA and central retinal thickness significantly improved compared with pretreatment values ($P = 0.008$ and 0.004, resp.). Immunoreactivity for S100 protein and glial fibrillary acidic protein, markers of astrocytes, was positive in the resected membrane tissues. *Conclusions*. These results suggest that epipapillary membrane is involved in the pathogenesis of some patients with cavitary optic disc anomaly-associated maculopathy as well as posterior hyaloid membrane. PPV with epipapillary membrane removal may be a useful treatment option for this maculopathy. This trial is registered with UMIN000011123.

1. Introduction

Optic disc pit (ODP) and morning glory disc disorders are congenital cavitary anomalies of the optic disc, which are associated with dysraphism of the optic fissure. Disc anomalies have common histopathologic characteristics: defects of the lamina cribrosa and the sclera, invagination of the retinal tissue into the excavation of the optic disc, attachment of the vitreous cortex and glial tissue to the invaginated retinal tissues, and presence of the subarachnoid space directly under the excavation site of the disc [1–3]. These disc anomalies can also involve retinal schisis extending from the optic disc to the posterior pole, with often

macular serous retinal detachment (SRD) [1, 3, 4]. However, the etiology that causes retinal schisis in these disc anomalies is not fully elucidated.

The posterior hyaloid membrane and the vitreous strand, which is possibly a remnant of the Cloquet's canal, are attached to the site with the pit [5–8]. In patients with ODP maculopathy without preoperative posterior vitreous detachment (PVD), indeed, retinal schisis is resolved in most cases after pars plana vitrectomy (PPV) with the generation of PVD, but without any internal limiting membrane peeling, retinal photocoagulation at the disc edge, or gas tamponade [9, 10]. Retinal schisis disappeared after spontaneous development of PVD [11]. These observations suggest that a certain communication between the retinal schisis and the vitreous cavity or subarachnoid space arose by which the posterior hyaloid membrane drew the vulnerable disc tissue [1, 12]. However, there were cases with no improvement or showing recurrence of the retinal schisis, even after PVD was made following PPV [9, 13, 14]. In case series with a long-term follow-up, a foveal reattachment rate after PPV with induction of PVD was 81% and internal limiting membrane (ILM) peeling was not associated with foveal reattachment [14]. Furthermore, the retinal schisis did not improve despite performing PPV in all cases with preoperative PVD [15]. A recent study reported surgical outcomes of PPV with creation of inner retinal fenestration [16]. Retinal schisis is resolved after PPV in almost all cases, even though both induction of PVD and ILM removal were not performed [16]. However, multicentered studies examining long-term outcomes of this new surgical procedure are needed. Thus, these observations suggest that there is another unidentified pathological mechanism other than the traction of the hyaloid membrane.

A recent study using spectral domain optical coherence tomography (SD-OCT) demonstrated that all eyes with ODP involved epipapillary membrane, which developed over time [17]. Although the membrane may be related to the pathogenesis of ODP maculopathy by dragging the disc, surgical outcomes of PPV with epipapillary membrane removal have previously been reported in only one case [18].

In patients with morning glory syndrome, a study using SD-OCT reported the detection of attached posterior hyaloid membrane and glial tissues at the excavation site of the disc and a good surgical outcome following PPV after the removal of these tissues [4]. This study suggests that the traction of the hyaloid membrane and/or glial tissues is involved in the pathogenesis of the morning glory syndrome.

Glaucomatous optic disc is an acquired cavitary anomaly of the optic disc. Though rarely, eyes with glaucoma involve retinal schisis, despite the absence of the pit within the disc [19–22]. Retinal schisis disappeared or improved after PPV with the generation of PVD in patients with retinoschisis associated with glaucoma without preoperative PVD [22]. Furthermore, retinal schisis was resolved following PPV with the removal of the glial tissue present on the disc in a patient with preoperative PVD [21]. These studies suggest that the posterior hyaloid membrane and/or glial tissue on the disc is related to the pathogenesis of retinoschisis associated with glaucoma. Taken together, previous findings suggest that traction force to the fragile optic disc of the posterior hyaloid membrane and/or epipapillary membrane is involved in the pathogenesis of maculopathy associated with congenital or acquired optic disc anomalies. Therefore, we hypothesized that PPV that removes not only the hyaloid membrane but also the epipapillary membrane would be effective for treating maculopathy associated with cavitary optic disc anomalies [23]. The purpose of this study was to evaluate the surgical outcomes of PPV with epipapillary membrane removal and to analyze histopathology of the resected membrane in order to examine the role of epipapillary membrane in patients with maculopathy associated with cavitary optic disc anomalies.

2. Methods

2.1. Patients. We retrospectively reviewed medical records of eight successive cavitary optic disc anomaly-associated maculopathy patients (eight eyes) that could be followed up for more than 6 months after PPV with epipapillary membrane removal. In addition to patients with maculopathy associated with congenital cavitary optic disc anomalies, we included patients with maculopathy associated with glaucoma as subjects of this study due to the following reasons: (1) this maculopathy has similar features with ODP maculopathy in anatomical vulnerability at the optic disc [1, 2, 24] and the area of retinal schisis; (2) we encountered successful postsurgical results in a patient with retinoschisis associated with glaucoma that underwent PPV with epipapillary membrane removal [21]. During the period extending from June 2009 to March 2015, we encountered nine patients with this syndrome at the vitreoretinal clinic of Hokkaido University Hospital. One case that was followed up for less than 6 months after surgery was excluded from this study. The current study was approved by the Ethics Committee of Hokkaido University Hospital (013-0098) and followed the tenets of the Declaration of Helsinki. Written informed consent was obtained from all patients after an explanation of the purpose and procedures of this study.

2.2. Surgical Procedures. All patients underwent standard three-port transconjunctival PPV using a 23- or 25-gauge trocar system. One surgeon (W.S.) performed PPV in all patients. The surgical procedures included the intentional generation of PVD except for patients with preoperative PVD, followed by vitreous gel excision to the equator using triamcinolone acetonide. In all cases, the ILM was peeled off in a range from the macular area to the margin of the optic disc, after being stained with Brilliant Blue G. Thereafter, the presence of the epipapillary membrane tissue was ascertained using triamcinolone acetonide and was carefully removed with the forceps under a high-magnification direct contact lens. Laser photocoagulation for the surrounding retina of the optic disc or intravitreal sulfur hexafluoride (SF_6) gas injection for macular retinal schisis/retinal detachment was not planned in all cases. Cataract surgery was concurrently performed at the time of PPV in six eyes. No patients suffered postoperative complications that could potentially affect OCT imaging during follow-up, such as hazy cornea, dislocated intraocular lens, or posterior capsule opacity.

2.3. Ophthalmic Examinations. On the initial visit, all patients underwent a complete ophthalmic examination including decimal best-corrected visual acuity (BCVA) with a Japanese standard Landolt visual acuity chart, color fundus photography, SD- and enhanced depth imaging (EDI-) OCT (RS-3000 and RS-3000 Advance with software version NAVIS-EX 1.3.7; NIDEK, Gamagori, Japan), and single-flash electroretinography (ERG). Fluorescein angiography was performed in all the eyes except for case 1. Central retinal thickness (CRT) using OCT was determined by manually measuring the distance between the inner limiting membrane and the retinal pigment epithelium at the fovea.

During follow-up, BCVA, SD-OCT, and EDI-OCT were performed at every visit. The changes in BCVA, morphology of the retina and optic disc on SD-OCT, and CRT were evaluated before and after PPV. Humphrey threshold 30-2 perimetry was performed for three patients with glaucoma pre- and postoperatively. We defined the presence of epipapillary membrane, when all of the following 3 requirements were met: (1) the presence of hyperreflective lesion lying on the optic disc, on preoperative OCT; (2) a material attached on the disc that the operator could visually recognize and remove during surgery; and (3) optic disc cupping on postoperative OCT that became deeper than that on preoperative OCT.

2.4. Immunohistochemistry. Membrane tissues on the optic disc excised during vitrectomy in cases 4 and 5 were fixed with 4% paraformaldehyde in the operating room. Formalin-fixed, paraffin-embedded tissue sections with a thickness of 5 μm were prepared. The slides were dewaxed, rehydrated, and rinsed in phosphate-buffered saline (PBS) twice for 10 min. Slides were submitted for hematoxylin-eosin staining and immunohistochemistry. As a pretreatment, microwave-based antigen retrieval was performed in 10 mM citrate buffer (pH 6.0). These slides were incubated with 3% hydrogen peroxide for 10 min and then with normal goat serum for 30 min. Sections were incubated with antiepiretinal membrane antigen (EMA) (monoclonal; dilution, 1:50; Dako, Japan), S100 (polyclonal; dilution, 1:50; Dako, Japan), and glial fibrillary acidic protein (GFAP) (monoclonal; dilution, 1:50; Dako, Japan) antibodies at 4°C overnight. Positive signals were visualized using diaminobendizine as a substrate. Slides were examined using a Keyence BZ-9000 (Keyence, Osaka, Japan) microscope.

2.5. Statistical Analysis. The BCVA was converted to the logarithm of the minimal angle of resolution (logMAR) scale for statistical analysis. Wilcoxon signed-rank test was used to compare mean values of logMAR BCVA and CRT before and after PPV. In all tests, $P < 0.05$ was considered significant.

3. Results

3.1. Patient Demographics. Table 1 summarizes the clinical features of eight patients with maculopathy associated with cavitary optic disc anomalies examined in the present study. Optic disc anomalies included ODP in three patients, glaucoma in three patients, morning glory anomaly in one patient, and coloboma of the optic disc in one patient. The male-to-female patient ratio was 3:1. All patients had unilateral pathology. The mean age at the initial visit was 62.5 ± 19.7 years (range: 20–82 years). The mean duration of clinical follow-up was 25.5 ± 14.2 months (range: 10–57 months). Systemic medical history revealed that two patients had well-controlled diabetes mellitus, one patient had systemic hypertension, and one patient had a breast cancer operation. One patient had already received topical latanoprost (case 6). Two patients were diagnosed with primary normal tension glaucoma on the initial visit, and treatment

with topical travoprost was then initiated (cases 7 and 8). No patient had a relevant family history. Clinical symptoms were blurred vision at the central area in seven patients and anorthopia in one patient.

3.2. Ophthalmic Findings. The mean preoperative refractive error was -0.03 ± 0.63 diopter. Slit-lamp examination showed no abnormal findings in the anterior segment of all patients and incipient cataract in five patients. The average intraocular pressure was 15.7 ± 4.0 mmHg (range: 11.3–21.0 mmHg) at the initial visit. Funduscopic examination revealed retinal elevations extending from the optic disc to the macular area in the affected eyes of all patients (Figures 1(a)–3(a), 5(a), and 6(a)). An optic disc coloboma without maculopathy (case 4) and morning glory disc anomaly with macular degeneration, suggesting the presence of a previous morning glory syndrome (case 5), were observed in each of the patients' fellow eye. Fluorescein angiography revealed initial hypofluorescence without late leakage of the dye in all eyes included. Infrared images of scanning laser ophthalmoscopy revealed hyporeflectivity that corresponded to the ODP and the morning glory anomaly, while hyperreflectivity corresponded to the glaucomatous disc cupping. Mean ocular axial length was 23.63 ± 0.87 mm (range: 22.63–25.30 mm). Single-flash electroretinography results were normal in all affected eyes.

3.3. Preoperative OCT Findings. SD- and EDI-OCT clearly revealed the presence of excavation of the optic disc including ODP (Figures 1(b), 2(b), 5(b), and 6(c)) in all except one eye (case 4) and retinal schisis extending from the optic disc to the macula (Figures 1(b), 2(b), 3(c), 3(d), 5(b), and 6(c)). Macular detachment was observed in five patients (62.5%). An epipapillary membrane was observed at the cavitary sites of the disc in all eyes, regardless of the presence or absence of preoperative PVD (Figures 1(b), 2(b), 3(d), 5(b), and 6(c)). In 3 of 4 eyes without preoperative PVD (cases 1, 2, and 5), the posterior hyaloid membrane was directly attached on the epipapillary membrane, invaginating into the cavitary sites of the disc (Figures 1(b), 2(b), and 5(b)). In four eyes (cases 2, 3, 5, and 7), tunnel-like hyporeflectivities, which suggested a communication between the retinal schisis and the disc, were observed either beneath the ILM (two cases, Figures 2(b) and 6(c)) or at the outer nuclear layer (two cases, Figure 5(b)) at the vicinity of the disc. In case 4, funduscopy and SD-OCT failed to detect the excavation beneath the epipapillary membrane (Figures 3(b) and 3(d)).

3.4. Intraoperative Findings. During surgery, PVD was intentionally induced in four eyes. In two ODP maculopathy patients (cases 1 and 2), even when PVD was artificially induced, the hyaloid membrane was attached on the epipapillary membrane, which was firmly fixed into the ODP (Figures 1(c)–1(e)). The presence of epipapillary membrane could be strongly suspected by triamcinolone acetonide that was injected intraoperatively and attached on the optic disc in all patients. In all eyes, no retinal tear was observed around the disc. The epipapillary membrane that was

TABLE 1: Clinical characteristics of patients with maculopathy associated with cavitary optic disc anomalies.

Case	Age/sex	Follow-up period (months)	Cause of maculopathy	Macular schisis	Macular RD	Preoperative PVD	Epipapillary membrane	Decimal BCVA		Central macular thickness (µm)			Others Findings
								Pre	Final	Pre	Post 6 M	Final	
1	20/M	23	Optic disc pit	+	+	−	+	0.7	1.2	747	309	251	PPV → MH → SF$_6$ gas injection → MH closed
2	24/M	10	Optic disc pit	+	+	−	+	0.4	0.9	848	309	284	Fellow eye: old morning glory syndrome
3	82/F	27	Optic disc pit	+	+	+	+	0.1	0.2	662	324	128	
4	70/F	57	Optic disc coloboma	+	−	+	+	0.4	0.8	448	244	231	Fellow eye: optic disc coloboma without maculopathy
5	68/M	15	Morning glory disc anomaly	+	+	−	+	0.5	0.8	585	623	460	
6	79/M	27	Glaucoma	+	−	+	+	0.6	1.0	444	374	326	VF defect remained unchanged postoperatively until 19 months
7	52/M	27	Glaucoma	+	+	−	+	0.3	1.0	1055	672	243	VF defect remained unchanged postoperatively
8	77/M	18	Glaucoma	+	−	+	+	0.8	1.0	771	759	404	VF defect remained unchanged postoperatively

RD: retinal detachment; PVD: posterior vitreous detachment; BCVA: best-corrected visual acuity; PPV: pars plana vitrectomy; MH: macular hole; VF: visual field.

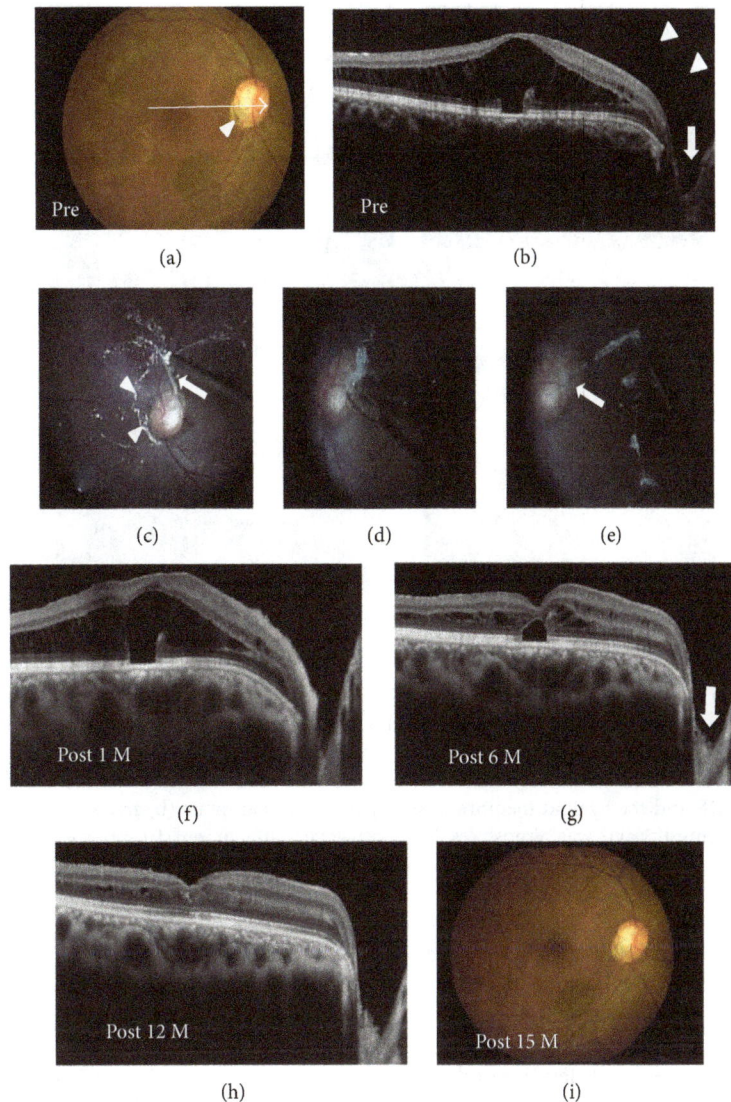

FIGURE 1: Photographs of the right eye in a 20-year-old optic disc pit (ODP) maculopathy patient without posterior vitreous detachment (PVD) (case 1). (a, b) Findings before surgery. Fundus photograph showed an ODP (a, arrowhead) and retinal elevation at the macular area (a). An arrow indicates an enhanced depth imaging optical coherence tomography (EDI-OCT) scan for the images shown in Figure 1. An EDI-OCT image revealed retinal schisis extending from the optic disc to the macula with foveal retinal detachment (b). The posterior hyaloid membrane (b, arrowheads) was attached toward the membrane that was present on the ODP (b, arrow). (c–e) Findings during pars plana vitrectomy with epipapillary membrane removal. When PVD was intentionally made, most of the hyaloid membrane was detached from the optic disc (c, arrowheads). However, a part of the membrane connected with the glial tissue on the disc (c, arrow). After making a complete PVD, the membrane tissue that remained on the ODP was grasped using forceps (d). The glial tissue was firmly attached, penetrating the ODP (e, arrow). (f–i) Postoperative OCT images. The retinal schisis gradually was reduced (f, g) and was resolved with foveal attachment 12 months after the surgery (h). The membrane tissue on the disc was also removed (g, arrow). Fundus photograph at 15 months after surgery shows the resolution of the retinal schisis (i).

present at the excavation sites of the disc was removed in all eyes. Intravitreal SF_6 gas injection was administered to a patient with peripheral iatrogenic retinal breaks (case 7).

3.5. Postoperative Findings. OCT revealed that the excavation of the optic disc became deeper than that of pretreatment after the surgery with the removal of the epipapillary membrane in all patients (Figures 1(g), 2(c), 4(c), 5(e), and 6(d)). The tunnel-like hyporeflectivities detected using OCT preoperatively became obscure from the early stage after

PPV (Figures 2(c) and 6(d)). During follow-up, macular schisis gradually decreased and finally showed complete resolution in almost all patients (Figures 1(h), 2(d), 4(d), 5(e), and 6(g)). Macular detachment was also resolved in four patients and was reduced in one patient (case 5). In one patient (case 4), OCT revealed the optic disc coloboma that was preoperatively concealed beneath the epipapillary membrane (Figures 4(c) and 4(e)). One patient (case 2) developed a macular hole, which was closed following SF_6 gas tamponade. None of the patients developed systemic or

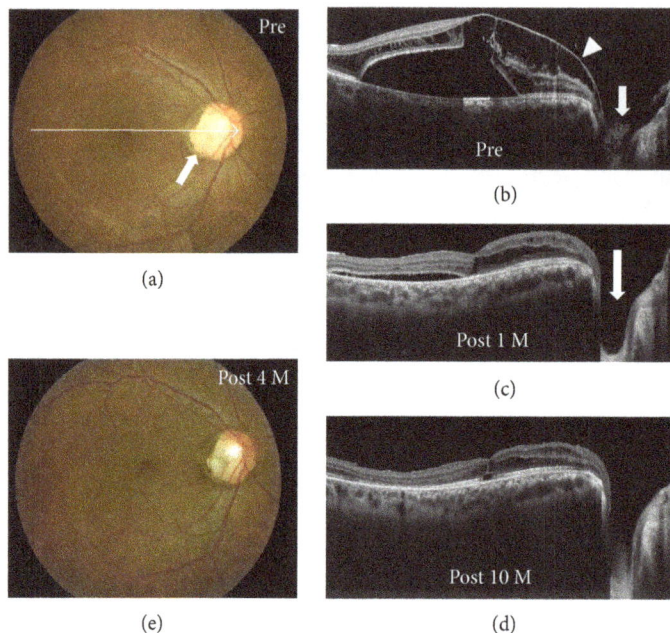

FIGURE 2: Photographs of the right eye in a 24-year-old optic disc pit (ODP) maculopathy patient without posterior vitreous detachment (case 2). (a) Fundus photograph before surgery showed an ODP (arrow) and macular retinal elevation. An arrow indicates enhanced depth imaging optical coherence tomography (EDI-OCT) scans for the images shown in Figure 2. (b–d) EDI-OCT images. Before surgery, retinal schisis extended from the optic disc to the macula with macular detachment (b). Glial tissue suggests that the Cloquet's canal (b, arrow) was also present, invaginating into the ODP and the hyaloid membrane attached to the glial tissue (b, arrowhead). The retinal schisis was reduced 1 month after pars plana vitrectomy (c) and was almost resolved with foveal attachment 10 months after surgery (d). The epipapillary membrane tissue was also removed (c, arrow). (e) The retinal elevation was reduced at four months after surgery.

other ocular complications. Of the three patients with glaucoma, the mean deviation values on the perimetry remained unchanged compared with the preoperative values during follow-up in two patients (cases 7 and 8), while it remained unchanged until 19 months after PPV but deteriorated after 22 months in one patient (case 6), suggesting a progression of glaucoma but not perioperative mechanical damage on the disc.

3.6. Changes of CRT and BCVA. The mean CRT in the included patients was reduced significantly ($P = 0.01$ and 0.004, resp.) from $674.8 \pm 235.0\,\mu m$ at pretreatment to $451.8 \pm 199.5\,\mu m$ six months after surgery and to $290.9 \pm 116.9\,\mu m$ at the final follow-up. BCVA at pretreatment was 0.5–0.9 in four eyes and 0.1–0.4 in the remaining four eyes. BCVA at the final follow-up was ≥ 1.0 in four eyes, 0.5–0.9 in three eyes, and 0.1–0.4 in one eye. Moreover, the mean logMAR value of the BCVA (0.12 ± 0.23) improved significantly compared with the pretreatment value (0.37 ± 0.31; $P = 0.008$).

3.7. Ophthalmic Pathology. The histology of the epipapillary membrane tissues resected in cases 4 and 5 revealed that spindle-shaped stromal cells were intermingled within the section (Figures 7(a) and 8(a)). Immunoreactivity for cytokeratin was not observed (Figures 7(b) and 8(b)). In contrast, immunoreactivity for S100 and GFAP was detected in the membrane (Figures 7(c), 7(d) and 8(c), 8(d)).

4. Discussion

In patients with maculopathy associated with congenital or acquired cavitary optic disc anomalies, we made the following observations: (1) an epipapillary membrane was observed in all patients via SD-OCT. (2) Maculoschisis was resolved with no recurrence regardless of the disease type or the presence or absence of preoperative PVD after PPV with epipapillary membrane removal in all patients. (3) The mean logMAR BCVA and CRT at the final follow-up significantly improved compared with pretreatment values. (4) Immunohistochemistry for GFAP and S100 proteins, which are markers for astrocytes, was positive in the resected membranes on the disc.

In all our patients without preoperative PVD, preoperative OCT revealed that the epipapillary membrane was present at the excavation sites of the disc, as shown in a recent study [17]. The hyaloid membrane was attached to not only the optic disc but also the epipapilary membrane in most of these patients. Moreover, we intraoperatively confirmed the connection between the epipapillary membrane and the hyaloid membrane, even though the latter was intentionally detached by PPV (Figures 1(c)–1(e)). The retinal schisis was resolved after PPV with the removal of both membranes, as shown in also a previously reported case [18]. In some patients with ODP maculopathy, actually, the retinal schisis did not improve or recur despite the PPV with only the removal of hyaloid membrane and/or ILM [9, 13, 14]. It is

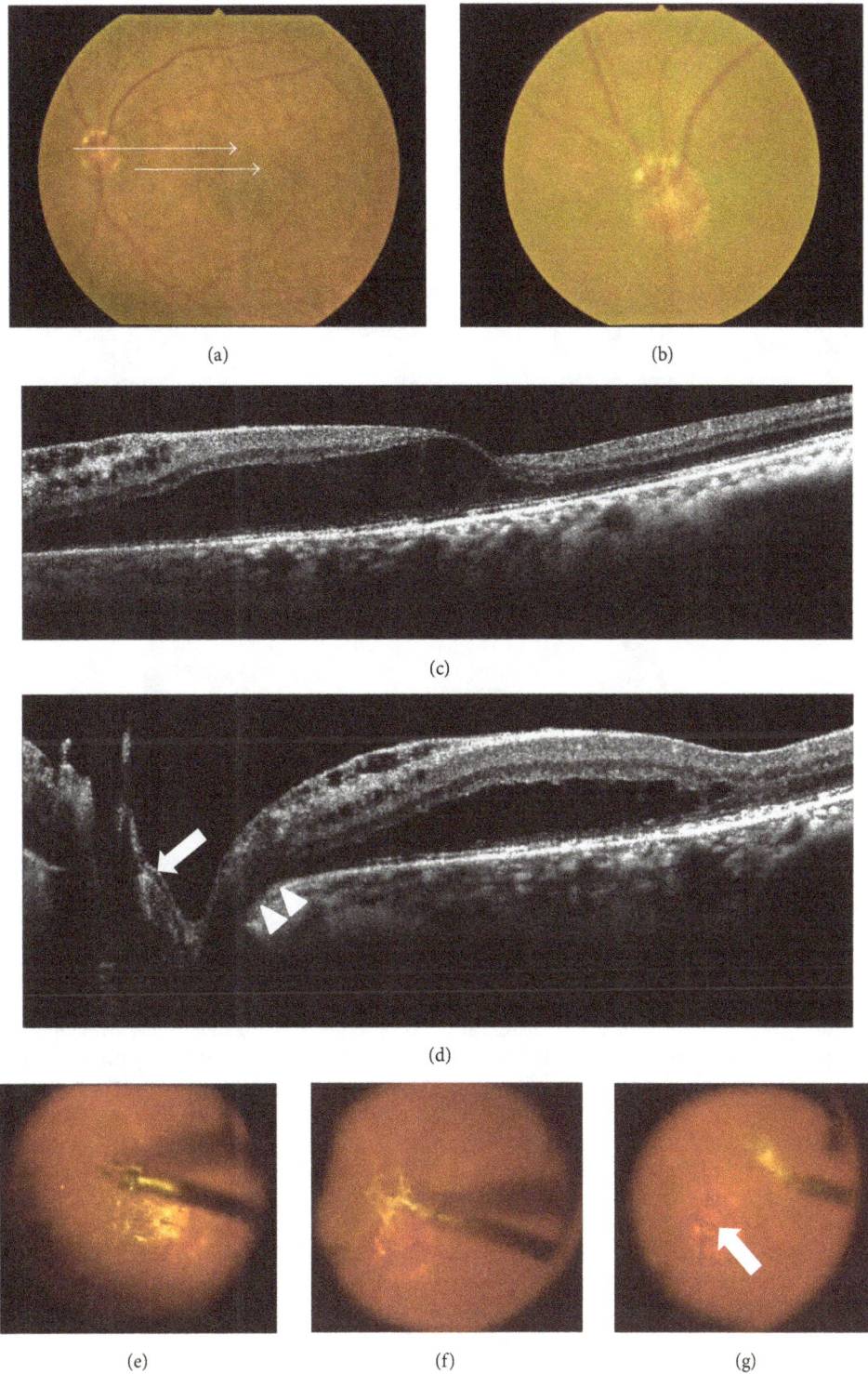

(a)   (b)

(c)

(d)

(e)   (f)   (g)

Figure 3: Photographs of the left eye in a 70-year-old patient with maculopathy in whom an optic disc coloboma became clear after surgery with epipapillary membrane removal (case 4). (a, b) Fundus photographs before surgery showing macular elevation (a) and a shallow cavitation in the center of the optic disc (b). Upper and lower arrows indicate the spectral domain optical coherence tomography (SD-OCT) scan in Figures 3(c) and 3(d), respectively (a). (c, d) SD-OCT images before surgery showing retinal schisis extending from the optic disc to the macula (c), with membrane tissue but with no obvious pit-like deep cavitation on the disc (d, arrow), and a shallow tunnel-like hyporeflective lesion directly connecting the retinal schisis to the disc (d, arrowheads). (e–g) Findings during pars plana vitrectomy. Internal limiting membrane (ILM) at the area from the macula to the surrounding of the disc was peeled (e). ILM connected the membrane tissue on the optic disc (f). When the epipapillary membrane tissue was removed, a pit-like concavity, which was hidden behind the tissue, appeared (g, arrow).

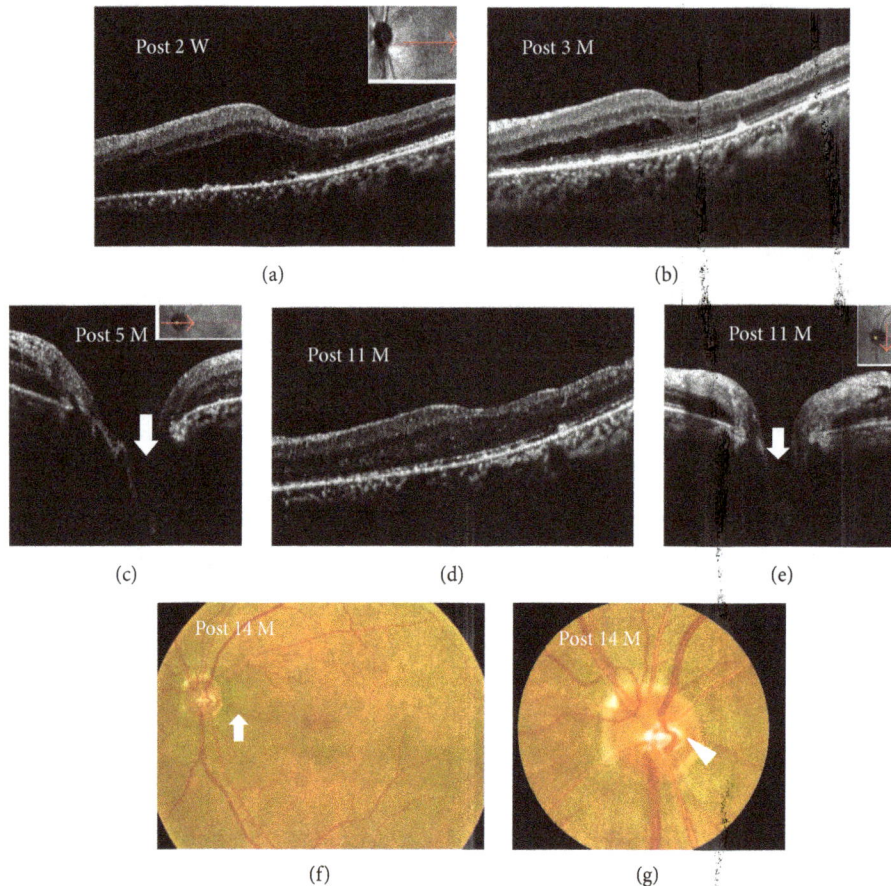

(a)

(b)

(c)

(d)

(e)

(f)

(g)

Figure 4: Findings after surgery in case 4. (a–e) Spectral domain optical coherence tomography images revealed that an optic disc coloboma (c, e, arrows) became clear after epipapillary membrane removal. Macular schisis also gradually decreased and was resolved 11 months after surgery (a, b, and d). (f, g) A retinal nerve fiber layer defect (f, arrow) corresponding to the coloboma (g, arrowhead) was evident together with the disappearance of the retinal schisis 14 months after surgery.

known that eyes with cavitary optic disc anomalies including ODP and glaucoma have congenital or acquired anatomical vulnerability at the optic disc in common [1, 2, 24]. Taken together, these results indicate that in some patients with cavitary optic disc anomaly-associated maculopathy without preoperative PVD, the epipapillary membrane, in concert with the hyaloid membrane, may play a role in the pathogenesis of the maculopathy by dragging these vulnerable disc tissues as the traction force to the disc. Postoperative resolution of the tunnel-like hyporeflectivity connecting the retinal schisis and the optic disc observed on preoperative OCT suggests a halt of the fluid flowing from the site with the disc anomalies to the retinal schisis.

It has been previously reported that ODP maculopathy patients with preoperative PVD are usually older, with no improvement of the retinal schisis and with deterioration of the BCVA postoperatively [15]. In this study, all patients with preoperative PVD had the epipapillary membrane on SD-OCT. Their retinal schisis and/or detachment was resolved after PPV with the removal of the epipapillary membrane. Furthermore, a tunnel-like hyporeflectivity connecting the schisis and the excavation site of the disc observed with SD-OCT preoperatively became obscured from the early stage after surgery [21]. Intrapapillary proliferation

was observed in all of 16 ODP maculopathy eyes [17]. The proliferation that sequentially developed was likely to cause the development of cavity within the pit [17]. Therefore, our current results suggest that the growth of the residual epipapillary membrane continues drawing the vulnerable disc tissues, even after PVD spontaneously occurred, and is involved in the pathogenesis of this maculopathy with preoperative PVD.

In the present study, ILM removal was performed in all patients included to prevent the occurrence of epiretinal membrane after surgery. The procedure might affect surgical outcomes. However, a previous report showed that retinoschisis was resolved in almost all patients by performing vitrectomy with intensional generation of PVD but without ILM removal [9]. In a study with a large number of patients with ODP maculopathy, moreover, there was no association between ILM peeling and improvement of the macular schisis [14]. This may be because it is difficult to release the traction of hyaloid and/or epipapillary membranes from the disc just by performing ILM removal. Therefore, we speculate that ILM removal would be restrictive for improvement of retinoschisis in this disease complex.

Furthermore, we detected GFAP and S100 proteins in the resected epipapillary membrane, suggesting the existence

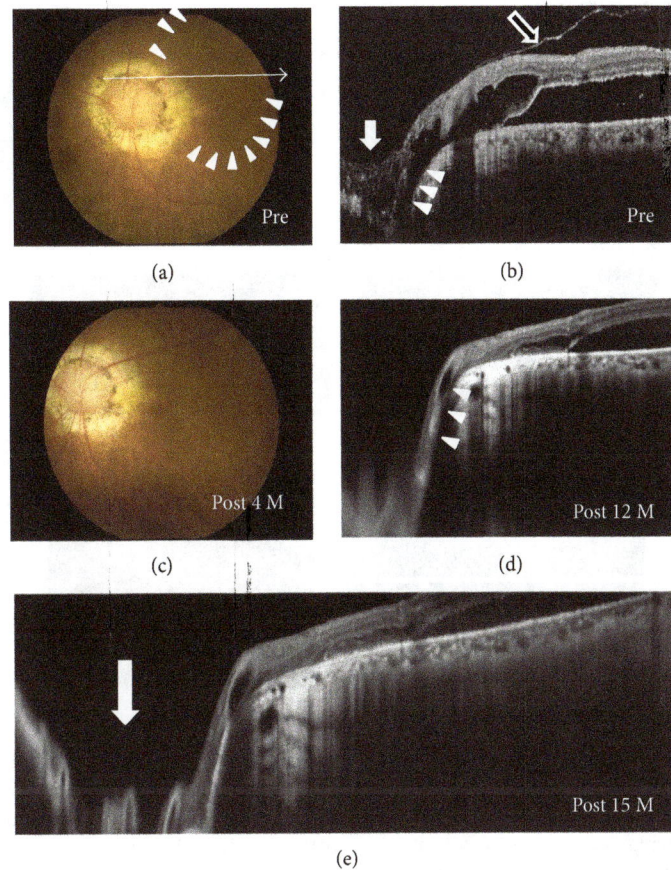

(a)   (b)

(c)   (d)

(e)

FIGURE 5: Photographs of the left eye in a 68-year-old patient with maculopathy associated with morning glory anomaly of the optic disc (case 5). (a, b) Preoperative images. Fundus photograph showed retinal detachment extending from the morning glory disc anomaly to the macula (a, arrowheads). Arrows indicate the optical coherence tomography (OCT) scan in Figure 5. A spectral domain OCT image showed retinal schisis with macular detachment and a tunnel-like hyporeflectivity extending from the retinal schisis toward the disc (b, arrowheads), suggesting a communication between the disc and retinal schisis (b). The hyaloid membrane (b, black arrow) was attached around the disc and on the epipapillary glial tissue (b, white arrow). (c) Macular detachment was reduced at 4 months after pars plana vitrectomy with epipapillary membrane removal. (d) Twelve months after surgery, an enhanced depth imaging OCT image revealed that the tunnel-like hyporeflectivity observed preoperatively was resolved with the reduction of the retinal schisis (arrowheads). (e) Fifteen months after surgery, retinal schisis was almost resolved and the optic disc cupping became deeper (arrow) than in pretreatment.

of astrocytes. Astrocytes are glial cells surrounding vessels or nerve fibers. Differentiated perinatally, they subsequently proliferate in the optic nerve and spread from the retinal nerve fiber layer to the neural retina at the periphery via the optic disc [25]. In the normal retina, astrocytes exist around the retinal ganglion cell layer; however, they penetrate deeper into retinal layers upon retinal detachment [26]. From our surgical and immunohistochemical results, we speculated that astrocytes migrated into deeper retinal layers following the onset of retinal schisis and/or detachment and subsequently migrated to the epipapillary membrane via a communication between the retinal schisis and the optic disc. Our histological observations may support that the epipapillary membrane relates to the pathogenesis of some patients with optic disc anomaly-associated maculopathy, although further research is required to verify our speculation.

In case 4, optic disc coloboma [23], which was hidden by the epipapillary membrane preoperatively, was found after PPV with membrane removal. Therefore, this case may be called occult optic disc coloboma-associated maculopathy. Cases with retinal schisis extending from the disc to the macula despite having funduscopically normal optic disc have been recently reported [27]. These cases had a predisposition to occur in emmetropic eyes of older patients and in the presence of preoperative PVD. These features were consistent with case 4 in the present study. However, the presence of the membrane tissue on the disc has not been examined yet in these idiopathic cases. Therefore, further studies are needed to examine the presence of the epipapillary membrane in cases with idiopathic foveomacular retinal schisis.

This pilot study has some limitations. This is a retrospective study, with a small number of patients; prospective studies with a larger number are needed to examine the outcome of our surgical procedure. Moreover, the surgical procedure shown in the present study has a possibility of causing optic nerve damage in eyes undergoing surgery, because S100 and GFAP being positive on immunohistochemistry of the resected epipapillary membranes were markers of not only

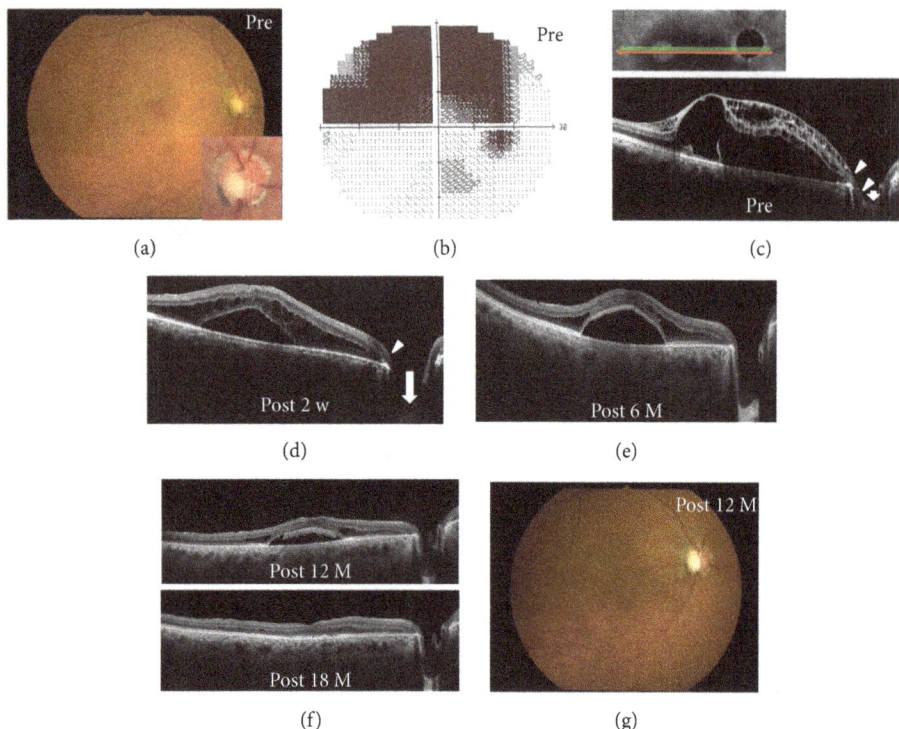

FIGURE 6: Photographs of the right eye in a 52-year-old patient with retinoschisis associated with glaucoma without posterior vitreous detachment (case 7). (a) Fundus photographs before surgery demonstrating retinal elevation, retinal folds extending from the macula to the optic disc, and glaucomatous optic disc cupping with nerve fiber layer defect but no obvious optic disc pit. (b) Humphrey threshold 30-2 perimetry before surgery showing decreased sensitivity at the Bjerrum area. (c–f) Horizontal scan images of enhanced depth imaging optical coherence tomography. An image before surgery showed retinal schisis with foveal detachment extending from the optic disc to the macula, the epipapillary membrane (c, arrow), and a shallow tunnel-like hyporeflectivity (c, arrowheads) directly connecting the retinal schisis and the 8 o' clock margin of the disc (c). The posterior hyaloid membrane was attached to the vicinty of the disc. Two weeks after pars plana vitrectomy, retinal schisis decreased with an obscure tunnel-like hyporeflectivity (d, arrowhead). The extent of the disc cupping was obviously deeper than preoperative one following the removal of the membrane tissue (d, arrow). Retinal schisis with macular detachment gradually decreased (d–f) and was completely resolved 18 months after surgery (f). (g) Fundus photograph showed the decrease of macular elevation at the macula but no optic disc pit at 12 months after surgery.

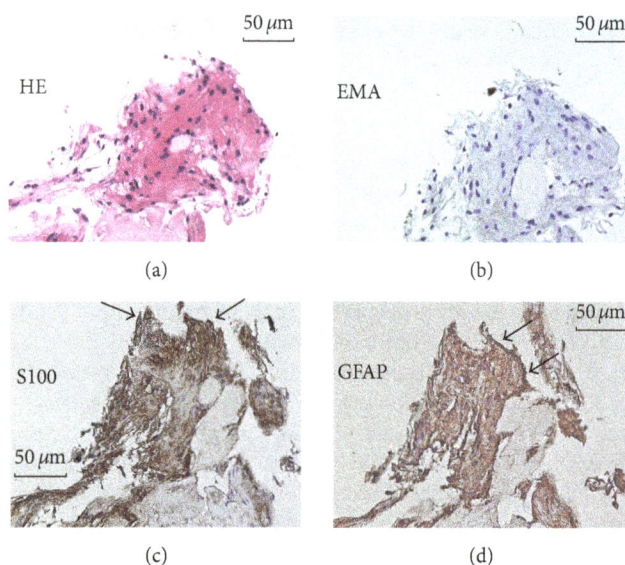

FIGURE 7: Histology (a) and immunohistochemistry (b–d) of a resected epipapillary membrane tissue in case 4. (a) Light micrograph demonstrating marked hyalinization. Spindle-shaped stromal cells were intermingled in the section (hematoxylin-eosin). (b) Immunochemistry for cytokeratin. Immunoreactivity was not observed. (c) Immunoreactivity for S100 was detected in the membrane (arrows). (d) Immunoreactivity for GFAP was strongly detected in the membrane (arrows).

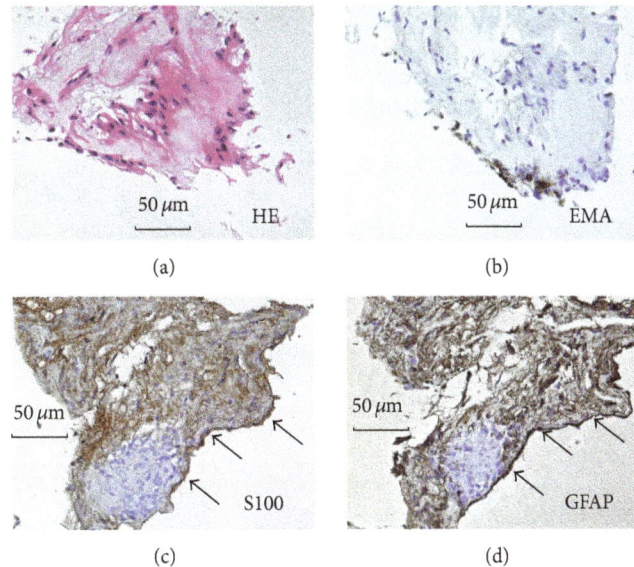

FIGURE 8: Histology (a) and immunohistochemistry (b–d) of a resected epipapillary membrane tissue in case 5. (a) Light micrograph showing marked hyalinization. Spindle-shaped stromal cells were intermingled in the section (hematoxylin-eosin). (b) Immunochemistry for cytokeratin. Immunoreactivity was not observed. (c) Immunoreactivity for S100 was strongly detected in the membrane (arrows). (d) Immunoreactivity for GFAP was strongly detected in the membrane (arrows).

astrocytes but also neural tissues of the optic disc. We confirmed that none of the three eyes with glaucomatous cupping showed any exacerbation in the visual field defects in the early stages after the surgery. Histological results of the resected membranes demonstrated a variety of cellular components, in addition to being positive for GFAP and S100, which were not consistent with neural fibers in the optic disc. The results suggest that the cells in the isolated membranes are astrocytes rather than neural tissues. When the surgeon performed the surgical procedure, careful operation handling was required in order not to injure the optic nerve head. Additionally, damage of the disc should be routinely monitored by performing perimetry before and after surgery.

5. Conclusions

Epipapillary membrane was preoperatively observed in all patients with maculopathy associated with cavitary optic disc anomalies. After PPV with epipapillary membrane removal, the retinal schisis was completely or almost resolved regardless of the disease type or the presence or absence of preoperative PVD, and the mean CMT and BCVA significantly improved. Markers for astrocytes were positive in the immunohistochemistry of the resected membranes on the disc. Our current data suggest that epipapillary membrane is involved in the pathogenesis of some patients with maculopathy associated with cavitary optic disc anomalies as well as posterior hyaloid membrane. PPV with epipapillary membrane removal may be a useful treatment option for patients with this disease complex. In the future, multicentered studies comparing surgical outcomes of PPV with or without epipapillary membrane removal are needed to verify the present results.

Conflicts of Interest

All authors have no financial disclosures. The authors declare that there is no conflict of interest regarding the publication of this paper.

References

[1] I. Georgalas, I. Ladas, G. Georgopoulos, and P. Petrou, "Optic disc pit: a review," *Graefe's Archive for Clinical and Experimental Ophthalmology*, vol. 249, no. 8, pp. 1113–1122, 2011.

[2] A. P. Ferry, "Macular detachment associated with congenital pit of the optic nerve head," *Archives of Ophthalmology*, vol. 70, no. 3, pp. 346–357, 1963.

[3] A. R. Irvine, J. B. Crawford, and J. H. Sullivan, "The pathogenesis of retinal detachment with morning glory disc and optic pit," *Retina*, vol. 6, no. 3, pp. 146–150, 1986.

[4] S. Chang, E. Gregory-Roberts, and R. Chen, "Retinal detachment associated with optic disc colobomas and morning glory syndrome," *Eye*, vol. 26, no. 4, pp. 494–500, 2012.

[5] A. Hirakata, T. Hida, T. Wakabayashi, and M. Fukuda, "Unusual posterior hyaloid strand in a young child with optic disc pit maculopathy: intraoperative and histopathological findings," *Japanese Journal of Ophthalmology*, vol. 49, no. 3, pp. 264–266, 2005.

[6] P. G. Theodossiadis, V. G. Grigoropoulos, J. Emfietzoglou, and G. P. Theodossiadis, "Vitreous findings in optic disc pit maculopathy based on optical coherence tomography," *Graefe's Archive for Clinical and Experimental Ophthalmology*, vol. 245, no. 9, pp. 1311–1318, 2007.

[7] T. Katome, Y. Mitamura, F. Hotta, A. Mino, and T. Naito, "Swept-source optical coherence tomography identifies connection between vitreous cavity and retrobulbar subarachnoid space in patient with optic disc pit," *Eye*, vol. 27, no. 11, pp. 1325-1326, 2013.

[8] T. Yokoi, Y. Nakayama, S. Nishina, and N. Azuma, "Abnormal traction of the vitreous detected by swept-source optical coherence tomography is related to the maculopathy associated with optic disc pits," *Graefe's Archive for Clinical and Experimental Ophthalmology*, vol. 254, no. 4, pp. 675–682, 2016.

[9] A. Hirakata, M. Inoue, T. Hiraoka, and B. W. McCuen II, "Vitrectomy without laser treatment or gas tamponade for macular detachment associated with an optic disc pit," *Ophthalmology*, vol. 119, no. 4, pp. 810–818, 2012.

[10] M. A. Abouammoh, S. M. Alsulaiman, V. S. Gupta et al., "Pars plana vitrectomy with juxtapapillary laser photocoagulation versus vitrectomy without juxtapapillary laser photocoagulation for the treatment of optic disc pit maculopathy: the results of the KKESH International Collaborative Retina Study Group," *British Journal of Ophthalmology*, vol. 100, no. 4, pp. 478–483, 2016.

[11] R. R. Gupta and N. Choudhry, "Spontaneous resolution of optic disc pit maculopathy after posterior vitreous detachment," *Canadian Journal of Ophthalmology*, vol. 51, no. 1, pp. e24–e27, 2016.

[12] E. Moisseiev, J. Moisseiev, and A. Loewenstein, "Optic disc pit maculopathy: when and how to treat? A review of the pathogenesis and treatment options," *International Journal of Retina Vitreous*, vol. 1, no. 1, p. 13, 2015.

[13] M. N. Coca, S. Tofigh, A. Elkeeb, and B. F. Godley, "Optic disc pit maculopathy recurring in the absence of vitreous gel," *JAMA Ophthalmology*, vol. 132, no. 11, pp. 1375-1376, 2014.

[14] J. S. Rayat, C. J. Rudnisky, C. Waite et al., "Long-term outcomes for optic disk pit maculopathy after vitrectomy," *Retina*, vol. 35, no. 10, pp. 2011–2017, 2015.

[15] M. Haruta, R. Kamada, Y. Umeno, and R. Yamakawa, "Vitrectomy for optic disc pit-associated maculopathy with or without preoperative posterior vitreous detachment," *Clinical Ophthalmology*, vol. 6, pp. 1361–1364, 2012.

[16] S. Ooto, R. A. Mittra, M. E. Ridley, and R. F. Spaide, "Vitrectomy with inner retinal fenestration for optic disc pit maculopathy," *Ophthalmology*, vol. 121, no. 9, pp. 1727–1733, 2014.

[17] J. Maertz, K. J. Mohler, J. P. Kolb et al., "Intrapapillary proliferation in optic disk pits: clinical findings and time-related changes," *Retina*, vol. 37, no. 5, pp. 906–914, 2017.

[18] M. Inoue, K. Shinoda, and S. Ishida, "Vitrectomy combined with glial tissue removal at the optic pit in a patient with optic disc pit maculopathy: a case report," *Journal of Medical Case Reports*, vol. 2, no. 1, p. 103, 2008.

[19] D. A. Hollander, M. E. Barricks, J. L. Duncan, and A. R. Irvine, "Macular schisis detachment associated with angle-closure glaucoma," *Archives of Ophthalmology*, vol. 123, no. 2, pp. 270–272, 2005.

[20] E. Z. Rath and S. Rumelt, "Acute visual loss due to serous retinal detachment from acquired optic pit may be a rare presentation of primary open-angle glaucoma," *Canadian Journal of Ophthalmology*, vol. 42, no. 2, pp. 339-340, 2007.

[21] S. Takashina, W. Saito, K. Noda, M. Katai, and S. Ishida, "Membrane tissue on the optic disc may cause macular schisis associated with a glaucomatous optic disc without optic disc pits," *Clinical Ophthalmology*, vol. 7, pp. 883–887, 2013.

[22] M. Inoue, Y. Itoh, T. Rii et al., "Macular retinoschisis associated with glaucomatous optic neuropathy in eyes with normal intraocular pressure," *Graefe's Archive for Clinical and Experimental Ophthalmology*, vol. 253, no. 9, pp. 1447–1456, 2015.

[23] N. Jain and M. W. Johnson, "Pathogenesis and treatment of maculopathy associated with cavitary optic disc anomalies," *American Journal of Ophthalmology*, vol. 158, no. 3, pp. 423–435, 2014.

[24] S. Kiumehr, S. C. Park, S. Dorairaj et al., "In vivo evaluation of focal lamina cribrosa defects in glaucoma," *Archives of Ophthalmology*, vol. 130, no. 5, pp. 552–559, 2012.

[25] H. Kolb, "Glial cells of the retina," *Webvision, The Organization of the Retina and Visual System*, 2016, May 18, http://webvision.med.utah.edu.

[26] G. Luna, P. W. Keeley, B. E. Reese, K. A. Linberg, G. P. Lewis, and S. K. Fisher, "Astrocyte structural reactivity and plasticity in models of retinal detachment," *Experimental Eye Research*, vol. 150, no. 9, pp. 4–21, 2016.

[27] I. Maruko, Y. Morizane, S. Kimura et al., "Clinical characteristics of idiopathic foveomacular retinoschisis," *Retina*, vol. 36, no. 8, pp. 1486–1492, 2016.

10

Surgical Synechiolysis of Iridocapsular Adhesion and Sulcus Placement of a Rigid Intraocular Lens on an Oversized Residual Capsular Rim

Jiao Lyu [ID],[1] Qi Zhang [ID],[1] Haiying Jin,[1] Tingyi Liang,[1] Jili Chen,[2] and Peiquan Zhao [ID][1]

[1]*Department of Ophthalmology, Xinhua Hospital, School of Medicine, Shanghai Jiao Tong University, Shanghai, China*
[2]*Shibei Hospital, Jing'an District, Shanghai, China*

Correspondence should be addressed to Peiquan Zhao; zhaopeiquan@xinhuamed.com.cn

Academic Editor: Lisa Toto

Purpose. To report the surgical outcomes of surgical synechiolysis of iridocapsular adhesion and sulcus placement of a polymethyl methacrylate scleral-sutured intraocular lens (IOL) in aphakic eyes with an oversized residual capsular rim. *Methods.* Eight aphakic eyes from eight consecutive patients were studied retrospectively. Synechiolysis was performed to maximally expose the residual capsulorhexis. Then, the rigid IOL was placed on the preserved capsulorhexis into the ciliary sulcus. *Results.* Synechiolysis of iridocapsular adhesion was achieved in all eight eyes intraoperatively. Six eyes had extensive dissection to facilitate IOL sulcus placement. Consequently, seven of the eight eyes had the IOL secured by the residual capsulorhexis, and the other eye had the IOL haptics supported by the narrow residual capsular rim. A visual acuity of 0.25 or above was achieved in four of eight patients, and a well-centered IOL was observed in seven of the eight eyes 26 to 53 months after surgery. A mild IOL decentration was detected in the eye whose capsular rim was not securing the IOL optic. *Conclusions.* A large-optic and rigid IOL in the sulcus is a feasible alternative when a sulcus-based IOL is considered for aphakic eyes with an oversized residual capsulorhexis. A preserved capsulorhexis after sufficient synechiolysis, which can secure the IOL optic intraoperatively, may yield better stability of the IOL position.

1. Introduction

Sulcus placement of a posterior chamber intraocular lens (PCIOL) is a surgical alternative to correct aphakia in the presence of a deficient or absent posterior capsule [1, 2]. The key characteristics for a sulcus-based PCIOL include (1) a large optic and tip-to-tip size for lateral stability; (2) long thin angulated haptics for iris clearance; and (3) an IOL made from a foldable material that allows for a smaller incision [1, 3]. However, a foldable IOL may not be appropriate for sulcus placement in aphakic eyes with an oversized residual capsular rim [1]. These aphakic eyes usually have experienced a complicated cataract surgery, an ocular trauma, or multiple intraocular surgical interventions, leaving an irregular or noncontinuous capsulorrhexis or vitrectorrhexis, iridolenticular synechia, fibrosis,

traction of ciliary process, and/or vitreoretinopathies. Thus, implantation of a sulcus-based PCIOL may involve synechiolysis, dissection of ciliary sulcus, insertion of a proper IOL on the preserved capsule tissue, and management of posterior segment comorbidities. Sulcus placement of a small size, relatively soft, foldable IOL may result in IOL decentration or dislocation, pigment dispersion syndrome, pigmentary glaucoma, or uveitis-glaucoma-hyphema syndrome [1, 4].

Surgical preservation of residual capsulorhexis and reconstruction of the ciliary sulcus are necessary for the stability of a sulcus IOL. Dissection techniques utilize a sharp dissection with a needle tip and capsulotomy vannas scissors or blunt dissection with viscoelastic material. However, it is difficult to achieve a 360° exposure of capsulorhexis almost to the ciliary sulcus, not to mention the removal of sticky fibrosis. Some surgeons avoid difficult synechiolysis manipulations and opt for transscleral fixation of a foldable PCIOL, implantation of an iris-claw IOL, or an anterior chamber IOL, irrespective of the residual capsulorhexis [5–7]. The disadvantages of each procedure should be considered before abandoning the idea of using a sulcus-based IOL. Transscleral fixation of an IOL requires intricate techniques and is occasionally associated with hypotony, IOL dislocation, and vitreoretinal complications [6]. Iris-claw IOLs can lead to chronic pigment release from the iris, inflammation, and pupil deformation [8]. Anterior chamber IOLs risk corneal endothelial cell decompensation in the long run [9].

Given these surgical dilemmas, we performed a combined procedure of a thorough synechiolysis using vitreoretinal instruments and a sulcus placement of a large-optic and rigid polymethyl methacrylate (PMMA) IOL, CZ70BD (Alcon, Fort Worth, TX, USA), in aphakic eyes with an oversized capsular rim in recent years. The CZ70BD IOL was originally designed for sulcus placement and has eyelets on haptics to facilitate suture fixation [10, 11]. We chose this lens for several reasons: (1) its favorable 7.0 mm optic size for an oversized capsular rim at a diameter close to 7 mm and its 12.5 mm tip-to-tip size; (2) tensile material for stability in the sulcus; and (3) long C-shaped haptics posteriorly angulated 5° to the optic to vault the optic from the iris. Herein, we present the visual and anatomic outcomes in a retrospective case series of aphakic eyes.

2. Methods

2.1. Patients and Methods. This study was conducted in accordance with the Declaration of Helsinki. All procedures were approved by the ethics committee of Xinhua Hospital, which is affiliated with Shanghai Jiao Tong University School of Medicine, Shanghai, China. Informed consent was obtained from all participants.

A retrospective chart review was performed on consecutive patients who had surgical synechiolysis and then sutureless sulcus placement of a CZ70BD IOL on the preserved large capsulorhexis at the Department of Ophthalmology, Xinhua Hospital, between 2013 and 2015. Clinical records were collected as follows: basic demographics, preoperative best corrected visual acuity, axial length and other available biometric parameters, horizontal white-to-white value (Lenstar LS900®, Haag Streit, Koeniz, Switzerland), preoperative ocular comorbidities, records of intraoperative procedures and videos, intraoperative or postoperative complications, postoperative best-corrected visual acuity, refractive status, and postoperative ophthalmic findings. IOL power calculations were performed using the SRK/T formula adjusted for sulcus fixation as follows: the sulcus IOL power was reduced by 0.5 diopter (D) from the chosen in-the-bag power in the IOL range 9.0 to 17.0 D, by 1.0 D from 17.5 to 28.0 D, and by 1.5 D above 28.0 D [12]. The target postoperative refraction was set as ± 0.5 D for adult emmetropia, at least −3.0 D overcorrection for highly myopic, and based on age for pediatric patients as described by Enyedi et al. [13].

2.2. Surgical Techniques. After topical or general anesthesia was administered, the surgical procedures began with two to three limbal side-port paracenteses to introduce in a 20 or 23 G anterior chamber maintainer and other instruments (Supplementary Materials, Video 1).

Figures 1–5 show intraoperative and anterior segment photographs and ultrasound biomicroscopy of patients 2 (Figure 1), 3 (Figure 2), 5 (Figure 3), 6 (Figure 4), and 7 (Figure 5). All patients had surgical synechiolysis to expose the capsulorhexis and then sulcus placement of an Alcon CZ70BD IOL on the oversized residual capsular rim. The arrow points to the capsular edge.

Figures 1(a)–1(d), 2(a), 3(a), and 5(a) show intraoperative photographs taken before the IOL was placed. The arrows point to the preserved capsular rim. Extensive surgical synechiolysis performed in patient 1 is shown in Figures 1(a)–(d). The 360° iridolenticular adhesion was dissected using a 27 G needle tip and 23 G vitreous scissors, and all fibrosis was removed by a vitreous cutter. After sufficient exposure of the capsulorhexis almost to the ciliary process, the foreign body embedded in the ciliary process appeared, and then it was grasped out smoothly. Synechiolysis procedures in Figures 2(a) and 3(a) also show the effect of dissection and preservation of residual capsule tissue.

Figure 4(a) shows the anterior segment photograph taken by a RetCam fundus imaging system (Clarity Medical Systems, Pleasanton, CA, USA).

Figures 2(b), 3(b), and 5(b) show intraoperative photographs taken after the IOL was placed in the sulcus. The IOL was well centered at the end of the surgery. The IOL optic was partly supported by the residual capsule.

Figures 1(e) and 3(c) show slit-lamp photographs showing that the IOL was well centered at the last visit.

Figure 4(b) shows the ultrasound biomicroscope photograph of patient 6 showing a well-positioned IOL 14 months postoperatively.

Surgical synechiolysis for focal adhesion started with dissection using a 27 G needle. Extensive and sticky iridolenticular adhesion from the pupillary margin almost to the ciliary process was separated using vitreoretinal scissors which moved tangentially to achieve 180° synechiolysis via one corneal paracentesis and then dissected toward the opposite direction via another corneal paracentesis for the other half sector of the synechia. Fibrosis of the iris and capsule was then removed with a vitrector.

Sutureless implantation of a CZ70BD IOL was attempted when sulcus placement of a foldable 3-piece PC IOL was not possible after evaluation of the oversized capsular rim. Following a superior fornix-based conjunctival flap and creation of a 7.5 × 2.0 mm rectangle-shaped sclerocorneal tunnel, starting 1 mm posterior to limbus, a CZ70BD IOL was then inserted into the anterior chamber through the wound with lens-insertion forceps. Passing through the tunnel, the optic was tilted slightly to facilitate sliding of the leading haptic onto the anterior capsular shelf. If necessary, this step was aided by a secondary instrument in the left hand, or iris retractors, which help to expose the underlying capsular edge. Following that, the

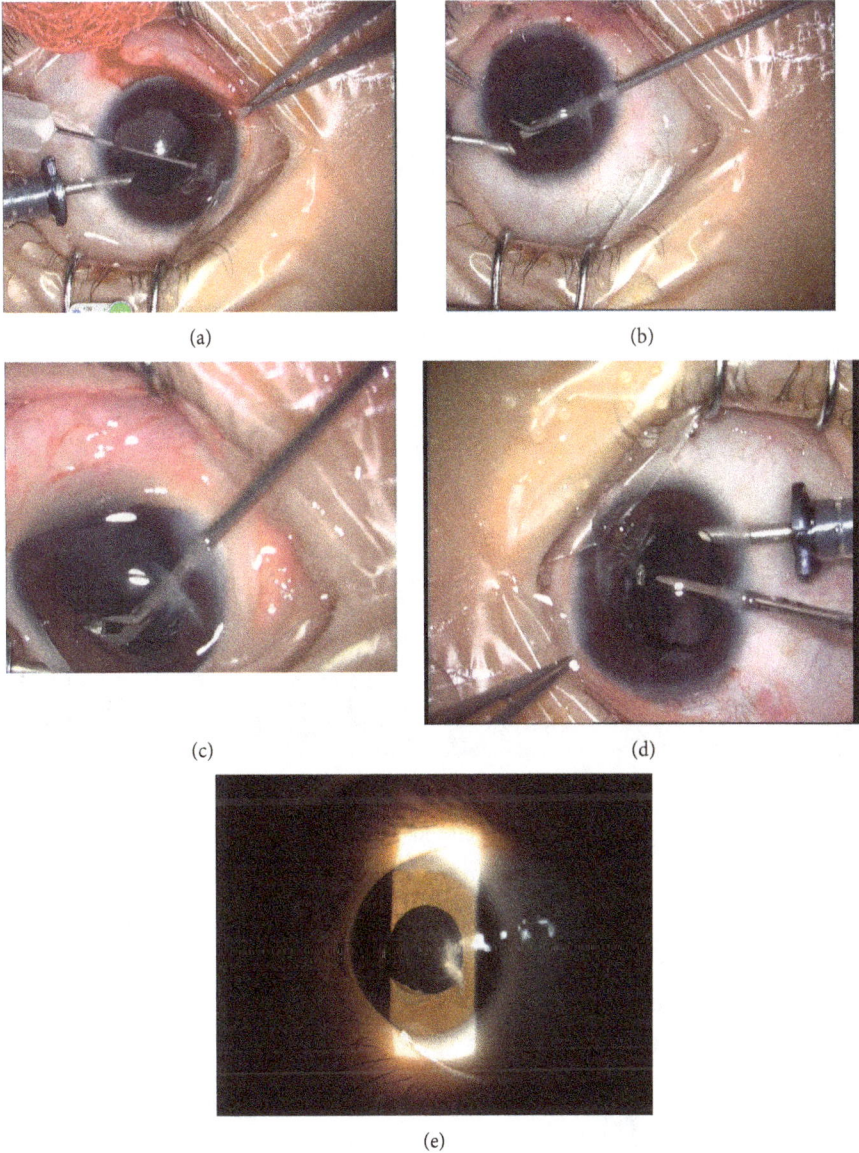

(a)

(b)

(c)

(d)

(e)

FIGURE 1

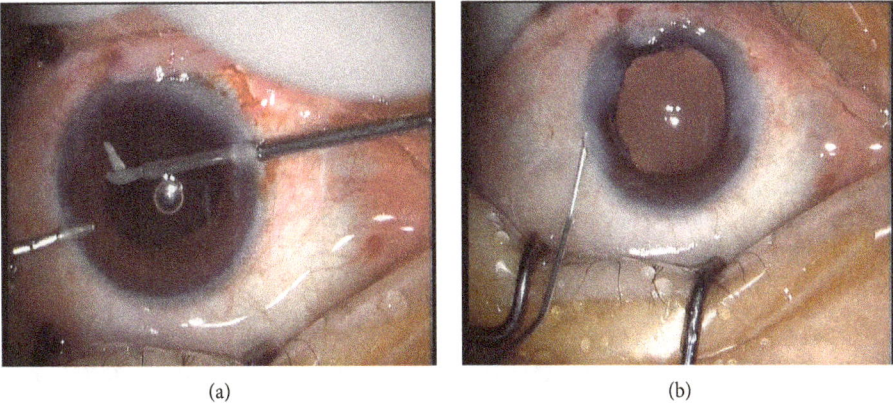

(a)

(b)

FIGURE 2

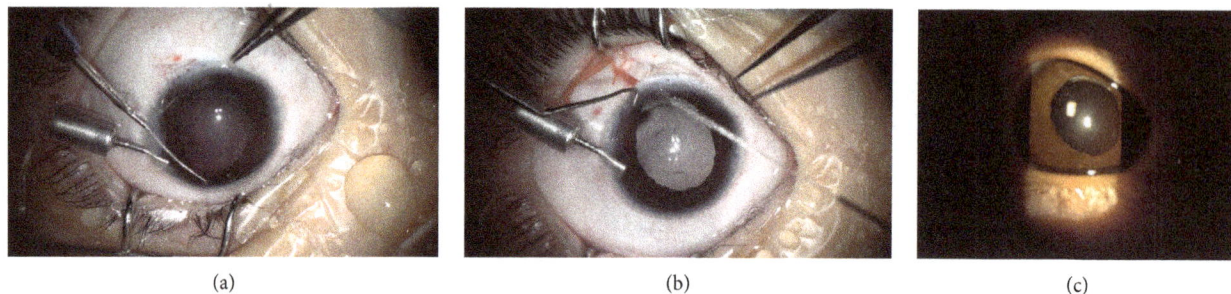

(a)   (b)   (c)

FIGURE 3

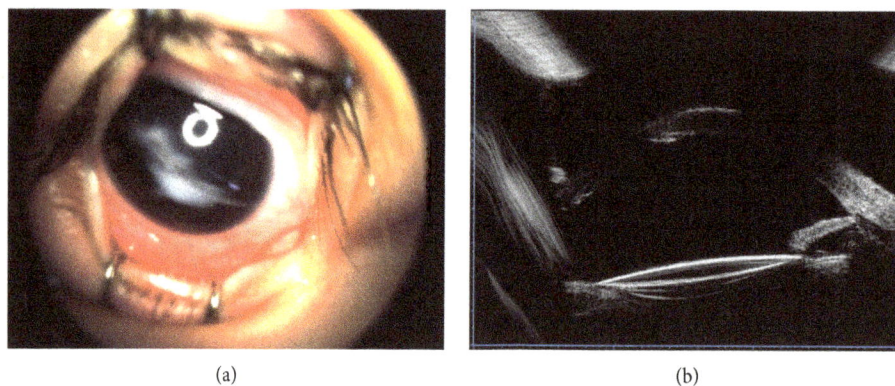

(a)   (b)

FIGURE 4

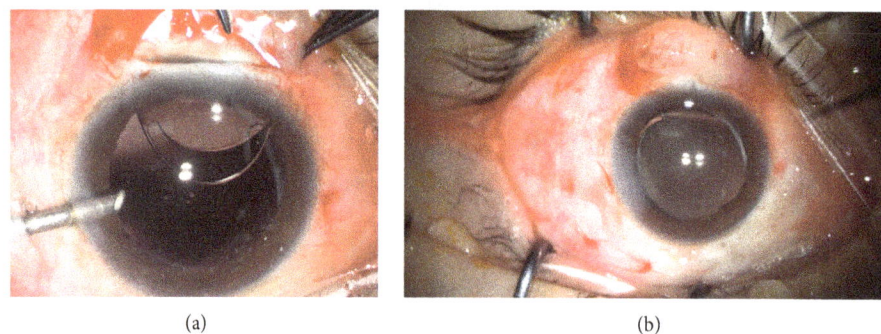

(a)   (b)

FIGURE 5

trailing haptic was oriented into the sulcus as the optic was gently rotated clockwise. If the residual capsular rim was extremely narrow, the IOL was initially inserted onto the anterior surface of the iris, followed by the introduction of the haptic onto the underlying capsular rim one after another. After gentle adjustment, the IOL was oriented in a centered and stable position, with the haptics riding on the wider part of the capsular rim. A suture for fixation was not performed as stabilization and centralization of the IOL was achieved intraoperatively. The scleral wound was then closed with 10-0 nylon-interrupted sutures. The anterior chamber maintainer was removed, and all the wounds were confirmed as tightly sealed. Finally, the conjunctiva and Tenon's fascia were closed over the wound and suture sites.

3. Results

Eight eyes from eight consecutive patients who underwent the surgical procedures were included in this study. The clinical characteristics of the patients are listed in Table 1. Seven patients had previously experienced anterior or total vitrectomy, and six patients had their cataract initially removed by lensectomy. Ocular comorbidities of the aphakic eyes were a corneal scar in four eyes, vitreoretinopathies in seven eyes, and posterior luxation of an originally sulcus-based three-piece foldable IOL (Canon-STAAR Preloaded IOL KS-3 (Ai) with a 6.0 mm optic and 12.5 mm tip-to-tip size) in one eye. The mean preoperative axial length was 22.92 ± 1.78 mm. Available horizontal white-to-white values ranged from 11.57 (patient 5) to 12.59 mm (patient 1).

TABLE 1: Patients characteristics and surgical outcomes.

Pt	Age (years)/gender	Eye	Preexisting condition	Surgical history (M/Y)	Secondary IOL implantation and concurrent surgeries (M/Y)	FU (M)	BCVA before/after OP(Chinese tumbling E chart)	AI (mm)/horizontal WTW	Prediction error	Astigmatism post (absolute value, diopters)	IOL position	Complication
1	7/M	R	Oversized vitrectorrhexis, corneal scar, ERM	Corneal laceration repair after penetrating injury (9/2012); lensectomy + PPV for cataract and VH (9/2012)	Extensive synechiolysis, sulcus placement of CZ70BD IOL (12/2012)	53	0.08/0.15	22.65/12.59	0.25	2.25	Mild decentration	None
2	7/M	R	Oversized vitrectorrhexis, corneal scar, ocular foreign body, preretinal hemorrhage	Corneal laceration repair after penetrating injury (1/2014); lensectomy + PPV for cataract and VH (1/2014)	Foreign body removal, PPV, extensive synechiolysis, sulcus placement of CZ70BD IOL (7/2014)	16	0.01/0.1	22.06/NA	−1.5	3	Centration	None
3	56/F	R	Oversized CCC	Phacoemulsification + PPV for cataract and VH caused by ocular contusion (4/2013)	Extensive synechiolysis, sulcus placement of CZ70BD IOL (10/2013)	44	0.3/0.5	23.01/12.39	−0.5	1.5	Centration	None
4	3/M	R	Oversized vitrectorrhexis, IOL dislocation	Lensectomy + anterior vitrectomy for congenital cataract (8/2011); sulcus implantation of a foldable IOL (9/2014)	Explanation of original IOL, synechiolysis, and sulcus placement of CZ70BD IOL (9/2014)	32	0.1/0.3	22.7/NA	−0.25	1.5	Centration	None
5	7/M	R	Oversized vitrectorrhexis, corneal opacity, PHPV, optic dysplasia	Lensectomy + anterior vitrectomy for combined PFV (7/2008)	Extensive synechiolysis, extraction of lens remnants, PPV, sulcus placement of CZ70BD IOL (6/2015)	28	0.1/0.25	21.6/11.57	−0.4	1.75	Centration	None

TABLE 1: Continued.

Pt	Age (years)/gender	Eye	Preexisting condition	Surgical history (M/Y)	Secondary IOL implantation and concurrent surgeries (M/Y)	FU (M)	BCVA before/after OP(Chinese tumbling E chart)	Al (mm)/horizontal WTW	Prediction error	Astigmatism post (absolute value, diopters)	IOL position	Complication
6	2.5/M	R	Oversized vitrectorrhexis, corneal scar	Corneal laceration repair + lensectomy + formation of anterior chamber after ocular blast injury (2/2013)	Extensive synechiolysis, limited vitrectomy, sulcus placement of CZ70BD IOL (6/2015)	26	CF/0.1	22.83/NA	−0.75	2.25	Centration	None
7	39/M	R	Oversized CCC, high myopia	Phacoemulsification + PPV + scleral buckling for RRD (12/2014)	Synechiolysis and sulcus placement of CZ70BD IOL (8/2015)	40	0.8/1.0	27.1/12.19 for horizontal and 12.42 for vertical	0.5	1	Centration	None
8	2/M	R	Oversized vitrectorrhexis, corneal scar	Corneal laceration repair after penetrating injury (7/2014); lensectomy + anterior vitrectomy for cataract (8/2014)	Extensive synechiolysis, sulcus placement of CZ70BD IOL (8/2015)	26	LP/CF	21.4/NA	0.75	1.75	Centration	None
Mean ± SD						33 ± 12		23 ± 2	−0.2 ± 0.7	1.9 ± 0.6		

AL, axial length; BCVA, best-corrected visual acuity; CCC, continuous curvilinear capsulorhexis; CF, counting fingers; ERM, epiretinal membrane; IOL, intraocular lens; LP, light perception; PFV, persistent fetal vasculature; PPV, pars plana vitrectomy; RRD, rhegmatogenous retinal detachment; VH, vitreous hemorrhage; M, male; F, female; R, right; IOL, intraocular lens; FU, follow-up visit period; M, months; Y, years; WTW, white-to-white.

Synechiolysis was performed in all 8 eyes of which 6 eyes received extensive dissections to re-expose the capsulorhexis and ciliary sulcus. The residual capsular rim was non-continuous and irregular. The size was approximately 7 mm in seven eyes (patients 2 to 8, Figure 1–5) and even larger in the other eye (patient 1), precluding sulcus placement of an ordinary foldable PC IOL with a 5.5 to 6.5 mm optic. The rigid IOL was placed in the sulcus onto the anterior capsular shelf. The IOL optic, especially the inferior part, was partly secured by a residual capsular rim in seven eyes. In the other eye, the residual capsular rim with a size beyond the IOL optic only supported the IOL haptics. Concurrent surgeries included pars plana vitrectomy in two eyes, limited limbal vitrectomy in one eye, foreign body removal in one eye, and explanation of the original dislocated IOL in one eye (Canon-STAAR Preloaded IOL KS-3 (Ai) placed in the sulcus).

The mean postoperative follow-up period was 33 ± 12 months. Reasonable visual improvement was achieved in all eyes and a best-corrected visual acuity above 0.25 was observed in four eyes. Mild IOL decentration toward the superior direction was detected one month after operation in patient 1 who had a horizontal white-to-white value of 12.59 mm and a capsular rim beyond the size of the IOL optic. Since the IOL position remained stable throughout the follow-up period, repositioning of the IOL was not attempted. For the other seven patients, care was taken to ensure that the IOL optic was partly supported by the residual capsular rim. Consequently, IOLs were well centered throughout the follow-up period (Figure 1–5, Table 1). In all patients, minor corneal edema with mild anterior chamber inflammation was resolved after the second week with the use of topical corticosteroids. A mild-to-moderate astigmatism was observed in five patients, and an irregular astigmatism at higher diopters was present in the other three patients with a preexisting corneal scar. The mean prediction refractive error calculation was negligible at six months after surgery. No eye experienced chronic corneal edema, elevated intraocular pressure, uveitis-glaucoma-hyphema syndrome, vitreous hemorrhage, or retinal detachment during the follow-up.

4. Discussion

We used a PMMA rigid CZ70BD IOL for sutureless ciliary sulcus placement in aphakic eyes with a large capsular rim preserved after synechiolysis. Taking advantage of the residual capsulorhexis, the ideal strategy for aphakic correction in these eyes was the sulcus placement of a PC IOL, which requires less intraocular manipulations, provides for optimal rehabilitation, and reduces intraocular injury.

The first issue for planning a sulcus-based IOL in these aphakic eyes was to reconstruct the ciliary sulcus and maximize the residual capsule support. A preoperative evaluation of sulcus anatomy and diameter by an ultrasound biomicroscope may be underpowered to predict the size of the residual capsular rim before a surgical synechiolysis. Furthermore, any retained adhesion between the iris and the lens capsule may compromise a centered sulcus placement of a PC IOL and result in lateral or anteroposterior instability. Thus, we incorporated various techniques to separate the adhesion between the capsule and iris almost to the ciliary sulcus. An indication for a sulcus-based PC IOL became apparent after the capsular rim was maximally preserved and exposed.

The choice of a sulcus-based PC IOL was considered. Common IOLs for the sulcus are summarized in Table 2. They differ in aspects of size and haptic angulation. In routine situations, we select a sulcus-fixated IOL as follows: (1). anterior capsulorhexis optic capture of a sulcus-fixated foldable intraocular lens on a continuous 5 to 5.5 mm diameter capsulorhexis; (2). a three-piece IOL on a capsulorhexis with a 6 to 6.5 mm diameter. However, in our cases, the oversized capsular rim with a diameter near 7 mm or even larger precluded sulcus placement of a commonly used foldable 3-piece IOL like Alcon MA 50 [3] or Canon-Staar AQ2010 V [1], owing to their 6.5 mm optic size and softness. Still, lateral instability has always been a concern for a soft foldable IOL in the sulcus if the optic cannot be captured under the oversized anterior capsulorhexis. Considering that the mean ciliary sulcus diameter was 12.51 ± 0.43 mm vertically and 12.19 ± 0.47 mm horizontally for cadaver emmetropes, a rigid PMMA IOL with a 12.5 to 13.0 mm overall size may be a better back-up alternative for the ciliary sulcus [1, 3, 14]. Although a CZ70BD IOL only has a 12.5 mm tip-to-tip size, we chose this IOL due to its large optic, rigidity, and posteriorly angulated haptics. In addition, the IOL has built-in eyelets on the haptics for extra suture fixation, which facilitates anchoring one or both haptics to the scleral wall in case of intraoperative IOL decentration. Other larger PMMA IOLs, such as the Alcon CR70BU with a larger overall size of 13.5 mm but without a posteriorly angulated optic, or the Alcon MC60BD with a relatively small optic size of 6.0 mm, were considered less suitable thus not chosen for sulcus placement in our cases.

Favorable visual and anatomic outcomes in our cases provide evidences that our surgical design was reasonable and unwanted intraoperative trauma was minimal. The implantation of IOL was done smoothly on the residual capsulorhexis into the ciliary sulcus when a thorough surgical synechiolysis had been achieved in a minimally invasive but effective way. To our knowledge, there are no clear guidelines regarding the minimum amount of the residual capsule necessary to support a PC IOL in the sulcus. Our experience indicated that IOL haptics should be oriented away from the narrow rim, and the optic, especially the inferior part, should be partly held by a capsular rim with a similar size to the optic. Caution should be taken for eyes with a larger anterior segment as well as a larger capsular rim. In this study, the positional stability of the IOL may be mainly attributed to the similar size of the residual capsular rim compared to the optic size. Superior decentration of the IOL in patient 1 was probably due to the lack of the capsular rim holding the optic and a larger sulcus beyond the tip-to-tip size of the IOL. In this case, suture fixation of one haptic of the IOL would be beneficial. Still, preoperative evaluations of the capsule support and white-to-white values are critical in patients with myopia for proper choice of a sulcus-based

TABLE 2: Representative types of IOLs used for sulcus placement in literatures [1, 3].

Type		Size, optic/overall (mm)	Haptic angulation
Foldable			
Three-piece silicone optic	Staar AQ 2010V	6.3/13.5	Yes
Three-piece acrylic	Alcon MA50	6.5/13.0	Yes
Three-piece acrylic	Alcon MA60AC	6.0/13.0	Yes
Rigid			
Single-piece PMMA	Alcon CZ70BD	7.0/12.5	Yes
Single-piece PMMA	Alcon MC60BD	6.0/13.5	Yes
Single-piece PMMA	Alcon CR70BU	7.0/13.5	No

IOL, intraocular lens; PMMA, polymethyl methacrylate.

IOL, as was the case for patient 7 in our study. Although impossible in our cases, capture of the IOL optic under the anterior capsulorhexis may be a better resolution for the possibility of rotation or lateral subluxation with IOLs placed in the sulcus [15]. Additionally, it was reported that a PC IOL can be integrated into the tissue of the ciliary sulcus, which otherwise may fixate the IOL in the long term [16].

A limitation of the method we used was the occurrence of more pronounced postoperative astigmatism in some patients, owing to a larger scleral tunnel for accommodation of the rigid IOL. In our experience, the surgically induced astigmatism for a 6–7 mm scleral tunnel ranged from 1.0 to 3.0 D. In our cases, a meticulous construction of the incision was made, and the refractive outcomes were acceptable. Three eyes with postoperative astigmatism over 2.0 D may have been partly due to preexisting corneal scars. In conclusion, sulcus placement of a large-optic and rigid CZ70BD IOL may be a reliable and feasible surgical alternative for aphakic correction in eyes with an oversized capsular rim, which is inadequate for a foldable IOL. A preserved capsular rim after surgical synechiolysis, which can partly secure the optic, may be an apparent indication for sutureless sulcus placement of the IOL. The long-term effect and stability of our method should be further evaluated. The comparison to other types of rigid IOLs placed in the sulcus requires further investigation.

Conflicts of Interest

The authors declare that there are no conflicts of interest regarding the publication of this article.

Authors' Contributions

Qi Zhang and Jiao Lyu contributed equally to the article.

Acknowledgments

The authors thank the participating patients and the medical staff of Xinhua Hospital, School of Medicine, Shanghai Jiao Tong University.

References

[1] D. F. Chang, S. Masket, K. M. Miller et al., "Complications of sulcus placement of single-piece acrylic intraocular lenses: recommendations for backup IOL implantation following posterior capsule rupture," *Journal of cataract and refractive surgery*, vol. 35, no. 8, pp. 1445–1458, 2009.

[2] S. Schulze, T. Bertelmann, and W. Sekundo, "Implantation of intraocular lenses in the ciliary sulcus," *Der Ophthalmologe: Zeitschrift der Deutschen Ophthalmologischen Gesellschaft*, vol. 111, no. 4, pp. 305–309, 2014.

[3] P. S. Kemp and T. A. Oetting, "Stability and safety of MA50 intraocular lens placed in the sulcus," *Eye*, vol. 29, no. 11, pp. 1438–1441, 2015.

[4] M. Mohebbi, S. A. Bashiri, S. F. Mohammadi et al., "Outcome of single-piece intraocular lens sulcus implantation following posterior capsular rupture during phacoemulsification," *Journal of Ophthalmic & Vision Research*, vol. 12, no. 3, pp. 275–280, 2017.

[5] A. Melamud, J. S. Topilow, L. Cai, and X. He, "Pars plana vitrectomy combined with either secondary scleral-fixated or anterior chamber intraocular lens implantation," *American Journal of Ophthalmology*, vol. 168, pp. 177–182, 2016.

[6] S. Yamane, S. Sato, M. Maruyama-Inoue, and K. Kadonosono, "Flanged intrascleral intraocular lens fixation with double-needle technique," *Ophthalmology*, vol. 124, no. 8, pp. 1136–1142, 2017.

[7] V. Galvis, A. Tello, N. I. Carreno, R. D. Berrospi, C. A. Nino, and M. O. Cuadros, "Aphakic iris-claw intraocular lens pseudophakic pseudoaccommodation," *Journal of Cataract and Refractive Surgery*, vol. 43, no. 1, p. 146, 2017.

[8] K. H. Kim and W. S. Kim, "Comparison of clinical outcomes of iris fixation and scleral fixation as treatment for intraocular lens dislocation," *American Journal of Ophthalmology*, vol. 160, no. 3, pp. 463–469 e461, 2015.

[9] A. Rey, I. Jurgens, A. Dyrda, X. Maseras, and A. Morilla, "Surgical outcome of late in-the-bag intraocular lens dislocation treated with pars plana vitrectomy," *Retina*, vol. 36, no. 3, pp. 576–581, 2016.

[10] D. Lockington, N. Q. Ali, R. Al-Taie, D. V. Patel, and C. N. McGhee, "Outcomes of scleral-sutured conventional and aniridia intraocular lens implantation performed in a university hospital setting," *Journal of Cataract & Refractive Surgery*, vol. 40, no. 4, pp. 609–617, 2014.

[11] M. A. Khan, O. P. Gupta, R. G. Smith et al., "Scleral fixation of intraocular lenses using gore-tex suture: clinical outcomes and safety profile," *British Journal of Ophthalmology*, vol. 100, no. 5, pp. 638–643, 2016.

[12] E. R Millar, D. Allen, and D. H. Steel, "Effect of anterior capsulorhexis optic capture of a sulcus-fixated intraocular lens on refractive outcomes," *Journal of Cataract and Refractive Surgery*, vol. 39, no. 6, pp. 841–844, 2013.

[13] L. B. Enyedi, M. W. Peterseim, S. F. Freedman, and E. G. Buckley, "Refractive changes after pediatric intraocular lens implantation," *American Journal of Ophthalmology*, vol. 126, no. 6, pp. 772–781, 1998.

Surgical Synechiolysis of Iridocapsular Adhesion and Sulcus Placement of a Rigid Intraocular Lens...

79

[14] J. Biermann, L. Bredow, D. Boehringer, and T. Reinhard, "Evaluation of ciliary sulcus diameter using ultrasound biomicroscopy in emmetropic eyes and myopic eyes," *Journal of Cataract & Refractive Surgery*, vol. 37, no. 9, pp. 1686–1693, 2011.

[15] J. S. Chang, J. C. Ng, and V. K. Chan, "Sulcus fixation of a 3-piece diffractive multifocal intraocular lens with and without optic capture in the anterior capsulorhexis," *Ophthalmology*, vol. 121, no. 1, pp. 429-430 e422, 2014.

[16] A. Ollerton, L. Werner, S. Strenk et al., "Pathologic comparison of asymmetric or sulcus fixation of 3-piece intraocular lenses with square versus round anterior optic edges," *Ophthalmology*, vol. 120, no. 8, pp. 1580–1587, 2013.

11

Application of Novel Drugs for Corneal Cell Regeneration

Sang Beom Han[ID],[1] **Yu-Chi Liu,**[2,3,4] **Karim Mohamed-Noriega**[ID],[5] **and Jodhbir S. Mehta**[ID][2,3,4]

[1]*Department of Ophthalmology, Kangwon National University Hospital, Kangwon National University, Chuncheon, Republic of Korea*
[2]*Singapore National Eye Centre, Singapore*
[3]*Singapore Eye Research Institute, Singapore*
[4]*Department of Ophthalmology, Yong Loo Lin School of Medicine, National University of Singapore, Singapore*
[5]*Department of Ophthalmology, Faculty of Medicine, University Hospital "Jose E. Gonzalez", Autonomous University of Nuevo Leon, Monterrey, NL, Mexico*

Correspondence should be addressed to Jodhbir S. Mehta; jodmehta@gmail.com

Academic Editor: Enrique Mencía-Gutiérrez

Corneal transplantation has been the only treatment method for corneal blindness, which is the major cause of reversible blindness. However, despite the advancement of surgical techniques for corneal transplantation, demand for the surgery can never be met due to a global shortage of donor cornea. The development of bioengineering and pharmaceutical technology provided us with novel drugs and biomaterials that can be used for innovative treatment methods for corneal diseases. In this review, the authors will discuss the efficacy and safety of pharmacologic therapies, such as Rho-kinase (ROCK) inhibitors, blood-derived products, growth factors, and regenerating agent on corneal cell regeneration. The promising results of these agents suggest that these can be viable options for corneal reconstruction and visual rehabilitation.

1. Introduction

Corneal blindness is one of the leading causes of reversible blindness worldwide [1]. Corneal transplantation has been the only method for the treatment of corneal blindness, of which penetrating keratoplasty has long been the major surgical procedure. More recently, partial thickness corneal transplantation, such as Descemet's stripping endothelial keratoplasty (DSEK), Descemet's membrane endothelial keratoplasty (DMEK), and deep anterior lamellar keratoplasty (DALK), has been gaining popularity due to better visual prognosis and reduced risk of rejection. However, a global shortage of donor corneal tissue makes it impossible to meet the demands for corneal transplantation with current cornea donation programs. In addition, despite the advancement of surgical techniques and devices, corneal transplantation is still associated with limitations, such as graft failure or rejection, difficulty of the surgical procedure, and complications including secondary glaucoma [2, 3].

Remarkable developments of novel biomaterials and stem cell-based tissue cultivation and expansion techniques during the past few decades might enable the mass production of synthetic corneal tissue and are expected to provide innovative treatment methods for corneal disease. Medical treatment using drugs, such as Rho-kinase (ROCK) inhibitors, blood-derived products, growth factors, and regenerating agent eye drops (RGTA), is also anticipated to have therapeutic potential. In this review, we aimed to provide information on the pharmacologic therapies for corneal cell regeneration using these drugs.

2. Rock Inhibitors

ROCK is a serine/threonine protein kinase that is activated by Rho and forms Rho/ROCK complex that regulates a variety of cellular functions, such as cell proliferation, differentiation, migration, contraction, and apoptosis [4, 5]. Therefore, the ROCK signaling pathway has drawn interest as a potential target for the treatment of diseases of multiple organs [4, 5]. Recent studies showed that the ROCK inhibitor might be an innovative therapeutic agent for various ocular diseases, particular for corneal endothelial decompensation [4]. Although corneal transplantation has been the only therapy for corneal endothelial dysfunction, studies indicate the potential of ROCK inhibitors as a less-invasive alternative to graft surgery [3].

2.1. ROCK Inhibitor for Corneal Endothelial Cell (CEC) Generation.

Okumura et al. [6] demonstrated that a selective ROCK inhibitor, Y-27632, promoted CEC proliferation and adhesion and suppressed its apoptosis, indicating that the topical ROCK inhibitor has been therapeutic for CEC regeneration [6]. An experimental study showed that a ROCK inhibitor facilitated the proliferation of CECs by the modulation of cyclin and p27; both are regulators of the G1/S transition [7]. Peh et al. [8] also revealed that Y-27632 increased cell proliferation. In their study, the effect of the ROCK inhibitor on the proliferation of CEC was significant only in the corneas from younger donors, suggesting that CECs from older corneas might lose the proliferation potential that could be activated by the ROCK inhibitor [8]. The findings of another study that Y-27632 had no effect on the proliferation of human CECs, although it facilitated corneal endothelial wound healing ex vivo and *in vitro*, support the assumption [9].

ROCK inhibitor eye drops enhanced corneal endothelial wound healing in a rabbit CEC injury model [6, 7, 10]. Topical ROCK inhibitor instillation also led to the facilitation of corneal endothelial wound healing and the recovery of corneal transparency in a primate CEC damage model [11]. Y-27632 was also shown to enhance the proliferation and adhesion and suppress the apoptosis of primate CECs cultured *in vitro* [6, 12]. Considering that primate CECs also have limited proliferative capacity, these results suggest that the ROCK inhibitor may have a therapeutic effect on human corneal endothelial dysfunction.

Okumura et al. [13] postulated that topical application of the ROCK inhibitor could facilitate the proliferation and migration of the residual CECs after acute corneal endothelial damage, thereby decreasing the risk of corneal endothelial decompensation [13]. A preliminary study showed that topical administration of the ROCK inhibitor resulted in the recovery of corneal transparency in 1-2 months in all 3 patients with postoperative acute corneal endothelial decompensation [3].

The ROCK inhibitor could be an alternative to corneal transplantation for Fuchs' endothelial corneal dystrophy (FECD). A human pilot study demonstrated that treatment with Y-27632 eye drops for patients with FECD resulted in the decrease in central corneal thickness and the recovery of corneal transparency in patients with corneal edema confined to the center, whereas the effect was not evident in those with diffuse corneal edema [3, 11, 14]. A recent case series study also revealed that descemetorhexis without graft surgery followed by topical ROCK inhibitor administration resulted in the restoration of corneal clarity and visual rehabilitation in patients with FECD [15].

2.2. ROCK Inhibitor for Tissue Engineering.

For the treatment of corneal endothelial decompensation, the following two strategies for tissue engineering appears to be promising [1]: transplantation of bioengineered corneal endothelial cell sheet and [2] direct injection of cultivated CEC suspension to the anterior chamber [3].

Experimental studies showed that the transplantation of cultivated CECs on a collagen sheet can result in the restoration of corneal transparency and reduction of corneal edema [16, 17]. However, manipulation of the fragile monolayer sheet in the anterior chamber is technically challenging and is associated with the risk of CEC loss [3].

Theoretically, direct injection of CECs into the anterior chamber might be simple and less invasive compared to CEC sheet transplantation. In addition, the preparation of cells for transplantation may be easier, without the need for an artificial substrate [3]. The risk of CEC damage during the procedure might also be reduced. As the CECs injected into the anterior chamber may not spontaneously attach to Descemet's membrane, methods for improving the adhesion of the injected CECs have been attempted, such as magnetic guidance of iron powder or superparamagnetic microspheres incorporated in the CECs [18–20].

Considering that the ROCK inhibitor was proven to promote CEC adhesion onto a substrate [12], it may be postulated that the ROCK inhibitor can be helpful for promoting the attachment of CECs injected into the anterior chamber. An experimental study using a rabbit corneal endothelial dysfunction model demonstrated that intracameral injection of rabbit CECs combined with Y-27632, followed by keeping each rabbit in the facedown position for 3 hr, achieved enhanced attachment of donor cells onto host Descemet's membrane and the restoration of corneal transparency [21], whereas CEC injection without the inclusion of Y-27632 led to persistent corneal edema [21].

Y-27632 also promoted the adhesion of intracamerally injected CECs onto Descemet's membrane in both rabbit and primate corneal endothelial decompensation models and upregulated the expression of functional proteins including Na+/K+ ATPase and ZO-1, thereby leading to the resolution of corneal edema [22]. Another study revealed that intracameral injection of either human or monkey CECs in combination with Y-27632 led to the regeneration of monkey corneal endothelium, suggesting that intracameral injection of cultivated human CECs combined with the ROCK inhibitor may be a plausible therapeutic option for corneal endothelial diseases [2]. Preliminary data from a human clinical study showed that cultured human CECs injected in conjunction with ROCK achieved improvement of corneal edema and visual acuity without any serious adverse effect [3]. Although the results appear to be promising, further prospective randomized studies with a long-term follow-up are necessary to evaluate the efficacy and safety of ROCK inhibitors for the treatment of corneal endothelial diseases [3].

2.3. Other Effects of ROCK Inhibitor on Corneal Regeneration.

The ROCK inhibitor was suggested to have additional effects that can be potentially applicable for corneal regeneration. Y-27632 was shown to promote both ex vivo and *in vitro* proliferation of limbal epithelial cell proliferation, suggesting it can be useful for the treatment of limbal stem cell deficiency [23]. Zhou et al. [24] also demonstrated that Y-27632 enhanced the cloning efficiency of limbal stem/progenitor cells by promoting their adhesion and capacity of reactive oxygen species scavenging in a rabbit model [24]. Y-27632 inhibited the transition of rabbit keratocyte to myofibroblast and modulated a wound healing process after a superficial lamellar keratectomy in a rabbit cornea [25]. Animal experimental studies revealed that ROCK inhibitors, fasudil and AMA0526, inhibited corneal neovascularization and opacity and facilitated corneal epithelial regeneration after corneal alkali burn [26, 27].

3. Blood-Derived Products

Application of blood-derived products for ocular surface diseases was first introduced in 1975 for 6 patients with chemical burns [28]. Since Tsubota et al. [29, 30] proved the efficacy and safety of autologous serum eye drops (ASE) for the treatment of dry eye disease (DED) and persistent epithelial defect (PED) [29, 30], studies have proven that blood-derived products are innovative therapeutic agents for various ocular surface disorders, such as DED [31], PED [32], neurotrophic keratitis [33], recurrent corneal erosion [34], and chemical burns [35].

3.1. Autologous Serum Eye Drops (ASE) [36]. ASE has a similar biochemical composition as human tears [37] and includes growth factors including epidermal growth factor (EGF) and transforming growth factor- (TGF-) β [38], chemokines, fibronectin, and various nutrients [38].

Consensus for the preparation method has never been established yet [37]. An *in vitro* experimental study indicated that an increased clotting time of 120 min or longer, a sharp centrifugation (3000g for 15 min), and dilution with balanced salt solution at 12.5–25% were optimal for corneal epithelial healing [39]. Clinically, 20% ASE is most frequently used to match the TGF-β concentration, which is 5 times higher in serum than in tears, to prevent delayed wound healing and promotion of corneal haze caused by TGF-β [30]. However, higher concentrations of ASE (50 to 100%) were also suggested to be effective and safe [40, 41]. A randomized prospective study showed that 100% ASE was more effective for the treatment of PED, Sjögren's syndrome (SS), and non-Sjögren DED than 50% ASE [42].

Randomized clinical studies revealed that ASE was more effective than conventional treatment for the improvement of both symptoms and signs of DED [43–45]. Kojima et al. [46] demonstrated that ASE suppressed apoptosis in the ocular surface epithelium and albumin contained in ASE recovered ocular surface damage [46]. ASE was superior to artificial tear in the improvement of dry eye signs after refractive surgery [47]. In addition, ASE can be a therapeutic option for PED refractory to conventional treatment [40, 48]. Schrader et al. [49] suggested that ASE combined with silicone hydrogel contact lenses might be helpful in recalcitrant PED [49]. Moreover, ASE was shown to be effective in facilitating reepithelialization of corneal graft after penetrating keratoplasty

[50]. It also promoted corneal epithelial healing in patients with neurotrophic keratitis and aniridic keratopathy [51, 52]. A prospective study with a long-term follow-up revealed that ASE was effective for the prevention of recurrence in patients with recurrent corneal erosion [53]. However, a review of five randomized clinical trials that compared AS versus artificial tears or saline in DED patients revealed that no evidence of a benefit was found after two weeks of treatment, although there might be some short-term effect on symptoms with AS compared with artificial tears [54]. Therefore, we also believe further well-designed, large-scale randomized controlled studies are warranted to evaluate the efficacy of AS [54]. The absence of preservatives and high nutrient level in ASE increases the risk of sample contamination [55, 56]. Therefore, attention should be paid for the signs of infection in patients using ASE [36]. Lagnado et al. [55] recommended that sample vials should be stored frozen at −20°C for up to 6 months, and each vial should be thawed and used for only 24 hours. A prospective randomized human study showed that containers equipped with a sterilizing filter can be used for up to 4 weeks without any increased risk of contamination [56]. The concentrations of growth factors in 20% ASE remained stable for up to 9 months when kept frozen at −20°C and up to 4 weeks when defrosted [57].

3.2. Allogeneic Serum Eye Drops (SE). Allogeneic SE from healthy donors can be advantageous in patients with fear or difficulty of blood sampling or coexisting blood disorders including anemia [58]. Moreover, it can also be a therapeutic option for patients with graft-versus-host disease (GVHD) or (SS), in which a considerable amount of proinflammatory cytokines could be included in their autologous serum [59]. Allogeneic SE can be prepared using the same protocol of ASE [58]. Because allogeneic SE includes anti-A and anti-B antibodies, it can theoretically cause an immune reaction against ABO antigens expressed on corneal and conjunctival epithelium [58]. Therefore, preparation of allogenic SE from ABO-identical donors or blood type AB donors is recommended [60, 61]. Studies demonstrated the efficacy of allogenic SE in DED, PED, neurotrophic keratitis, GVHD, and exposure keratopathy [60, 62, 63], indicating its potential as a viable alternative to ASE [36].

3.3. Umbilical Cord Serum Eye Drops (UCSE). UCSE samples can be prepared using umbilical cord blood collected during delivery [36]. Rigorous screening for blood-borne infections is mandatory prior to donation [36, 58]. UCSE can also be a therapeutic option for patients with blood disorders or systemic inflammatory diseases, in which ASE is contraindicated [58]. Although allogeneic serum does have the same advantage, UCS contains a higher level of growth factors, neurotrophic factors, and essential tear components compared to allogeneic serum [31, 33, 64]. Moreover, compared to allogeneic serum, a substantially larger amount of UCSE can be obtained with a single sampling from one donor and can be distributed to multiple patients [58]. As UCS contains high levels of neurotrophic factors such as substance P (SP), insulin-like growth factor- (IGF-) 1, and nerve growth factor (NGF) [32, 33], as well as growth factors including EGF and TGF-β [64], it is conceivably helpful for corneal nerve regeneration and epithelial healing. Studies have revealed that UCSE accelerated the recovery of PED and neurotrophic keratitis recalcitrant to conventional treatment [32, 33]. UCSE was shown to be more effective than ASE for the improvement of symptoms and signs of DED, particularly in severe cases associated with GVHD and SS [64, 65]. UCSE was superior to artificial tear in treating recurrent corneal erosions and reducing its recurrence [34]. In ocular chemical burn, UCSE resulted in faster corneal epithelial healing and milder corneal opacity compared to ASE or artificial tears [35]. UCSE is also shown to decrease early corneal haze and improve ocular surface parameters after laser epithelial keratomileusis (LASEK) [66].

3.4. Platelet-Derived Plasma Preparations. Platelet-derived plasma preparations contain a large amount of growth factors and cytokines [36, 58] and have been successfully used in maxillofacial and orthopedic surgery as well as in regenerative medicine for the promotion of tissue healing [67]. Various preparations have been developed, such as plasma rich in growth factors (PRGF), platelet-rich plasma (PRP), and platelet lysate [58]. PRGF is obtained by the filtration of plasma supernatants after centrifugation of the whole blood [68]. PRP is a plasma with increased concentrations of platelets obtained with an additional centrifugation of the whole blood [69]. Platelet lysate is collected by inducing platelet lysis and release of growth factors including platelet-derived growth factor (PDGF) using PRP [70].

Kim et al. [71] demonstrated that PRP was superior to ASE in the treatment of PED. PRGF was also suggested to be useful for the healing of PED [72]. PRP was shown to be effective for the improvement of both symptoms and signs of DED [73]. Plasma lysate was suggested to be helpful for the treatment of DED associated with GVHD or SS [74, 75]. PRP was also superior to conventional treatment for the recovery of visual acuity and corneal transparency in patients with ocular chemical injury [76]. In addition, PRP is potentially available for a biomaterial for ocular surface reconstruction [77, 78].

4. Growth Factors for Corneal Diseases

4.1. Nerve Growth Factor (NGF). NGF facilitates corneal epithelial healing, which is mediated by the cleavage of β4 integrin and the upregulation of matrix metalloproteinase-9 [79]. Topical administration of NGF was shown to be effective in neurotrophic keratitis refractory to conventional treatment [80–82]. NGF is also expected to be effective for the treatment of diabetic keratopathy, as it could alleviate inflammation and apoptosis of corneal cells that can occur in diabetes mellitus [83].

Topical NGF was also shown to have a beneficial effect for postoperative corneal wound healing [80]. Cellini et al. [84] demonstrated that topical NGF was superior to artificial tear for corneal reconstruction after cataract. Animal experimental studies revealed that topical application of NGF accelerated restoration of corneal sensitivity and promoted cornea

epithelial proliferation and nerve regeneration after laser in situ keratomileusis (LASIK) or photorefractive keratectomy (PRK) [85–87].

4.2. Substance P (SP) and Insulin-Like Growth Factor- (IGF-) 1. A randomized prospective study revealed that topical SP and IGF-1 combination therapy was useful for the prevention of superficial punctate keratopathy after cataract surgery in diabetic patients [88]. SP was shown to promote an epithelial healing process in diabetic cornea and attenuate hyperosmotic stress-induced apoptosis of corneal epithelial cells through the neurokinin-1 receptor signaling pathway [89, 90]. IGF-1 also facilitated the regeneration of corneal surface ultrastructure and nerves after LASIK in rabbit eyes [91].

4.3. Vascular Endothelial Growth Factor (VEGF). VEGF can facilitate the functional and anatomical recovery after peripheral nerve damage [92]. Guaiquil et al. [93] demonstrated that VEGF-B treatment selectively promoted nerve regeneration and restored sensory and trophic functions of injured corneal nerves, suggesting that it might have a therapeutic potential for peripheral corneal nerve injury [93].

An experimental study revealed that the expression of endogenous VEGF-B was attenuated in regenerated corneal epithelium in a diabetic mouse model, whereas supplementation of exogenous VEGF-B accelerated corneal nerve regeneration [94].

4.4. Other Grow Factors. An animal study showed that pigment epithelial-derived factor, in conjunction with docosahexaenoic acid, might be effective for the treatment of DED caused by corneal nerve damage and neurotrophic keratitis [95]. Topical administration of neuroprotectin D1 was also shown to attenuate inflammation and facilitate nerve regeneration after corneal damage in a rabbit model [96]. Ciliary neurotrophic factor was shown to be able to activate corneal epithelial stem/progenitor cells and promote the corneal nerve regeneration and epithelial recovery, suggesting its therapeutic potential for diabetic keratopathy and limbal stem cell deficiency [97]. A randomized clinical study demonstrated that basic fibroblast growth factor promoted corneal epithelial healing after PRK, indicating it could be a therapeutic option for delayed healing [98].

4.5. Regenerating Agent Eye Drops (RGTAs). RGTA (OTR4120 Cacicol20®; Théa, Clermont-Ferrand, France) is a carboxymethyl dextran sulfate polymer bioengineered to replace heparan sulfate, which is an important factor both for matrix proteins and for growth factors [99, 100]. Thus, RGTA is conceivably helpful for restoring equilibrium in cellular microenvironment [99, 101]. It is also expected to be useful for corneal wound healing, and several studies have shown promising results [99–107].

Experimental studies using a rabbit corneal burn model and a clinical case series study suggested that RGTA might be an innovative agent for promoting corneal regeneration and attenuating ocular surface inflammation by reducing oxidative, proteolytic, and nitrosative corneal damage [104, 108, 109]. A clinical pilot study also revealed the efficacy of RGTA for corneal ulcers and dystrophies refractory

TABLE 1: Effect and possible application of the novel drugs.

Drug	Effect	Possible application
ROCK inhibitor	Corneal endothelial cell regeneration	Topical eye drops for recovery of corneal clarity in corneal endothelial dysfunction
	Promotion of corneal endothelial cell adhesion	Adjuvant therapy for the corneal endothelial cell injection
Blood-derived products	Promotion of healing of ocular surface epithelium	Recovery of persistent epithelial defect or neurotrophic keratitis
		Promoting ocular surface regeneration and prevention of corneal haze after ocular chemical injury or keratorefractive surgery
Growth factors	Facilitation of corneal epithelial healing and nerve regeneration	Treatment of persistent epithelial defect or neurotrophic keratitis
		Topical eye drops for diabetic keratopathy
		Recovery of cornea epithelium and nerve after keratorefractive surgery
RGTA*	Promotion of corneal regeneration and attenuation of ocular surface inflammation	Treatment of persistent epithelial defect or neurotrophic keratitis
		Recovery of corneal epithelium after corneal cross-linking
		Corneal recovery after keratorefractive surgery

*RGTA: regenerating agent eye drops.

to conventional treatment [105]. A prospective clinical study demonstrated that RGTA might be effective and safe for the treatment of neurotrophic keratitis [106]. Chappelet et al. [101] recently showed that RGTA could be useful for the treatment of a PED after bacterial keratitis [101].

RGTA ophthalmic solution was also reported to facilitate corneal epithelial healing after corneal cross-linking (CXL) by reconstruction of the extracellular matrix in the corneal wound area [99, 100]. A randomized clinical trial demonstrated that RGTA might be superior to topical hyaluronic acid for corneal wound recovery after CXL in patients with keratoconus [103].

In animal excimer laser models, topical RGTA reduced corneal haze and promoted nerve regeneration, suggesting that it could be a useful option for the restoration of corneal microarchitecture after keratorefractive surgery [102, 107].

5. Conclusion

In this review paper, we have introduced a number of research papers that have demonstrated the efficacy of pharmacologic therapies, such as ROCK inhibitors, blood-derived products, growth factors, and RGTA on corneal cell regeneration. The promising results of these studies suggest that these agents can be viable options to aid corneal cell regeneration.

In summary, the ROCK inhibitor can promote the regeneration of CECs and its adhesion to Descemet's membrane. Thus, it can be used as a topical eye drops for the treatment of corneal endothelial dysfunction. It can also be used as an adjuvant therapy for CEC injection to AC. Blood-derived products can promote healing of ocular surface epithelium. Hence, it can be used for PED or neurotrophic keratitis. It can also be used for promoting ocular surface reconstruction and prevention of corneal opacity after ocular chemical injury. Growth factors promote the recovery of cornea epithelium and nerve; thus, these drugs can especially be helpful for PED, neurotrophic keratitis, and diabetic keratopathy. As RGTA facilitates corneal regeneration and attenuates ocular surface inflammation, it can be indicated for corneal regeneration after corneal CXL. It can also be helpful for the treatment of PDE or neurotrophic keratitis. The recovery of corneal epithelium and nerve after keratorefractive surgery can be facilitated by blood-derived products, growth factors, and RGTA (Table 1).

Although these therapeutic agents are innovative, further prospective randomized studies are needed for the verification of the efficacy and safety of the drugs [3]. Further studies are also required for the development of novel therapeutic agents for corneal cell regeneration.

Conflicts of Interest

None of the authors have a proprietary interest in the study or financial interests to disclose.

Acknowledgments

This study was supported by 2017 Research Grant from Kangwon National University.

References

[1] J. P. Whitcher, M. Srinivasan, and M. P. Upadhyay, "Corneal blindness: a global perspective," *Bulletin of the World Health Organization*, vol. 79, no. 3, pp. 214–221, 2001.

[2] N. Okumura, Y. Sakamoto, K. Fujii et al., "Rho kinase inhibitor enables cell-based therapy for corneal endothelial dysfunction," *Scientific Reports*, vol. 6, no. 1, article 26113, 2016.

[3] N. Okumura, S. Kinoshita, and N. Koizumi, "Application of Rho kinase inhibitors for the treatment of corneal endothelial diseases," *Journal of Ophthalmology*, vol. 2017, Article ID 2646904, 8 pages, 2017.

[4] R. Nourinia, S. Nakao, S. Zandi, S. Safi, A. Hafezi-Moghadam, and H. Ahmadieh, "ROCK inhibitors for the treatment of ocular diseases," *British Journal of Ophthalmology*, vol. 102, no. 1, 2017.

[5] N. Koizumi, N. Okumura, M. Ueno, and S. Kinoshita, "New therapeutic modality for corneal endothelial disease using Rho-associated kinase inhibitor eye drops," *Cornea*, vol. 33, Supplement 11, pp. S25–S31, 2014.

[6] N. Okumura, N. Koizumi, M. Ueno et al., "Enhancement of corneal endothelium wound healing by Rho-associated kinase (ROCK) inhibitor eye drops," *British Journal of Ophthalmology*, vol. 95, no. 7, pp. 1006–1009, 2011.

[7] N. Okumura, S. Nakano, E. D. P. Kay et al., "Involvement of cyclin D and p27 in cell proliferation mediated by ROCK inhibitors Y-27632 and Y-39983 during corneal endothelium wound healing," *Investigative Ophthalmology & Visual Science*, vol. 55, no. 1, pp. 318–329, 2014.

[8] G. S. L. Peh, K. Adnan, B. L. George et al., "The effects of Rho-associated kinase inhibitor Y-27632 on primary human corneal endothelial cells propagated using a dual media approach," *Scientific Reports*, vol. 5, no. 1, p. 9167, 2015.

[9] A. Pipparelli, Y. Arsenijevic, G. Thuret, P. Gain, M. Nicolas, and F. Majo, "ROCK inhibitor enhances adhesion and wound healing of human corneal endothelial cells," *PLoS One*, vol. 8, no. 4, article e62095, 2013.

[10] N. Okumura, N. Koizumi, M. Ueno et al., "The new therapeutic concept of using a rho kinase inhibitor for the treatment of corneal endothelial dysfunction," *Cornea*, vol. 30, Supplement 1, pp. S54–S59, 2011.

[11] N. Okumura, N. Koizumi, E. D. P. Kay et al., "The ROCK inhibitor eye drop accelerates corneal endothelium wound healing," *Investigative Ophthalmology & Visual Science*, vol. 54, no. 4, pp. 2493–2502, 2013.

[12] N. Okumura, M. Ueno, N. Koizumi et al., "Enhancement on primate corneal endothelial cell survival in vitro by a ROCK inhibitor," *Investigative Ophthalmology & Visual Science*, vol. 50, no. 8, pp. 3680–3687, 2009.

[13] N. Okumura, S. Kinoshita, and N. Koizumi, "The role of rho kinase inhibitors in corneal endothelial dysfunction," *Current Pharmaceutical Design*, vol. 23, no. 4, pp. 660–666, 2017.

[14] N. Koizumi, N. Okumura, M. Ueno, H. Nakagawa, J. Hamuro, and S. Kinoshita, "Rho-associated kinase inhibitor eye drop treatment as a possible medical treatment for Fuchs corneal dystrophy," *Cornea*, vol. 32, no. 8, pp. 1167–1170, 2013.

[15] G. Moloney, C. Petsoglou, M. Ball et al., "Descemetorhexis without grafting for Fuchs endothelial dystrophy-supplementation with topical ripasudil," *Cornea*, vol. 36, no. 6, pp. 642–648, 2017.

[16] N. Koizumi, Y. Sakamoto, N. Okumura et al., "Cultivated corneal endothelial cell sheet transplantation in a primate model," *Investigative Ophthalmology & Visual Science*, vol. 48, no. 10, pp. 4519–4526, 2007.

[17] T. Mimura, S. Yamagami, S. Yokoo et al., "Cultured human corneal endothelial cell transplantation with a collagen sheet in a rabbit model," *Investigative Ophthalmology & Visual Science*, vol. 45, no. 9, pp. 2992–2997, 2004.

[18] T. Mimura, N. Shimomura, T. Usui et al., "Magnetic attraction of iron-endocytosed corneal endothelial cells to Descemet's membrane," *Experimental Eye Research*, vol. 76, no. 6, pp. 745–751, 2003.

[19] T. Mimura, S. Yamagami, T. Usui et al., "Long-term outcome of iron-endocytosing cultured corneal endothelial cell transplantation with magnetic attraction," *Experimental Eye Research*, vol. 80, no. 2, pp. 149–157, 2005.

[20] I. H. Ma, L. W. Chen, W. H. Tu, C. J. Lu, C. J. Huang, and W. L. Chen, "Serum components and clinical efficacies of autologous serum eye drops in dry eye patients with active

and inactive Sjogren syndrome," *Taiwan Journal of Ophthalmology*, vol. 7, no. 4, pp. 213–220, 2017.

[21] T. Mimura, S. Yamagami, S. Yokoo et al., "Sphere therapy for corneal endothelium deficiency in a rabbit model," *Investigative Ophthalmology & Visual Science*, vol. 46, no. 9, pp. 3128–3135, 2005.

[22] N. Okumura, N. Koizumi, M. Ueno et al., "ROCK inhibitor converts corneal endothelial cells into a phenotype capable of regenerating *in vivo* endothelial tissue," *The American Journal of Pathology*, vol. 181, no. 1, pp. 268–277, 2012.

[23] C. C. Sun, H. T. Chiu, Y. F. Lin, K. Y. Lee, and J. H. S. Pang, "Y-27632, a ROCK inhibitor, promoted limbal epithelial cell proliferation and corneal wound healing," *PLoS One*, vol. 10, no. 12, article e0144571, 2015.

[24] Q. Zhou, H. Duan, Y. Wang, M. Qu, L. Yang, and L. Xie, "ROCK inhibitor Y-27632 increases the cloning efficiency of limbal stem/progenitor cells by improving their adherence and ROS-scavenging capacity," *Tissue Engineering. Part C: Methods*, vol. 19, no. 7, pp. 531–537, 2013.

[25] M. Yamamoto, A. J. Quantock, R. D. Young et al., "A selective inhibitor of the Rho kinase pathway, Y-27632, and its influence on wound healing in the corneal stroma," *Molecular Vision*, vol. 18, pp. 1727–1739, 2012.

[26] P. Zeng, R. B. Pi, P. Li et al., "Fasudil hydrochloride, a potent ROCK inhibitor, inhibits corneal neovascularization after alkali burns in mice," *Molecular Vision*, vol. 21, pp. 688–698, 2015.

[27] D. Sijnave, T. Van Bergen, K. Castermans et al., "Inhibition of Rho-associated kinase prevents pathological wound healing and neovascularization after corneal trauma," *Cornea*, vol. 34, no. 9, pp. 1120–1129, 2015.

[28] R. A. Ralph, M. G. Doane, and C. H. Dohlman, "Clinical experience with a mobile ocular perfusion pump," *Archives of Ophthalmology*, vol. 93, no. 10, pp. 1039–1043, 1975.

[29] K. Tsubota, E. Goto, S. Shimmura, and J. Shimazaki, "Treatment of persistent corneal epithelial defect by autologous serum application," *Ophthalmology*, vol. 106, no. 10, pp. 1984–1989, 1999.

[30] K. Tsubota, E. Goto, H. Fujita et al., "Treatment of dry eye by autologous serum application in Sjogren's syndrome," *British Journal of Ophthalmology*, vol. 83, no. 4, pp. 390–395, 1999.

[31] K. C. Yoon, S. K. Im, Y. G. Park, Y. D. Jung, S. Y. Yang, and J. Choi, "Application of umbilical cord serum eyedrops for the treatment of dry eye syndrome," *Cornea*, vol. 25, no. 3, pp. 268–272, 2006.

[32] K. C. Yoon, H. Heo, I. Y. Jeong, and Y. G. Park, "Therapeutic effect of umbilical cord serum eyedrops for persistent corneal epithelial defect," *Korean Journal of Ophthalmology*, vol. 19, no. 3, pp. 174–178, 2005.

[33] K. C. Yoon, I. C. You, S. K. Im, T. S. Jeong, Y. G. Park, and J. Choi, "Application of umbilical cord serum eyedrops for the treatment of neurotrophic keratitis," *Ophthalmology*, vol. 114, no. 9, pp. 1637–1642.e2, 2007.

[34] K. C. Yoon, W. Choi, I. C. You, and J. Choi, "Application of umbilical cord serum eyedrops for recurrent corneal erosions," *Cornea*, vol. 30, no. 7, pp. 744–748, 2011.

[35] N. Sharma, M. Goel, T. Velpandian, J. S. Titiyal, R. Tandon, and R. B. Vajpayee, "Evaluation of umbilical cord serum therapy in acute ocular chemical burns," *Investigative Ophthalmology & Visual Science*, vol. 52, no. 2, pp. 1087–1092, 2011.

[36] N. G. Soni and B. H. Jeng, "Blood-derived topical therapy for ocular surface diseases," *British Journal of Ophthalmology*, vol. 100, no. 1, pp. 22–27, 2015.

[37] G. Geerling, S. Maclennan, and D. Hartwig, "Autologous serum eye drops for ocular surface disorders," *British Journal of Ophthalmology*, vol. 88, no. 11, pp. 1467–1474, 2004.

[38] C. Yamada, K. E. King, and P. M. Ness, "Autologous serum eyedrops: literature review and implications for transfusion medicine specialists," *Transfusion*, vol. 48, no. 6, pp. 1245–1255, 2008.

[39] L. Liu, D. Hartwig, S. Harloff, P. Herminghaus, T. Wedel, and G. Geerling, "An optimised protocol for the production of autologous serum eyedrops," *Graefe's Archive for Clinical and Experimental Ophthalmology*, vol. 243, no. 7, pp. 706–714, 2005.

[40] B. H. Jeng and W. J. Dupps Jr, "Autologous serum 50% eyedrops in the treatment of persistent corneal epithelial defects," *Cornea*, vol. 28, no. 10, pp. 1104–1108, 2009.

[41] K. Lekhanont, P. Jongkhajornpong, L. Choubtum, and V. Chuckpaiwong, "Topical 100% serum eye drops for treating corneal epithelial defect after ocular surgery," *BioMed Research International*, vol. 2013, Article ID 521315, 7 pages, 2013.

[42] Y. K. Cho, W. Huang, G. Y. Kim, and B. S. Lim, "Comparison of autologous serum eye drops with different diluents," *Current Eye Research*, vol. 38, no. 1, pp. 9–17, 2013.

[43] B. A. Noble, R. S. Loh, S. MacLennan et al., "Comparison of autologous serum eye drops with conventional therapy in a randomised controlled crossover trial for ocular surface disease," *British Journal of Ophthalmology*, vol. 88, no. 5, pp. 647–652, 2004.

[44] T. Kojima, R. Ishida, M. Dogru et al., "The effect of autologous serum eyedrops in the treatment of severe dry eye disease: a prospective randomized case-control study," *American Journal of Ophthalmology*, vol. 139, no. 2, pp. 242–246, 2005.

[45] A. R. C. Celebi, C. Ulusoy, and G. E. Mirza, "The efficacy of autologous serum eye drops for severe dry eye syndrome: a randomized double-blind crossover study," *Graefe's Archive for Clinical and Experimental Ophthalmology*, vol. 252, no. 4, pp. 619–626, 2014.

[46] T. Kojima, A. Higuchi, E. Goto, Y. Matsumoto, M. Dogru, and K. Tsubota, "Autologous serum eye drops for the treatment of dry eye diseases," *Cornea*, vol. 27, Supplement 1, pp. S25–S30, 2008.

[47] T. Noda-Tsuruya, N. Asano-Kato, I. Toda, and K. Tsubota, "Autologous serum eye drops for dry eye after LASIK," *Journal of Refractive Surgery*, vol. 22, no. 1, pp. 61–66, 2006.

[48] A. C. Poon, G. Geerling, J. K. Dart, G. E. Fraenkel, and J. T. Daniels, "Autologous serum eyedrops for dry eyes and epithelial defects: clinical and in vitro toxicity studies," *British Journal of Ophthalmology*, vol. 85, no. 10, pp. 1188–1197, 2001.

[49] S. Schrader, T. Wedel, R. Moll, and G. Geerling, "Combination of serum eye drops with hydrogel bandage contact lenses in the treatment of persistent epithelial defects," *Graefe's Archive for Clinical and Experimental Ophthalmology*, vol. 244, no. 10, pp. 1345–1349, 2006.

[50] Y. M. Chen, F. R. Hu, J. Y. Huang, E. P. Shen, T. Y. Tsai, and W. L. Chen, "The effect of topical autologous serum on graft re-epithelialization after penetrating keratoplasty," *American Journal of Ophthalmology*, vol. 150, no. 3, pp. 352–359.e2, 2010.

[51] Y. Matsumoto, M. Dogru, E. Goto et al., "Autologous serum application in the treatment of neurotrophic keratopathy," *Ophthalmology*, vol. 111, no. 6, pp. 1115–1120, 2004.

[52] J. S. Lopez-Garcia, L. Rivas, I. Garcia-Lozano, and J. Murube, "Autologous serum eyedrops in the treatment of aniridic keratopathy," *Ophthalmology*, vol. 115, no. 2, pp. 262–267, 2008.

[53] N. G. Ziakas, K. G. Boboridis, C. Terzidou et al., "Long-term follow up of autologous serum treatment for recurrent corneal erosions," *Clinical & Experimental Ophthalmology*, vol. 38, no. 7, pp. 683–687, 2010.

[54] Q. Pan, A. Angelina, M. Marrone et al., "Autologous serum eye drops for dry eye," *Cochrane Database of Systematic Reviews*, vol. 2, article CD009327, 2017.

[55] R. Lagnado, A. J. King, F. Donald, and H. S. Dua, "A protocol for low contamination risk of autologous serum drops in the management of ocular surface disorders," *British Journal of Ophthalmology*, vol. 88, no. 4, pp. 464-465, 2004.

[56] J. S. Lopez-Garcia and I. Garcia-Lozano, "Use of containers with sterilizing filter in autologous serum eyedrops," *Ophthalmology*, vol. 119, no. 11, pp. 2225–2230, 2012.

[57] J. S. Lopez-Garcia, I. Garcia-Lozano, L. Rivas, N. Ramírez, M. T. Méndez, and R. Raposo, "Stability of growth factors in autologous serum eyedrops after long-term storage," *Current Eye Research*, vol. 41, no. 3, pp. 1–7, 2016.

[58] G. Giannaccare, P. Versura, M. Buzzi, L. Primavera, M. Pellegrini, and E. C. Campos, "Blood derived eye drops for the treatment of cornea and ocular surface diseases," *Transfusion and Apheresis Science*, vol. 56, no. 4, pp. 595–604, 2017.

[59] P. A. Stenwall, M. Bergstrom, P. Seiron et al., "Improving the anti-inflammatory effect of serum eye drops using allogeneic serum permissive for regulatory T cell induction," *Acta Ophthalmologica*, vol. 93, no. 7, pp. 654–657, 2015.

[60] L. H. Harritshoj, C. Nielsen, H. Ullum, M. B. Hansen, and H. O. Julian, "Ready-made allogeneic ABO-specific serum eye drops: production from regular male blood donors, clinical routine, safety and efficacy," *Acta Ophthalmologica*, vol. 92, no. 8, pp. 783–786, 2014.

[61] K. G. Badami and M. McKellar, "Allogeneic serum eye drops: time these became the norm?," *British Journal of Ophthalmology*, vol. 96, no. 8, pp. 1151-1152, 2012.

[62] C. C. Chiang, W. L. Chen, J. M. Lin, and Y. Y. Tsai, "Allogeneic serum eye drops for the treatment of persistent corneal epithelial defect," *Eye*, vol. 23, no. 2, pp. 290–293, 2009.

[63] K. S. Na and M. S. Kim, "Allogeneic serum eye drops for the treatment of dry eye patients with chronic graft-versus-host disease," *Journal of Ocular Pharmacology and Therapeutics*, vol. 28, no. 5, pp. 479–483, 2012.

[64] K. C. Yoon, H. Heo, S. K. Im, I. C. You, Y. H. Kim, and Y. G. Park, "Comparison of autologous serum and umbilical cord serum eye drops for dry eye syndrome," *American Journal of Ophthalmology*, vol. 144, no. 1, pp. 86–92.e2, 2007.

[65] K. C. Yoon, I. Y. Jeong, S. K. Im, Y. G. Park, H. J. Kim, and J. Choi, "Therapeutic effect of umbilical cord serum eyedrops for the treatment of dry eye associated with graft-versus-host disease," *Bone Marrow Transplantation*, vol. 39, no. 4, pp. 231–235, 2007.

[66] K. C. Yoon, H. J. Oh, J. W. Park, and J. Choi, "Application of umbilical cord serum eyedrops after laser epithelial

keratomileusis," *Acta Ophthalmologica*, vol. 91, no. 1, pp. e22–e28, 2013.

[67] B. H. Choi, C. J. Im, J. Y. Huh, J. J. Suh, and S. H. Lee, "Effect of platelet-rich plasma on bone regeneration in autogenous bone graft," *International Journal of Oral and Maxillofacial Surgery*, vol. 33, no. 1, pp. 56–59, 2004.

[68] E. Anitua, M. de la Fuente, F. Muruzabal, A. Riestra, J. Merayo-Lloves, and G. Orive, "Plasma rich in growth factors (PRGF) eye drops stimulates scarless regeneration compared to autologous serum in the ocular surface stromal fibroblasts," *Experimental Eye Research*, vol. 135, pp. 118–126, 2015.

[69] S. T. Tanidir, N. Yuksel, O. Altintas, D. K. Yildiz, E. Sener, and Y. Caglar, "The effect of subconjunctival platelet-rich plasma on corneal epithelial wound healing," *Cornea*, vol. 29, no. 6, pp. 664–669, 2010.

[70] L. Liu, D. Hartwig, S. Harloff et al., "Corneal epitheliotrophic capacity of three different blood-derived preparations," *Investigative Ophthalmology & Visual Science*, vol. 47, no. 6, pp. 2438–2444, 2006.

[71] K. M. Kim, Y. T. Shin, and H. K. Kim, "Effect of autologous platelet-rich plasma on persistent corneal epithelial defect after infectious keratitis," *Japanese Journal of Ophthalmology*, vol. 56, no. 6, pp. 544–550, 2012.

[72] S. Lopez-Plandolit, M. C. Morales, V. Freire, J. Etxebarría, and J. A. Durán, "Plasma rich in growth factors as a therapeutic agent for persistent corneal epithelial defects," *Cornea*, vol. 29, no. 8, pp. 843–848, 2010.

[73] J. L. Alio, A. E. Rodriguez, R. Ferreira-Oliveira, D. Wróbel-Dudzińska, and A. A. Abdelghany, "Treatment of dry eye disease with autologous platelet-rich plasma: a prospective, interventional, non-randomized study," *Ophthalmology and Therapy*, vol. 6, no. 2, pp. 285–293, 2017.

[74] S. Pezzotta, C. Del Fante, L. Scudeller, M. Cervio, E. R. Antoniazzi, and C. Perotti, "Autologous platelet lysate for treatment of refractory ocular GVHD," *Bone Marrow Transplantation*, vol. 47, no. 12, pp. 1558–1563, 2012.

[75] A. M. Fea, V. Aragno, V. Testa et al., "The effect of autologous platelet lysate eye drops: an in vivo confocal microscopy study," *BioMed Research International*, vol. 2016, Article ID 8406832, 10 pages, 2016.

[76] A. Panda, M. Jain, M. Vanathi, T. Velpandian, S. Khokhar, and T. Dada, "Topical autologous platelet-rich plasma eyedrops for acute corneal chemical injury," *Cornea*, vol. 31, no. 9, pp. 989–993, 2012.

[77] J. L. Alio, A. E. Rodriguez, and L. M. Martinez, "Bovine pericardium membrane (tutopatch) combined with solid platelet-rich plasma for the management of perforated corneal ulcers," *Cornea*, vol. 32, no. 5, pp. 619–624, 2013.

[78] J. L. Alio, A. E. Rodriguez, L. M. Martinez, and A. L. Rio, "Autologous fibrin membrane combined with solid platelet-rich plasma in the management of perforated corneal ulcers: a pilot study," *JAMA Ophthalmology*, vol. 131, no. 6, pp. 745–751, 2013.

[79] T. Blanco-Mezquita, C. Martinez-Garcia, R. Proenca et al., "Nerve growth factor promotes corneal epithelial migration by enhancing expression of matrix metalloprotease-9," *Investigative Ophthalmology & Visual Science*, vol. 54, no. 6, pp. 3880–3890, 2013.

[80] A. Lambiase, M. Sacchetti, and S. Bonini, "Nerve growth factor therapy for corneal disease," *Current Opinion in Ophthalmology*, vol. 23, no. 4, pp. 296–302, 2012.

[81] F. R. Ghosheh, F. Cremona, B. D. Ayres et al., "Indications for penetrating keratoplasty and associated procedures, 2001-2005," *Eye & Contact Lens*, vol. 34, no. 4, pp. 211–214, 2008.

[82] S. Bonini, A. Lambiase, P. Rama, G. Caprioglio, and L. Aloe, "Topical treatment with nerve growth factor for neurotrophic keratitis," *Ophthalmology*, vol. 107, no. 7, pp. 1347–1351, 2000.

[83] J. H. Park, S. S. Kang, J. Y. Kim, and H. Tchah, "Nerve growth factor attenuates apoptosis and inflammation in the diabetic cornea," *Investigative Ophthalmology & Visual Science*, vol. 57, no. 15, pp. 6767–6775, 2016.

[84] M. Cellini, E. Bendo, G. O. Bravetti, and E. C. Campos, "The use of nerve growth factor in surgical wound healing of the cornea," *Ophthalmic Research*, vol. 38, no. 4, pp. 177–181, 2006.

[85] M. J. Joo, K. R. Yuhan, J. Y. Hyon et al., "The effect of nerve growth factor on corneal sensitivity after laser in situ keratomileusis," *Archives of Ophthalmology*, vol. 122, no. 9, pp. 1338–1341, 2004.

[86] S. Esquenazi, H. E. P. Bazan, V. Bui, J. He, D. B. Kim, and N. G. Bazan, "Topical combination of NGF and DHA increases rabbit corneal nerve regeneration after photorefractive keratectomy," *Investigative Ophthalmology & Visual Science*, vol. 46, no. 9, pp. 3121–3127, 2005.

[87] K. Ma, N. Yan, Y. Huang, G. Cao, J. Deng, and Y. Deng, "Effects of nerve growth factor on nerve regeneration after corneal nerve damage," *International Journal of Clinical and Experimental Medicine*, vol. 7, no. 11, pp. 4584–4589, 2014.

[88] N. Chikamoto, T. Chikama, N. Yamada, T. Nishida, T. Ishimitsu, and A. Kamiya, "Efficacy of substance P and insulin-like growth factor-1 peptides for preventing postsurgical superficial punctate keratopathy in diabetic patients," *Japanese Journal of Ophthalmology*, vol. 53, no. 5, pp. 464–469, 2009.

[89] L. Yang, G. Di, X. Qi et al., "Substance P promotes diabetic corneal epithelial wound healing through molecular mechanisms mediated via the neurokinin-1 receptor," *Diabetes*, vol. 63, no. 12, pp. 4262–4274, 2014.

[90] L. Yang, W. Sui, Y. Li et al., "Substance P inhibits hyperosmotic stress-induced apoptosis in corneal epithelial cells through the mechanism of Akt activation and reactive oxygen species scavenging via the neurokinin-1 receptor," *PLoS One*, vol. 11, no. 2, article e0149865, 2016.

[91] C. Wang, Y. Peng, S. Pan, and L. Li, "Effect of insulin-like growth factor-1 on corneal surface ultrastructure and nerve regeneration of rabbit eyes after laser in situ keratomileusis," *Neuroscience Letters*, vol. 558, pp. 169–174, 2014.

[92] Z. Pan, S. Fukuoka, N. Karagianni, V. H. Guaiquil, and M. I. Rosenblatt, "Vascular endothelial growth factor promotes anatomical and functional recovery of injured peripheral nerves in the avascular cornea," *The FASEB Journal*, vol. 27, no. 7, pp. 2756–2767, 2013.

[93] V. H. Guaiquil, Z. Pan, N. Karagianni, S. Fukuoka, G. Alegre, and M. I. Rosenblatt, "VEGF-B selectively regenerates injured peripheral neurons and restores sensory and trophic functions," *Proceedings of the National Academy of Sciences of the United States of America*, vol. 111, no. 48, pp. 17272–17277, 2014.

[94] G. Di, X. Zhao, X. Qi et al., "VEGF-B promotes recovery of corneal innervations and trophic functions in diabetic mice," *Scientific Reports*, vol. 7, article 40582, 2017.

[95] J. He, M. S. Cortina, A. Kakazu, and H. E. P. Bazan, "The PEDF neuroprotective domain plus DHA induces corneal nerve regeneration after experimental surgery," *Investigative Ophthalmology & Visual Science*, vol. 56, no. 6, pp. 3505–3513, 2015.

[96] M. S. Cortina, J. He, T. Russ, N. G. Bazan, and H. E. P. Bazan, "Neuroprotectin D1 restores corneal nerve integrity and function after damage from experimental surgery," *Investigative Ophthalmology & Visual Science*, vol. 54, no. 6, pp. 4109–4116, 2013.

[97] Q. Zhou, P. Chen, G. Di et al., "Ciliary neurotrophic factor promotes the activation of corneal epithelial stem/progenitor cells and accelerates corneal epithelial wound healing," *Stem Cells*, vol. 33, no. 5, pp. 1566–1576, 2015.

[98] A. Meduri, P. Aragona, P. L. Grenga, and A. M. Roszkowska, "Effect of basic fibroblast growth factor on corneal epithelial healing after photorefractive keratectomy," *Journal of Refractive Surgery*, vol. 28, no. 3, pp. 220–223, 2012.

[99] K. Gumus, M. G. Guerra, S. H. de Melo Marques, S. Karakücük, and D. Barritault, "A new matrix therapy agent for faster corneal healing and less ocular discomfort following epi-off accelerated corneal cross-linking in progressive keratoconus," *Journal of Refractive Surgery*, vol. 33, no. 3, pp. 163–170, 2017.

[100] G. D. Kymionis, D. A. Liakopoulos, M. A. Grentzelos et al., "Effect of the regenerative agent poly(carboxymethylglucose sulfate) on corneal wound healing after corneal cross-linking for keratoconus," *Cornea*, vol. 34, no. 8, pp. 928–931, 2015.

[101] M. A. Chappelet, D. Bernheim, C. Chiquet, and F. Aptel, "Effect of a new matrix therapy agent in persistent epithelial defects after bacterial keratitis treated with topical fortified antibiotics," *Cornea*, vol. 36, no. 9, pp. 1061–1068, 2017.

[102] I. Alcalde, A. Inigo-Portugues, N. Carreño, A. C. Riestra, and J. M. Merayo-Lloves, "Effects of new biomimetic regenerating agents on corneal wound healing in an experimental model of post-surgical corneal ulcers," *Archivos de la Sociedad Española de Oftalmología*, vol. 90, no. 10, pp. 467–474, 2015.

[103] A. M. Bata, K. J. Witkowska, P. A. Wozniak et al., "Effect of a matrix therapy agent on corneal epithelial healing after standard collagen cross-linking in patients with keratoconus: a randomized clinical trial," *JAMA Ophthalmology*, vol. 134, no. 10, pp. 1169–1176, 2016.

[104] F. Brignole-Baudouin, J. M. Warnet, D. Barritault, and C. Baudouin, "RGTA-based matrix therapy in severe experimental corneal lesions: safety and efficacy studies," *Journal Français d'Ophtalmologie*, vol. 36, no. 9, pp. 740–747, 2013.

[105] C. K. Chebbi, K. Kichenin, N. Amar et al., "Pilot study of a new matrix therapy agent (RGTA OTR4120) in treatment-resistant corneal ulcers and corneal dystrophy," *Journal Français d'Ophtalmologie*, vol. 31, no. 5, pp. 465–471, 2008.

[106] M. Guerra, S. Marques, J. Q. Gil et al., "Neurotrophic keratopathy: therapeutic approach using a novel matrix regenerating agent," *Journal of Ocular Pharmacology and Therapeutics*, vol. 33, no. 9, pp. 662–669, 2017.

[107] M. Xeroudaki, B. Peebo, J. Germundsson, P. Fagerholm, and N. Lagali, "RGTA in corneal wound healing after transepithelial laser ablation in a rabbit model: a randomized, blinded, placebo-controlled study," *Acta Ophthalmologica*, vol. 94, no. 7, pp. 685–691, 2016.

[108] R. P. J. Arvola, A. Robciuc, and J. M. Holopainen, "Matrix regeneration therapy: a case series of corneal neurotrophic ulcers," *Cornea*, vol. 35, no. 4, pp. 451–455, 2016.

[109] J. Cejkova, C. Olmiere, C. Cejka, P. Trosan, and V. Holan, "The healing of alkali-injured cornea is stimulated by a novel matrix regenerating agent (RGTA, CACICOL20): a biopolymer mimicking heparan sulfates reducing proteolytic, oxidative and nitrosative damage," *Histology and Histopathology*, vol. 29, no. 4, pp. 457–478, 2014.

12

Clinical Features and Surgical Outcomes of Posterior Segment Intraocular Foreign Bodies in Children in East China

Ting Zhang,[1,2] **Hong Zhuang,**[1,2] **Keyan Wang** ⓘ**,**[1,2] **and Gezhi Xu** ⓘ[1,2]

[1]*Department of Ophthalmology, Eye, Ear, Nose and Throat Hospital, Fudan University, Shanghai 200031, China*
[2]*Shanghai Key Laboratory of Visual Impairment and Restoration, Eye, Ear, Nose and Throat Hospital, Fudan University, Shanghai 200031, China*

Correspondence should be addressed to Keyan Wang; drwangky@gmail.com

Academic Editor: Enrico Peiretti

Purpose. To report the long-term follow-up results of posterior segment intraocular foreign body (IOFB) removal in children and to determine the prognostic factors for visual outcome. *Methods.* Design: retrospective, noncomparative, interventional case series; a single tertiary care center study. Participants or samples: eleven eyes (11 patients) under 16 years of age with posterior segment IOFB injuries from May 2014 to November 2017. Main outcome measures: clinical features of injury, visual acuity, and complications. *Results.* The mean age was 6.8 years, and the mean follow-up was 20.2 months. The main IOFB sources were accidental penetration of the eye by materials in the playground (6 cases) or by pencil lead at school (4 cases). The mean IOFB size was 3.8 (range 1–6) mm. At the last visit, the visual acuities were 20/40 or better in 40.0% of patients and better than 20/200 in 70.0%. Poor visual outcome was correlated with intraoperative rhegmatogenous retinal detachment ($P = 0.0083$). Postoperative complications included elevated transient intraocular pressure, retinal redetachment, and secondary glaucoma. *Conclusions.* The clinical features of pediatric posterior segment IOFBs suggest insufficient awareness of such injuries both on the playground and at school. Visual outcomes from surgical treatment were relatively favorable in this series.

1. Introduction

Ocular trauma is a leading cause of noncongenital monocular blindness in children, and it imposes a significant economic burden on society [1]. In adults, intraocular foreign bodies (IOFBs) account for approximately one-third of open globe injuries and most commonly affect the posterior segment of the eye [2, 3]. They generally occur at workplaces. The most common IOFB is metallic pieces produced from hammering. Foreign body injuries are also common in children [4]; however, there are few reports of IOFBs in patients aged < 16 years. Here, we report the clinical features and surgical outcomes in consecutive pediatric patients with posterior segment IOFBs who visited the Eye, Ear, Nose and Throat Hospital of Fudan University, the largest tertiary referral eye center in East China that handles almost all IOFB cases in this region.

2. Methods

2.1. Data Collection. This was a retrospective study designed to assess the characteristics and surgical outcomes of posterior segment IOFB injuries in children and possible prognostic factors for visual outcome. The posterior segment is the back two-thirds of the eye that includes the vitreous, retina, choroid, and optic nerve. Inclusion criteria were consecutive patients aged less than 16 years who were admitted to the Eye, Ear, Nose and Throat Hospital between January 2014 and December 2017 for posterior segment IOFB injuries. Exclusion criteria were patients older than 16 years or patients with only anterior segment or intraorbital foreign bodies. Patients with suspected IOFB preoperatively were also excluded with no final evidence of IOFB after imaging test or surgical treatment. The study was conducted in accordance with the principles of the Declaration of Helsinki and approved by the Ethics Committee of the Eye,

Ear, Nose and Throat Hospital. Informed consent was obtained from each patient's parents.

At presentation to the hospital, a detailed medical history was collected from each child and their guardians, and each child underwent a complete ophthalmologic examination including assessment of visual acuity (VA), pupillary reflex evaluation, slit-lamp examination, and fundus examination. The interval between IOFB injury and surgery, type of injury, number of IOFBs, IOFB type and size, entry site of the IOFB, concomitant ocular injuries, presence of endophthalmitis, IOFB extraction route, and details of vitrectomy were recorded. Computed tomography (CT) of the orbits without contrast was performed preoperatively to confirm and localize the IOFBs. Helical CT was performed through the orbits in three planes (axial, sagittal, and coronal) with slice thickness of 0.75 mm. If the primary wound entry had already been closed, B scan ultrasonography was also used to confirm and localize the IOFB and evaluate the vitreous and retina. Ultrasound biomicroscopy was used to evaluate the IOFBs if CT indicated the presence of an IOFB in the ciliary body. The International Society of Ocular Trauma Classification [5, 6] and Birmingham Eye Trauma Terminology [7] systems were applied in the present study. The Ocular Trauma Score (OTS) predictions were compared with the actual visual outcomes, as performed by Yu Wai Man and Steel [8].

Postoperative follow-up visits were scheduled at 1, 7, and 14 days and 1, 2, 3, 6, 12, 24, and 36 months after surgery for each patient and included VA testing, intraocular pressure measurement, and a comprehensive ophthalmic examination. VA values obtained from the Snellen eye test were converted into the logarithm of the mean angle of resolution (logMAR) units for analysis. The VAs for hand motion, light perception, and no light perception were assigned logMAR values of 2.6, 3, and 4, respectively. Follow-up was scheduled after any additional surgeries.

The diagnosis of endophthalmitis was based on the clinical findings of presence of corneal edema, anterior chamber cells, hypopyon, and inflammation in the vitreous. The diagnosis of panophthalmitis was based on the ophthalmic examination findings of presence of corneal edema, hypopyon, severe vitritis, and edema of the eye walls, as well as an obvious elevation in white blood cell counts. Topical levofloxacin 0.5% and tobramycin 0.3% eye drops were applied preoperatively every 30 minutes to eyes with suspected infection. Intravitreal injections of ceftazidime (2.25 mg/0.1 ml) and vancomycin (1 mg/0.1 ml) were administered to eyes with endophthalmitis after the initial surgery to remove the IOFB. Intravenous ceftazidime (50 mg/kg twice daily) was administered for 3 days postoperatively to patients with endophthalmitis or panophthalmitis. The white blood cell count of patients with panophthalmitis was measured every other day until it decreased to within the normal range. The antibiotic therapy was adjusted accordingly when microorganisms were detected in cultures of vitreous samples or extracted IOFBs. Patients with no signs of infection did not receive intravitreal or systemic antibiotics. Topical prednisolone acetate 0.1% and levofloxacin 0.5% eye drops three times daily for 4 weeks postoperatively were prescribed for all eyes.

2.2. Surgical Procedures. All patients with IOFBs received surgical treatment within 1 day after admission to our hospital. Conventional three-port 20-gauge pars plana vitrectomy (PPV) was performed. An undiluted vitreous sample from eyes with suspected endophthalmitis was obtained at initiation of PPV for Gram staining and culture. Media opacities including hyphema, hypopyon, or traumatic cataract were removed prior to performing core vitrectomy. If the IOFB was suspended in the vitreous gel, adhesions surrounding the IOFB were dissected around the perimeter, and the IOFB was then extracted via scleral or limbal incision. After removal of an intravitreal IOFB, artificial posterior vitreous detachment was performed. However, if there were significant signs of vitritis or retinitis, excision of the hyaloid face was performed with extreme caution or even deferred for subsequent surgery. If retinal impact sites were present, with or without the IOFBs embedded in the impact sites, vitreous-retina adhesion around these areas was eliminated thoroughly, and the area around the retinal impact sites was treated with laser photocoagulation before removal of the IOFB.

The extraction strategy for the IOFBs was determined preoperatively, based mainly on the size and composition of the IOFB. Ferromagnetic IOFBs were removed bimanually using an intraocular magnet and forceps. Nonferrous or organic IOFBs were removed using foreign body forceps, and heavier-than-water liquid was introduced if necessary to protect the macula. Where possible, smaller foreign bodies were removed after enlargement of the sclerotomy site. Large IOFBs were removed via a new limbal incision.

After extraction, the IOFB was sent for microbiological culture, the limbal incision or enlarged scleral incision was sutured, and a complete retinal examination using scleral depression was conducted. If rhegmatogenous retinal detachment (RRD) was present, PPV using perfluoropropane or silicone oil tamponade was performed. The decision to use gas or oil tamponade was made by the surgeon, based on issues including the severity of endophthalmitis and the number and location of retinal breaks. The postoperative face-down position could not be accomplished by the children and thus was not mandatory. Removal of the silicone oil was scheduled for 3 months after the primary vitrectomy. Aphakic eyes with a postoperative VA better than 20/200 received intraocular lens implantation at least 3 months after successful vitrectomy.

Evisceration was indicated in cases of panophthalmitis. The cornea was excised completely following peritomy, and the intraocular contents and IOFB were removed using an evisceration spoon. The IOFB was sent for microbiological culture to detect pathogens, and the contents of the eye were sent for histopathological examination. Any remaining pigment was removed by scrubbing with cotton-tipped applicators soaked in 95% alcohol. Irrigation was then performed to remove the residual pigment and alcohol. A scleral shell was envelope-sutured, Tenon's capsule was closed, and the conjunctiva was sutured with burying of the knots. A conformer was then placed inside the eyelid. A hydroxyapatite implant was planned at least 3 months after the infection had subsided.

TABLE 1: Demographic characteristics of subjects with posterior segment IOFBs.

Subject	Sex	Age (years)	Eye	Interval between accident and surgery (days)	Initial VA	Nature of IOFB	IOFB size (mm)	Location of IOFB	Distance of IOFB to limbus (mm)
1	F	2	OS	2	NA	Pencil tip	5*1*1	Ciliary body	5
2	M	10	OD	0.5	20/200	Wood from playground	2*2*1.5	Vitreous	14
3	F	5	OD	1	HM	Pencil tip	2*2*1	Retina	16
4	M	9	OD	5	20/63	Iron from playground	4*2*2	Retina	13
5	M	6	OD	50	20/20	Pencil tip	3*2*1	Ciliary body	6
6	M	6	OS	1	NLP	Stone in mud, from exploding fireworks	6*6*4	Vitreous	15
7	M	12	OD	0.5	20/160	Iron from playground	5*3*3	Retina	16
8	F	6	OD	1	20/200	Pencil tip	2*2*1	Vitreous	16
9	M	8	OS	2	LP	Plastic pieces of fireworks	3*2*1, 6*5*1	Anterior chamber, vitreous	16
10	F	8	OS	5	HM	Iron from hairpin	4*2*2	Vitreous	13
11	M	3	OD	6	NA	Iron from playground	3*1*1	Vitreous	5

IOFB: intraocular foreign body; VA: visual acuity; OS: left eye; OD: right eye; NA: not available; HM: hand motion; NLP: no light perception; LP: light perception.

TABLE 2: Ocular injuries and OTS in subjects with posterior segment IOFBs.

Subject	Wound entrance	Length of wound (mm)	Anterior chamber and iris	Cataract	Vitreous opacity	Retina	OTS
1	Cornea	1	—	Y	Endophthalmitis	RRD[a]	NA
2	Cornea	3	—	Y	Endophthalmitis	—	3
3	Cornea	5	Iris incarceration	Y	Vitreous hemorrhage	Retinal hole	3
4	Cornea	2	Iris penetration	Y	—	Retinal hole	4
5	Sclera	NA	—	—	—	—	5
6	Cornea	10	Hypopyon, iris dialysis	Y	Panophthalmitis	—	1
7	Sclera	3	—	Y	Vitreous hemorrhage	Retinal hole	4
8	Cornea	5.5	Iris incarceration	Y	—	Retinal hole	4
9	Cornea/sclera	7	Iris incarceration	Y	Endophthalmitis	—	1
10	Cornea	2	Hypopyon	Y	Endophthalmitis	RRD[†]	1
11	Cornea	3	—	Y	—	—	NA

IOFB: intraocular foreign body; OTS: ocular trauma score; RRD: rhegmatogenous retinal detachment; NA: not available. [†]Injury during IOFB removal.

2.3. Statistical Analysis.

2.3. Statistical Analysis. Statistical analysis was performed using SPSS for Macintosh (version 21, SPSS Inc., Chicago, IL, USA). Fisher's exact test was used for comparisons of categorical variables. The preoperative and postoperative best-corrected visual acuity (BCVA) values were compared using the nonparametric Wilcoxon matched-pairs signed-rank test. A two-tailed P value < 0.05 was considered to indicate statistical significance in all tests.

3. Results

Eleven eyes in seven boys (63.6%) and 4 girls (36.4%; mean age 6.8 ± 3.0 years; range 2–12) were included in the study (Table 1). The most common causes of IOFB were accidental penetration of the eye by various materials in the playground (6 patients) and by pencil lead at school (4 patients).

The median interval from injury to IOFB removal was 2 days (mean 6.7, range 0.5–50) This was irrespective of the presence of vitritis (2.1 ± 1.7 days in 5 eyes with endophthalmitis or panophthalmitis versus 10.6 ± 19.4 days in 6 eyes with no signs of infection; $P = 0.18$).

All injuries were type C IOFB according to the International Society of Ocular Trauma classification system and the OTS score was evaluated for each patient (Table 2).

The entry site was zone I in eight eyes (72.7%) and zone II in three eyes (27.3%). Ten eyes (90.9%) had traumatic cataracts, four eyes (36.4%) had retinal tears, four eyes (36.4%) had suspected endophthalmitis, two eyes (18.2%) had vitreous hemorrhage, and one eye had panophthalmitis (9.1%) at presentation.

The OTS was available in 9 children. As shown in Table 3, the OTS predicted visual survival (LP or better) in 6 out of 8 children and no vision (NPL or enucleation) in 1 out of 1 child. Its sensitivity to predict visual survival and specificity to predict no vision was 75.0% and 100%, respectively. Similarly, the OTS predicted minimal to severe visual loss (20/20 to 3/60) in 6 out of 7 children and profound visual loss (worse than 3/60) in 2 out of 2 children. Its sensitivity to predict minimal to severe visual loss and specificity to predict profound vision loss was 85.7% and 100%, respectively.

The IOFBs were located in the retina in three eyes (27.3%), ciliary body in two eyes (18.2%), and vitreous in six eyes (54.5%). The composition of the IOFB was iron in four eyes, graphite in four eyes, wood in one eye, stone in one eye, and plastic (two pieces) from a fireworks explosion in one eye. In the eye with panophthalmitis, the IOFB was a stone thrown up with mud by exploding fireworks.

TABLE 3: Comparison of the ocular trauma score (OTS) predictions with the actual visual outcomes.

		Actual visual outcomes	
		Vision survival	No vision
OTS predictions	Vision survival (LP or better)	6	0
	No vision (NLP or enucleation)	2	1
		Minimal to severe vision loss	Profound vision loss
	Minimal to severe vision loss (20/20~3/60)	6	0
	Profound vision loss (worse than 3/60)	1	2

OTS: ocular trauma score; LP: light perception; NLP: no light perception.

TABLE 4: Surgeries, complications, and follow-up of subjects with posterior segment IOFBs.

Subject	Primary surgery	IOFB extraction route	Additional surgery	Complications	Final VA	Follow-up (months)
1	LC, PPV, SO	Planar	Retinotomy, SO (3 times)	Glaucoma, RRD	LP	42
2	LC, PPV	Planar	IOL implantation	—	20/25	35
3	LC, PPV, C_3F_8,	Planar	IOL implantation	—	20/32	26
4	LC, PPV, C_3F_8,	Planar	IOL implantation	IOP increase	20/100	22
5	Anterior PPV	Planar	—	—	20/20	22
6	Evisceration	Evisceration	Hydroxyapatite implantation	—	NLP	22
7	LC, PPV, C_3F_8,	Planar	RGP	IOP increase	20/100	20
8	LC, PPV	Planar	IOL implantation	—	20/32	13
9	LC, PPV	Limbal	RGP	—	20/40	9
10	LC, PPV	Limbal	SO removal	IOP increase	HM	8
11	Anterior PPV	Planar	—	—	NA	3

LC: lensectomy; PPV: pars planar vitrectomy; SO: silicone oil tamponade; RRD: rhegmatogenous retinal detachment; VA: visual acuity; LP: light perception; NLP: no light perception; HM: hand motion; IOL: intraocular lens; IOP: intraocular pressure; C_3F_8: perfluoropropane; RGP: rigid gas-permeable lens; NA: not available.

The IOFBs were removed via the scleral incision in PPV in 8 (72.3%) of 11 eyes, via limbal incision after extraction to the anterior chamber in 2 eyes (18.2%), and by evisceration in 1 eye (9.1%). A single IOFB was present in 10 eyes (90.9%) and multiple IOFBs in 1 eye (9.1%). The size of the IOFB varied from $2 \times 2 \times 1$ mm to $6 \times 6 \times 4$ mm, and the mean length was 3.8 ± 1.5 mm.

As shown in Table 4, cataract extraction combined with PPV, anterior PPV, and evisceration of the eye were performed in eight eyes (72.3%), two eyes (18.2%), and one eye (9.1%), respectively. In all cases, the IOFBs were removed during the initial surgery. Seven eyes underwent additional surgeries to treat complications, remove silicone oil, or restore VA; of these seven eyes, four underwent secondary implantation of an intraocular lens, one underwent implantation of a hydroxyapatite prosthesis, one underwent four procedures for recurrent retinal detachment, and one underwent simple silicone oil removal. Two eyes were prescribed rigid gas-permeable contact lenses after removal of the corneal sutures. Seven eyes with a postoperative VA better than 20/200 were treated for amblyopia.

The mean follow-up period was 20.2 (range 3–42) months. Preoperative and final VA data were available for 9 and 10 eyes, respectively (Tables 1 and 4). The mean preoperative and final VAs were 1.37 ± 1.35 (range 0–4) logMAR and 1.04 ± 1.37 (range 0–4) logMAR, respectively ($P = 0.20$). Vision improved in five eyes, did not change in three eyes, and worsened in one eye. Regarding final VA in the 10 eyes for which final VA data were available, 7 and 4 had final VAs of 20/200 or better and 20/40 or better, respectively.

Cultures of vitreous samples or extracted IOFBs were positive in only two eyes (one for *Staphylococcus epidermidis* and one for *Bacillus cereus*). Retinal tears caused by IOFB impact occurred in four eyes and retinal detachment during IOFB removal in another two eyes. Postoperative complications included a transient increase in intraocular pressure in three eyes and recurrence of retinal detachment and secondary glaucoma in one eye. None of the patients experienced sympathetic ophthalmia during the follow-up period.

The predictors of the final VA are summarized in Table 5. Children with intraoperative RRD had a worse visual recovery than did children with no retinal detachment (Fisher's exact test, $P = 0.0083$). Factors such as presence of vitritis, culture results, or IOFB location were not predictors of the final VA.

4. Discussion

IOFBs are seen most often in adults and most frequently occur at work sites [3]. However, IOFBs in children are not rare, especially in China. No epidemiological study on the incidence of pediatric IOFBs has been conducted in China. Our hospital, the Eye, Ear, Nose and Throat Hospital of Fudan University, is the largest tertiary referral eye center in East China, and almost all IOFB cases in this region are treated here. Here, we report retrospective interventional follow-up results from 11 children with posterior IOFBs. To our knowledge, this is the first retrospective case series of IOFBs in patients aged < 16 years.

We found that IOFB injuries in children occurred most commonly in the playground, where six children were injured by IOFBs composed of iron, wood, plastic, or stone. One child

TABLE 5: Predictors of final visual outcomes in subjects with posterior segment IOFBs.

Variable	VA ≥ 20/200	VA < 20/200	P value (Fisher's exact test)
Presence of vitritis			
Endophthalmitis or panophthalmitis	2	3	0.1667
None	5	0	—
RRD			
Presence	0	3	0.0083
Absence	7	0	—
Vitreous or IOFB culture			
Positive	1	1	1.000
Negative	6	2	—
Location of IOFB			
Vitreous	3	2	1.000
Retina or ciliary body	4	1	—

VA: visual acuity; RRD: rhegmatogenous retinal detachment; IOFB: intraocular foreign body.

developed panophthalmitis 1 day after he lit a firework buried in a pile of stones in the playground, an injury that could have been prevented by parental supervision or by wearing protective glasses. To our surprise, our study revealed school as the next most common site for IOFB injury. Four eyes of four children were penetrated by sharp pencils, and the graphite lead remained in the eye after the pencil was removed, which is rarely seen in adults with IOFB. In fact, ocular injuries caused by pencils are not rare in children and include penetration of the eye wall, traumatic cataract, endophthalmitis, and pencil lead retained in the anterior chamber [9] or posterior segment. Pencil fragments left in the eye after orbital or orbitocranial penetrating injuries can even be life and vision threatening [10]. Insufficient awareness of such injuries at school may be the cause of these preventable accidents.

IOFBs were composed of plastic, wood, or pencil lead in six eyes in our study. This supports the suggestion that 50% of IOFBs are not detectable on plain radiographs and is in agreement with the recommendations of other reports that thin-slice CT of the orbits might be preferable [11, 12].

The IOFB was pencil lead in four of the present patients, and was located in the ciliary body in one eye, retina in one eye, and vitreous in one eye. It is debatable whether an IOFB of graphite pencil lead should be removed. Its main component, graphite, can remain inert in the eye for long periods [13]. Indeed, there were no signs of an inflammatory reaction in three cases in our study, even in one case with pencil lead that had remained in the ciliary body for 50 days. However, pencil lead is composed of a mixture of graphite, wax, clay, and animal fat, and potential toxicity due to the other components may lead to progressive damage to ocular structures [14, 15]. Therefore, we removed all pencil lead IOFBs from the eyes in our study, and three of these eyes had a final VA better than 20/30; prognosis was poor in only one eye, as a result of concomitant endophthalmitis and RRD.

During the follow-up period, the VA improved in 5 (of 9) children, and 7 (of 9) children had a final VA better than 20/100. In our study, the OTS sensitivity and specificity to predict visual outcomes was high, which may provide prognostic information in children with open globe injuries, consistent with other studies [16, 17].

The presence of RRD during surgery was a predictor of VA. RRD can be induced during vitrectomy, especially in the presence of severe vitritis and retinitis [3]. Surgical manipulation during extraction of the IOFBs can also lead to dialysis of the ora serrata and thus RRD. In addition, artificial posterior vitreous detachment was difficult in these pediatric patients, as the vitreous gel adheres very tightly to the optic disc, macula, and retinal vasculatures, which could explain the recurrent RRD in one of our patients. Therefore, the surgeon's experience and cautious maneuvers may influence the final prognosis of pediatric patients with IOFBs.

The limitations of this study included the relatively small sample size and lack of a control group, preventing the performance of some statistical analyses and obtaining statistically significant differences. Thus, more studies with larger sample sizes are warranted.

In conclusion, the clinical features of pediatric posterior segment IOFBs were unique, including the IOFB composition and the setting where the injury occurred. The visual prognosis was favorable in this case series, and a poor visual outcome was associated with retinal detachment during removal of IOFB.

Conflicts of Interest

The authors declare that they have no conflicts of interest.

Authors' Contributions

Ting Zhang and Hong Zhuang contributed equally to this work.

Acknowledgments

This research was supported by the National Natural Science Foundation of China (81700861) and the grant from Science and Technology Commission of Shanghai Municipality (16411953700).

References

[1] X. Li, M. A. Zarbin, and N. Bhagat, "Pediatric open globe injury: a review of the literature," *Journal of Emergencies, Trauma, and Shock*, vol. 8, no. 4, pp. 216–223, 2015.

[2] C. M. Greven, N. E. Engelbrecht, M. M. Slusher, and S. S. Nagy, "Intraocular foreign bodies: management, prognostic factors, and visual outcomes," *Ophthalmology*, vol. 107, no. 3, pp. 608–612, 2000.

[3] D. Loporchio, L. Mukkamala, K. Gorukanti, M. Zarbin, P. Langer, and N. Bhagat, "Intraocular foreign bodies: a review," *Survey of Ophthalmology*, vol. 61, no. 5, pp. 582–596, 2016.

[4] J. J. Sinikumpu and W. Serlo, "Confirmed and suspected foreign body injuries in children during 2008-2013: a hospital-based single center study in Oulu University Hospital," *Scandinavian Journal of Surgery*, vol. 106, no. 4, pp. 350–355, 2017.

[5] D. J. Pieramici, P. Sternberg Jr., T. M. Aaberg Sr. et al., "A system for classifying mechanical injuries of the eye (globe). The Ocular Trauma Classification Group," *American Journal of Ophthalmology*, vol. 123, no. 6, pp. 820–831, 1997.

[6] F. Kuhn, R. Maisiak, L. Mann, V. Mester, R. Morris, and C. D. Witherspoon, "The ocular trauma score (OTS)," *Ophthalmology Clinics of North America*, vol. 15, no. 2, pp. 163–165, 2002.

[7] F. Kuhn, R. Morris, and C. D. Witherspoon, "Birmingham eye trauma terminology (BETT): terminology and classification of mechanical eye injuries," *Ophthalmology Clinics of North America*, vol. 15, no. 2, pp. 139–143, 2002.

[8] C. Yu Wai Man and D. Steel, "Visual outcome after open globe injury: a comparison of two prognostic models–the ocular trauma score and the classification and regression tree," *Eye*, vol. 24, no. 1, pp. 84–89, 2010.

[9] A. Amritanand, S. S. John, S. S. Philip, D. John, and S. David, "Unusual case of a graphite foreign body in the anterior chamber," *Clinics and Practice*, vol. 1, no. 3, p. 73, 2011.

[10] W. K. Cho, A. C. Ko, H. Eatamadi et al., "Orbital and orbitocranial trauma from pencil fragments: role of timely diagnosis and management," *American Journal of Ophthalmology*, vol. 180, pp. 46–54, 2017.

[11] A. B. Dass, P. J. Ferrone, Y. R. Chu, M. Esposito, and L. Gray, "Sensitivity of spiral computed tomography scanning for detecting intraocular foreign bodies," *Ophthalmology*, vol. 108, no. 12, pp. 2326–2328, 2001.

[12] S. N. Patel, P. D. Langer, M. A. Zarbin, and N. Bhagat, "Diagnostic value of clinical examination and radiographic imaging in identification of intraocular foreign bodies in open globe injury," *European Journal of Ophthalmology*, vol. 22, no. 2, pp. 259–268, 2012.

[13] Y. Honda and K. Asayama, "Intraocular graphite pencil lead without reaction," *American Journal of Ophthalmology*, vol. 99, no. 4, pp. 494-495, 1985.

[14] N. Hamanaka, T. Ikeda, N. Inokuchi, S. Shirai, and Y. Uchihori, "A case of an intraocular foreign body due to graphite pencil lead complicated by endophthalmitis," *Ophthalmic Surgery and Lasers*, vol. 30, no. 3, pp. 229–231, 1999.

[15] E. R. Han, W. R. Wee, J. H. Lee, and J. Y. Hyon, "A case of retained graphite anterior chamber foreign body masquerading as stromal keratitis," *Korean Journal of Ophthalmology*, vol. 25, no. 2, pp. 128–131, 2011.

[16] Y. Uysal, F. M. Mutlu, and G. Sobaci, "Ocular trauma score in childhood open-globe injuries," *Journal of Trauma: Injury, Infection, and Critical Care*, vol. 65, no. 6, pp. 1284–1286, 2008.

[17] M. M. Schorkhuber, W. Wackernagel, R. Riedl, M. R. Schneider, and A. Wedrich, "Ocular trauma scores in paediatric open globe injuries," *British Journal of Ophthalmology*, vol. 98, no. 5, pp. 664–668, 2014.

13

Outcomes of Descemet Membrane Endothelial Keratoplasty for Vitrectomized Eyes with Sutured Posterior Chamber Intraocular Lens

Norihiro Yamada,[1] Takahiko Hayashi ⓘ,[1,2,3,4,5] Kentaro Yuda,[2,3,4] Toshiki Shimizu,[2,3] Itaru Oyakawa ⓘ,[6] Hidenori Takahashi,[5] and Naoko Kato[1]

[1]Department of Ophthalmology, Saitama Medical University Hospital, Saitama, Japan
[2]Department of Ophthalmology, Yokohama City University Hospital, Yokohama, Japan
[3]Department of Ophthalmology, Yokohama Minami Kyosai Hospital, Yokohama, Japan
[4]Kikuna Yuda Eye Clinic, Yokohama, Japan
[5]Department of Ophthalmology, Jichi Medical University, Tochigi, Japan
[6]Department of Ophthalmology, Heart Life Hospital, Okinawa, Japan

Correspondence should be addressed to Takahiko Hayashi; takamed@gmail.com

Academic Editor: Karim Mohamed-Noriega

Purpose. To evaluate the clinical outcomes of Descemet membrane endothelial keratoplasty (DMEK) for vitrectomized eyes that underwent pars plana vitrectomy (PPV) and transscleral-sutured intraocular lens (IOL) implantation. *Methods.* In this retrospective study, DMEK cases were reviewed from medical records and divided into two groups: the eyes after PPV and transscleral-sutured IOL implantation (vitrectomized group) and the eyes with in-the-bag IOL implantation (control group) prior to DMEK. The main outcome measures included time of graft unfolding during surgery and best spectacle-corrected visual acuity (BSCVA), central corneal thickness (CCT), and endothelial cell density (ECD) at 1, 3, and 6 months after the DMEK. *Results.* Twenty-three eyes (vitrectomized group, $n = 8$; control group, $n = 15$) in 23 patients were included in this study. The unfolding time was significantly longer in the vitrectomized group than in the control group ($P < 0.001$). Postoperative BSCVA was worse in the vitrectomized group (0.16 ± 0.15) than in the control group (-0.06 ± 0.06; $P = 0.017$). The improvement in BSCVA was negatively correlated with the patients' age and frequency of previous surgeries. *Conclusions.* Despite the longer graft unfolding time and limited visual recovery, DMEK should be applicable to vitrectomized eyes with transscleral-sutured IOL implantation.

1. Introduction

Descemet membrane endothelial keratoplasty (DMEK) is a new method of corneal endothelial keratoplasty introduced by Melles et al. [1], which allows rapid recovery of visual acuity and minimizes immunological rejection [1–5]. The surgical steps in DMEK include careful graft preparation, safe graft insertion into the anterior chamber, recognition of graft orientation, smooth graft unfolding, and successful graft attachment in the anterior chamber by air or gas tamponade [6–13].

The eyes that are most suitable for DMEK are thought to be pseudophakic bicameral eyes with normal anterior chamber depth. When DMEK is performed on an eye containing a sutured intraocular lens (IOL), the IOL should be properly centered within the lens capsule, providing an intact iris-IOL diaphragm. Although the indications of DMEK have been widely expanded to many endothelial disorders, the eyes with iris abnormalities or sutured IOL are thought to be unsuitable for DMEK [14–18], because the graft might be lost through the peripheral iris defect or the interspace between the iris and fixed IOL [18].

Vitrectomized eyes are further challenging because the absence of vitreous pressure during surgery requires unfolding and attaching the graft using air, which is difficult. Previous reports indicated that higher rates of postoperative graft dislocation were observed following DMEK for vitrectomized eyes and required rebubbling, resulting in a higher incidence of primary graft failure [15, 18]. However, some eyes develop bullous keratopathy that requires suturing of IOLs as well as pars plana vitrectomy (PPV) prior to endothelial keratoplasty.

The purpose of the present study was to determine the clinical outcomes, postoperative complications, and features of DMEK in the eyes that underwent previous PPV and transscleral-sutured IOLs.

2. Material and Methods

2.1. Participants. This was a retrospective study, and the study protocol was approved by the Institutional Review Board of Yokohama Minami Kyosai Hospital (approval number 29_03_05) and Saitama Medical University (approval number 17-032). The research followed the tenets of the Declaration of Helsinki. Patients with bullous keratopathy who underwent DMEK at the Yokohama Minami Kyosai Hospital and Saitama Medical University Hospital from January 2016 to December 2016 and who were followed up for more than 6 months were retrospectively analyzed. In this analysis, the eyes were classified into two groups based on the status of the IOL. The "vitrectomized" group consisted of patients with eyes that underwent PPV and transscleral-sutured IOL implantation before DMEK. The control group consisted of patients who had routine IOL implantation before DMEK. The eyes that underwent previous trabeculectomy or penetrating keratoplasty or had a history of birth injury or endotheliitis were excluded. Patients who did not agree with this study or could not be followed up were not included.

2.2. Surgical Procedure

2.2.1. Donor Preparation. BBG 250® (BBG; Sigma-Aldrich, St. Louis, MO, USA) was dissolved in balanced saline solution (BSS® or BSS-plus®; Alcon, Osaka, Japan) to 0.1% (*w/v*). All grafts were peeled as described previously. BBG (0.1%, *w/v*) was used to stain the graft edges during peeling. A punch was gently placed on the endothelial surface to indent a circle 7.75, 8.0, or 8.25 mm in diameter. Subsequently, 1.0 and 1.5 mm- diameter dermatological biopsy punches (Kai Industries, Seki, Japan) were used to place asymmetric marks on the edges of the identified circles [19]. Donor grafts thus marked were stained with 0.1% (*w/v*) BBG (1.0 mg/mL) for 1 min and stored in BSS prior to insertion, 30 min later [20]. Because unfolding time depends on donor age, we usually selected donors over 60 years old.

2.2.2. Surgical Techniques. All surgeries were performed under local anesthesia. After establishing retrobulbar anesthesia and Nadbath facial nerve block, two paracenteses and a 2.8 mm upper corneal or corneoscleral incision were made for the recipient cornea. Peripheral iridotomy was performed at the 6 o'clock position to prevent a postoperative pupillary block. The donor membrane graft, stained with 0.1% (*w/v*) BBG (1.0 mg/mL), was placed into an IOL injector (model WJ-60M; Santen Pharmaceuticals, Osaka, Japan) and inserted into the anterior chamber.

The inserted graft was unfolded using a noncontact technique by shallowing the anterior chamber [13]. In the vitrectomized group, if shallowing the anterior chamber was difficult, a small amount of air was also injected between the host cornea and donor graft, and the rolled up donor graft was subsequently unfolded. After the graft was unfolded, additional air was added slowly underneath the graft from the center, and the rolled graft was gradually attached to the host cornea. The folded edges of the graft were additionally stretched using "bubble-bumping maneuver" [13]. In cases of severe bullous keratopathy, we used the chandelier illumination technique during DMEK surgery via the pars plana approach [21]. After the correct orientation was confirmed, the anterior chamber was filled with air to adhere the graft to the host cornea. Fifteen minutes later, the air was partially replaced with BSS. Finally, 0.4 mg of betamethasone (Rinderon®; Shionogi, Osaka, Japan) was subconjunctivally administered in 1.5% (*w/v*) levofloxacin eye drops (Cravit®; Santen Pharmaceuticals).

Postoperative medications included 1.5% (*w/v*) levofloxacin (Cravit) and 0.1% (*w/v*) betamethasone sodium phosphate (Sanbetasone®; Santen Pharmaceuticals) commencing at four times daily for 3 months and tapering thereafter.

2.2.3. Postoperative Follow-Up and Examinations. In addition to the standard ophthalmic examination, the best spectacle-corrected visual acuity (BSCVA), corneal endothelial cell density (ECD), central corneal thickness (CCT), and graft adaptation were evaluated both preoperatively and for up to 6 months postoperatively in all eyes. BSCVA was measured as decimal visual acuity and was converted to a logarithm of the minimum angle of resolution (LogMAR) values. Graft adaptation was assessed with both slit-lamp microscopy and an anterior segment OCT (SS1000; Tomey, Nagoya, Japan). Corneal thickness was measured by corneal tomography (SS1000; Tomey). When progressive graft detachment occurred near the central area, a rebubbling procedure was performed as described previously [22]. Preoperative ECD values were retrieved from donor eye bank records, and postoperative ECD values were measured with the aid of a specular microscope (FA3509; Konan Medical, Nishinomiya, Japan). Spectral-domain optical coherence tomography (RS 3000; Nidek, Japan) was performed 1, 3, and 6 months after DMEK. When CME was diagnosed postoperatively, topical bromfenac (Bronuck®, Senju, Pharmaceutical Co., Osaka, Japan) and sub-Tenon injection of triamcinolone acetonide (MaQaid®; Wakamoto Pharmaceutical Co., Tokyo, Japan) were immediately applied.

2.2.4. Graft Unfolding Time. The graft unfolding time was evaluated using surgical videos and compared between the two groups. The time from the first tap used to unfold the tissue to the start of air injection underneath the graft was measured and defined as the unfolding time.

TABLE 1: Patient characteristics before surgery.

	Vitrectomized group	Control group	P^*
Number of eyes	8	15	
Sex (male/female)	5/3	3/12	0.051^*
Age	72.8 ± 10.5	74.1 ± 5.1	$0.906^{\dagger}$
Eye (R/L)	3/5	7/8	0.632^*
BSCVA (LogMAR)	1.15 ± 0.60	0.98 ± 0.52	$0.795^{\dagger}$
CCT (μm)	765 ± 63	722 ± 88	$0.194^{\dagger}$
Frequency of previous surgeries	3.11 ± 0.78	1	**<0.001**

BSCVA: best spectacle-corrected visual acuity; CCT: central corneal thickness; L: left; LogMAR: logarithm of the minimal angle of resolution; R: right. $^*\chi^2$ test (comparison between two groups); †unpaired t-test.

2.2.5. Statistical Analysis. The Wilcoxon test or paired t-test was used to compare values preoperatively and postoperatively, as appropriate. The Mann–Whitney U test or unpaired t-test was used to compare values between the two groups, as appropriate. Due to the distribution of unfolding times, they were compared using the two-sided Student's t-test after logarithmic transformation. The male/female and right/left ratios were compared using the chi-square test. To explore related factors, multiple regression analysis with stepwise variable selection (minimum Bayesian information criterion, increasing number of variables) was performed. All analyses were performed using JMP Pro Software version 11.2.0 (SAS Institute, Cary, NC, USA). A P value < 0.05 was considered statistically significant.

3. Results

3.1. Patients. Twenty-three eyes in 23 patients (8 men and 15 women) were considered eligible for the study. Eight eyes came from the vitrectomized group, and the other fifteen eyes came from the control group. Ages ranged from 52 to 82 years (mean, 73.8 years). Preoperative patient profiles of the two groups are summarized in Table 1.

In the present study, the frequency of previous surgeries prior to DMEK was 3.11 ± 0.78 in the vitrectomized group. In contrast, only phacoemulsification and simultaneous IOL implantation were performed in the control group. The comparison between the two groups was statistically significant ($P < 0.001$).

3.1.1. Vitrectomized Group. Eight eyes had previously undergone PPV and transscleral-sutured IOL implantation (vitrectomized group). Five of the eight eyes showed an aphakic state derived from complicated cataract surgeries, one eye underwent phacoemulsification and aspiration for pseudoexfoliation syndrome, and two eyes underwent intracapsular cataract extraction. These latter three eyes revealed pseudoexfoliation corneal endotheliopathy. One of the three eyes underwent aspiration for congenital cataract during childhood, after which the patient used a hard contact lens for a long time. Another eye was implanted with an IOL that was

subluxated, which required the extraction of the lens and the secondary implantation of a new lens.

In three eyes, bullous keratopathy was caused by vitreoretinal surgeries; two had undergone pars plana vitrectomy for rhegmatogenous retinal detachment with silicone oil injection, while one had pars plana vitrectomy with silicone oil injection for endophthalmitis after cataract surgery. Detailed patient profiles of the vitrectomized group are summarized in Table 2.

3.1.2. Control Group. Fifteen eyes underwent routine cataract surgery with in-the-bag IOL implantation prior to DMEK (control group). Six eyes had Fuchs' corneal endothelial dystrophy, nine had iatrogenic bullous keratopathy, six underwent argon laser iridotomy, and three were subjected to phacoemulsification and IOL implantation.

3.2. Visual Acuity. In the vitrectomized group, BSCVA improved from 1.15 ± 0.60 preoperatively to 0.37 ± 0.19 at 1 month, 0.28 ± 0.15 at 3 months, and 0.16 ± 0.15 at 6 months. In the control group, BSCVA improved from 0.98 ± 0.52 preoperatively to 0.20 ± 0.23 at 1 month, 0.07 ± 0.12 at 3 months, and -0.06 ± 0.06 at 6 months. A statistically significant improvement in BSCVA was obtained in the vitrectomized group at all observation points ($P = 0.011$ at 1 month, 0.005 at 3 months, and 0.003 at 6 months). A statistically significant improvement of BSCVA was also obtained in the control group at all observation points ($P = 0.002$ at 1 month, 0.001 at 3 months, and 0.001 at 6 months). The BSCVA in the control group was significantly better than that in the vitrectomized group at all the examination points ($P = 0.795$ preoperatively, 0.032 at 1 month, 0.007 at 3 months, and 0.017 at 6 months; Figure 1).

3.3. Central Corneal Thickness. In the vitrectomized group, the CCT decreased from $764.5 \pm 62.7 \mu m$ preoperatively to $529.5 \pm 56.6 \mu m$ at 1 month, 520.6 ± 51.6 at 3 months, and 513.3 ± 43.3 at 6 months. In the control group, the CCT decreased from $722.0 \pm 88.8 \mu m$ preoperatively to $555.9 \pm 64.8 \mu m$ at 1 month, 507.3 ± 53.7 at 3 months, and 513.8 ± 52.9 at 6 months. A statistically significant improvement in CCT was observed in each group at all examination points ($P < 0.001$, Wilcoxon rank sum test in both groups). There was no significant difference in CCT between the two groups at any examination point. The P values were 0.194 preoperatively, 0.136 at 1 month, 1.0 at 3 months, and 0.810 at 6 months.

3.4. Corneal Endothelial Cell Density. In the vitrectomized group, the donor corneal ECD decreased from 2629 ± 303 cells/mm^2 preoperatively to 1728 ± 429 cells/mm^2 at 1 month, 1620 ± 414 cells/mm^2 at 3 months, and 1548 ± 401 cells/mm^2 at 6 months postoperatively ($40.7 \pm 11.2\%$ less than the preoperative value of the donor graft). In the control group, the donor corneal ECD decreased from 2707 ± 238 cells/mm^2 preoperatively to 2021 ± 466 cells/mm^2 at 1 month, 1837 ± 440 cells/mm^2 at 3 months, and 1679 ± 419 cells/mm^2 at 6 months postoperatively ($38.2 \pm 18.6\%$ less than the preoperative value of the donor graft). There was no significant difference in ECD between the two groups at

TABLE 2: Profiles of the enrolled patients (vitrectomized group).

Case	Sex	Age	OD/OS	Etiology for PPV	Previous surgeries	Preop BSCVA	Preop CCT (μm)	Treatment before DMEK
1	F	79	OD	PEX	PEA, PPV + IOLs	20/2000	793	
2	M	79	OS	PEX	ICCE, PPV + IOLs	20/1000	724	
3	F	74	OS	PEX	ICCE + PPV + IOLs, DSAEK	20/200	836	ASR
4	F	52	OS	Extended CL wearing	Cataract aspiration, PPV + IOLs	20/50	672	
5	F	64	OS	Dropped IOL	PPV + IOLs	20/2000	734	ASR
6	F	56	OS	RRD	PPV + SOi, SOr + IOLs	20/50	757	
7	M	79	OD	RRD	PPV + SOi, SOr + IOLs	20/500	939	ASR
8	M	74	OD	Endophthalmitis	PPV + IOLr + SOi, SOr + IOLs	20/100	658	ASR

ASR: anterior segment reconstruction; BSCVA: best spectacle-corrected visual acuity; CCT: central corneal thickness; DMEK: Descemet membrane endothelial keratoplasty; ICCE: intracapsular cataract extraction; IOLr: removal of intraocular lens; IOLs: transscleral-sutured posterior chamber intraocular lens implantation; OD: right eye; OS: left eye; PEA: phacoemulsification and aspiration; PEX: pseudoexfoliation syndrome; PPV: pars plana vitrectomy; Preop: preoperative; RRD: rhegmatogenous retinal detachment; SOi: silicone oil injection; SOr: silicon oil extraction.

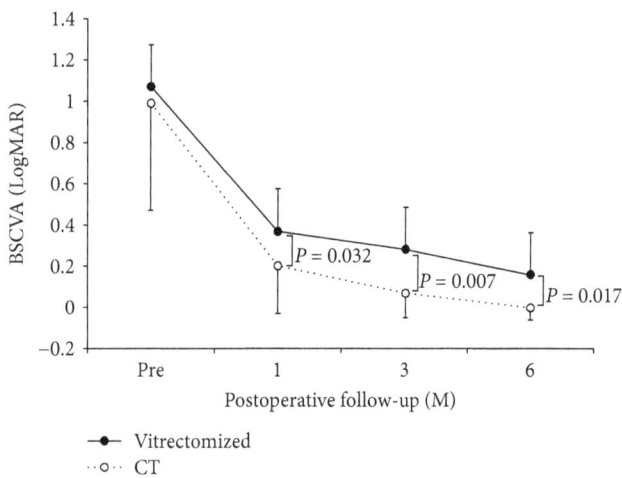

FIGURE 1: Changes in best spectacle-corrected visual acuity (BSCVA). Statistically significant improvement in BSCVA was seen in the vitrectomized group ($P = 0.011$ at 1 month, 0.005 at 3 months, and 0.003 at 6 months; Wilcoxon rank sum test). In the control group, a statistically significant improvement of BSCVA was seen at all observation points ($P = 0.002$ at 1 month, 0.001 at 3 months, and 0.001 at 6 months; Wilcoxon rank sum test). There was also a statistically significant difference in BSCVA between the two groups at all postoperative examinations ($P = 0.795$ preoperatively, 0.032 at 1 month, 0.007 at 3 months, and 0.017 at 6 months; Mann–Whitney U test). Vitrectomized: vitrectomized group; CI: confidence interval; CT: control group.

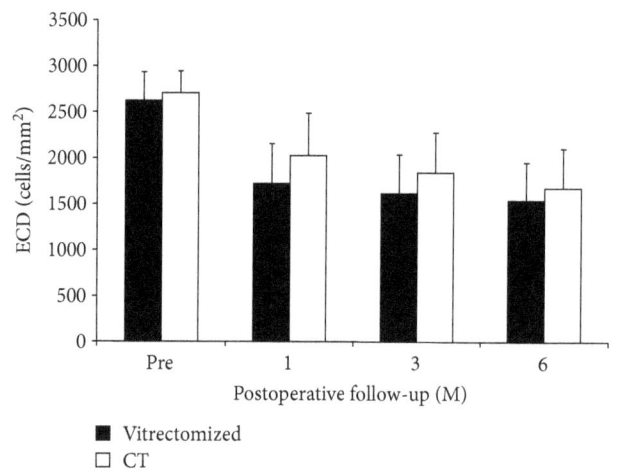

FIGURE 2: Changes in endothelial cell density (ECD). In the vitrectomized group, the donor corneal ECD decreased from 2629 ± 303 cells/mm^2 preoperatively to 1548 ± 401 cells/mm^2 at 6 months postoperatively ($40.7 \pm 11.2\%$ less than the preoperative value of the donor graft). In the control group, the donor corneal ECD decreased from 2707 ± 238 cells/mm^2 at preoperative point to 1679 ± 419 cells/mm^2 at 6 months postoperatively ($38.2 \pm 18.6\%$ less than the preoperative value of the donor graft). There was no significant difference in ECD between the two groups at any pre- and postoperative points (P value = 0.832 preoperatively, 0.136 at 1 month, 0.259 at 3 months, and 0.526 at 6 months; Mann–Whitney U test). Vitrectomized: vitrectomized group; CI; confidence interval; CT; control group.

any pre- and postoperative points (Figure 2). The P values were 0.832 preoperatively, 0.136 at 1 month, 0.259 at 3 months, and 0.526 at 6 months.

3.5. Graft Unfolding Time. The geometric mean of the graft unfolding time was 19.0 min in the vitrectomized group (95% confidence interval (CI), 13.4–24.7) and 7.1 min in the control group (95% CI, 3.2–10.9). The graft unfolding time was significantly longer in the vitrectomized group than the control group ($P < 0.001$; Figure 3).

3.6. Complications after DMEK. None of the eyes showed intraoperative complications. Rebubbling for partial detachment was required in two eyes (25.0%) of the vitrectomized group and in four eyes (26.7%) of the control group; no significant difference between the two groups was observed ($P = 0.554$). CME was present in four eyes (50.0%) in the vitrectomized group and two eyes (13.3%) in the control group ($P = 0.081$). In all affected eyes, the CME resolved with topical bromfenac and sub-Tenon injection of

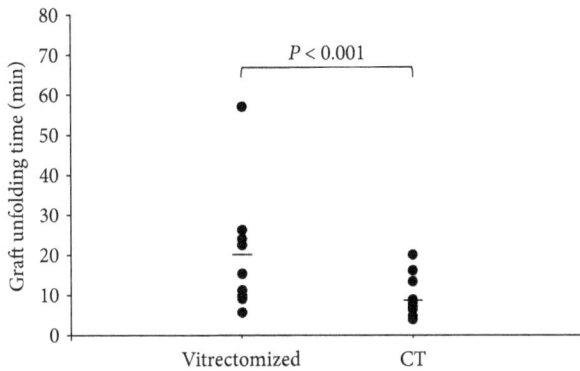

FIGURE 3: Comparison of graft unfolding time. Graft unfolding time was significantly longer in the vitrectomized group than in the control group (*$P < 0.001$). The geometric mean graft unfolding time (indicated with bars) was 19.0 min in the vitrectomized group and 7.1 min in the control group. Vitrectomized: vitrectomized group; CI; confidence interval; CT; control group.

triamcinolone acetonide. The mean BSCVA at 6 months after DMEK was 0.11 ± 0.12 in the eyes without CME and 0.037 ± 0.14 in the eyes with CME ($P = 0.30$).

3.7. BSCVA Prognosis-Related Factors. For BSCVA prognosis, we performed multiple regression analysis after stepwise variable selection. We used BSCVA at 6 months after DMEK as the response variable, and age, anterior chamber depth before DMEK, axial length, frequency of previous surgeries, graft unfolding time, and baseline BSCVA were examined as explanatory variables. The results are summarized in Table 3. After stepwise selection, age (estimated value $- 0.006$, $P = 0.007$) and frequency of previous surgeries (estimated value $= 0.015$, $P < 0.001$) were obtained as significant factors.

4. Discussion

The present investigation indicated that DMEK could be successfully performed in vitrectomized eyes with transscleral-sutured IOL, even though the graft unfolding times were significantly longer in the vitrectomized eyes. BSCVA was significantly improved in both groups, and postoperative CCT, ECD, and complication rates were comparable between the two groups.

In vitrectomized eyes, unfolding the graft can be challenging because the anterior chamber becomes shallow. Indeed, the geometric mean of the graft unfolding time was 19.0 min in the vitrectomized group, significantly longer than that of the control group (7.1 min; $P < 0.001$). This result is consistent with previous findings [23]. Yoeruek et al. reported 55% rebubbling rates after DMEK for postvitreous surgery, while 10% showed iatrogenic primary graft failure in the immediate postoperative period [15]. Weller et al. reported that graft detachments were observed in 45.8% of cases [14]. These previous findings indicate that longer manipulation to unfold the graft may cause more endothelial damage to the transplanted grafts. Fortunately, there was no primary graft failure, and the rebubbling

TABLE 3: Multiple regression analysis for correlates of postoperative best spectacle-corrected visual acuity (BSCVA).

Predictor	Estimated value	SE	P value
Age	0.00061	0.0021	**0.009**
AXL	Unselected		0.95
ACD	Unselected		0.26
Frequency of previous surgeries	0.11	0.016	**<0.001**
Unfolding time	Unselected		0.95
CME	Unselected		0.45
Preoperative BSCVA	Unselected		0.68

SE: standard error; AXL: axial length; ACD: anterior chamber depth; CME: cystoid macular edema. Multivariate analysis was constructed after stepwise variable selection (BIC, forward method).

rates were 22.2% in the vitrectomized group and 26.7% in the controls, with no group difference. Similarly, the ratio of ECD decrease at 6 months after DMEK was comparable between the two groups, with $40.7 \pm 11.2\%$ in the vitrectomized group and $38.2 \pm 18.6\%$ in the control group. These results indicate that careful preparation and manipulation during surgery might have contributed to successful DMEK even in the vitrectomized eyes.

The results suggest some important points for performing DMEK on the eyes that have undergone transscleral-sutured IOL implantation combined with PPV. First, an intact iris-IOL diaphragm is necessary. In such eyes, anterior segment reconstruction by suturing the iris could be necessary before DMEK. In the present investigation, we performed anterior segment reconstruction in four of the eight eyes in the vitrectomized group. Second, the position of the transscleral-sutured IOL is important. If the intraocular lens was sutured far posterior from the iris, the graft could be lost into the interspace between the iris and IOL or fall into the vitreous cavity [24]. Careful preoperative selection of the eyes and appropriate anterior segment reconstruction are thus necessary for successful DMEK.

Although the postoperative BSCVA significantly improved in both the vitrectomized and the control groups, it was also significantly lower in the vitrectomized group than in the control group. To clarify the underlying cause for this difference, we performed multiple regression analysis after stepwise variable selection for BSCVA prognosis, and the results showed that the patients' age and the frequency of the previous surgeries were highly related to the postoperative BSCVA. Similar findings that the visual acuity of younger patients tended to improve have also been reported after other ocular surgeries, such as cataract surgery and vitrectomy for macular hole [25–27]. Several factors, including unrecognized or subclinical comorbidity, age-related changes in macular function, and the tendency to perceive functional impairment irrespective of vision in elderly people, could have contributed to these differences [28].

Another important factor affecting postoperative BSCVA was the frequency of previous surgeries. Postoperative BSCVA has been reported to be worse for previous repeated intraocular surgeries including penetrating keratoplasty,

Boston keratoplasty, and PPV [29–31]. Repeated surgeries may cause persistent inflammation, elevated intraocular pressure, and/or insufficient ocular circulation, resulting in deteriorated retinal function. Moreover, precisely centering the IOL can be difficult for the eyes with transscleral-sutured IOL, also contributing to BSCVA impairment. However, this aspect was not evaluated in the present study. The worse BSCVA in the vitrectomized group compared with the control group may thus be caused by various factors.

Flanary et al. reported that the incidence of CME was 8.0% (7 among 88 eyes) after staged DMEK that was performed within 6 months after cataract surgery and 7.1% (6 among 85 eyes) in solitary DMEK performed more than 6 months after cataract surgery [32]. According to a cohort study by Heinzelmann et al., 13% of the eyes developed a single episode of CME during the follow-up time after DMEK [33]. In the current study, the incidence of development of CME was similar to that of previous reports in the control group (13.3%), but much higher in the vitrectomized group (50.0%), although there was no significant difference between the two groups. Furthermore, CME occurrence was not significantly correlated with postoperative BSCVA (0.110 versus 0.037, resp.; $P = 0.300$). We speculate that this is probably because we applied topical bromfenac and sub-Tenon injection of triamcinolone acetonide immediately upon the detection of CME postoperatively. However, further studies are still needed to ascertain the influence of CME on the final visual outcome after DMEK.

Our findings indicate that we could obtain comparable outcomes with respect to the mean ECD and complication rates using DMEK for typical pseudophakic nonvitrectomized eyes. Moreover, DMEK could produce excellent visual outcomes and low rejection rates. Even in complex cases such as vitrectomized eyes, we observed impressive visual recovery after DMEK. In fact, the BSCVA in one case improved from 20/200 to 20/50, despite the fact that the patient had been limited to 20/100 after previous DSAEK. Caution should be exercised in the selection of the candidates, including presurgical preparation such as creating an intact iris-IOL diaphragm. Careful postoperative evaluation of the occurrence of CME and its immediate treatment may also contribute to improvement of the surgical outcomes.

5. Conclusion

In conclusion, DMEK can improve visual function in the eyes that underwent previous PPV and transscleral-sutured IOL implantation.

Conflicts of Interest

The authors declare that there is no conflict of interest regarding the publication of this paper.

Authors' Contributions

Norihiro Yamada and Takahiko Hayashi contributed equally to this work.

References

[1] G. R. J. Melles, T. S. Ong, B. Ververs, and J. van der Wees, "Descemet membrane endothelial keratoplasty (DMEK)," *Cornea*, vol. 25, no. 8, pp. 987–990, 2006.

[2] T. Tourtas, K. Laaser, B. O. Bachmann, C. Cursiefen, and F. E. Kruse, "Descemet membrane endothelial keratoplasty versus Descemet stripping automated endothelial keratoplasty," *American Journal of Ophthalmology*, vol. 153, no. 6, pp. 1082–1090.e2, 2012.

[3] A. Anshu, M. O. Price, and F. W. Price Jr., "Risk of corneal transplant rejection significantly reduced with Descemet's membrane endothelial keratoplasty," *Ophthalmology*, vol. 119, no. 3, pp. 536–540, 2012.

[4] T. Hayashi, S. Yamagami, K. Tanaka et al., "Immunologic mechanisms of corneal allografts reconstituted from cultured allogeneic endothelial cells in an immune-privileged site," *Investigative Ophthalmology & Visual Science*, vol. 50, no. 7, pp. 3151–3158, 2009.

[5] M. Ang, M. R. Wilkins, J. S. Mehta, and D. Tan, "Descemet membrane endothelial keratoplasty," *British Journal of Ophthalmology*, vol. 100, no. 1, pp. 15–21, 2016.

[6] I. Dapena, L. Ham, K. Droutsas, K. van Dijk, K. Moutsouris, and G. R. J. Melles, "Learning curve in Descemet's membrane endothelial keratoplasty: first series of 135 consecutive cases," *Ophthalmology*, vol. 118, no. 11, pp. 2147–2154, 2011.

[7] E. C. Hamzaoglu, M. D. Straiko, Z. M. Mayko, C. S. Sales, and M. A. Terry, "The first 100 eyes of standardized Descemet stripping automated endothelial keratoplasty versus standardized Descemet membrane endothelial keratoplasty," *Ophthalmology*, vol. 122, no. 11, pp. 2193–2199, 2015.

[8] J. R. Nussbaumer, S. Alloju, and W. Chamberlain, "Clinical outcomes of Descemet membrane endothelial keratoplasty during the surgeon learning curve versus Descemet stripping endothelial keratoplasty performed at the same time," *Journal of Clinical & Experimental Ophthalmology*, vol. 7, no. 5, 2016.

[9] C. Monnereau, R. Quilendrino, I. Dapena et al., "Multicenter study of Descemet membrane endothelial keratoplasty: first case series of 18 surgeons," *JAMA Ophthalmology*, vol. 132, no. 10, pp. 1192–1198, 2014.

[10] F. Arnalich-Montiel, A. Pérez-Sarriegui, and A. Casado, "Impact of introducing 2 simple technique modifications on the Descemet membrane endothelial keratoplasty learning curve," *European Journal of Ophthalmology*, vol. 27, no. 1, pp. 16–20, 2016.

[11] M. Ang, J. S. Mehta, S. D. Newman, S. B. Han, J. Chai, and D. Tan, "Descemet membrane endothelial keratoplasty: preliminary results of a donor insertion pull-through technique using a donor mat device," *American Journal of Ophthalmology*, vol. 171, pp. 27–34, 2016.

[12] T. Hayashi, I. Oyakawa, and N. Kato, "Techniques for learning Descemet membrane endothelial keratoplasty for eyes of Asian patients with shallow anterior chamber," *Cornea*, vol. 36, no. 3, pp. 390–393, 2017.

[13] I. Dapena, K. Moutsouris, K. Droutsas, L. Ham, K. van Dijk, and G. R. Melles, "Standardized "no-touch" technique for Descemet membrane endothelial keratoplasty," *Archives of Ophthalmology*, vol. 129, no. 1, pp. 88–94, 2011.

[14] J. M. Weller, T. Tourtas, and F. E. Kruse, "Feasibility and outcome of Descemet membrane endothelial keratoplasty in complex anterior segment and vitreous disease," *Cornea*, vol. 34, no. 11, pp. 1351–1357, 2015.

[15] E. Yoeruek, G. Rubino, T. Bayyoud, and K. U. Bartz-Schmidt, "Descemet membrane endothelial keratoplasty in vitrectomized eyes: clinical results," *Cornea*, vol. 34, no. 1, pp. 1–5, 2015.

[16] N. Sorkin, A. Einan-Lifshitz, Z. Ashkenazy et al., "Enhancing Descemet membrane endothelial keratoplasty in postvitrectomy eyes with the use of pars plana infusion," *Cornea*, vol. 36, no. 3, pp. 280–283, 2017.

[17] H. Yazu, T. Yamaguchi, M. Dogru, N. Ishii, Y. Satake, and J. Shimazaki, "Descemet-stripping automated endothelial keratoplasty in eyes with transscleral-sutured intraocular lenses," *Journal of Cataract & Refractive Surgery*, vol. 42, no. 6, pp. 846–854, 2016.

[18] V. S. Liarakos, L. Ham, I. Dapena et al., "Endothelial keratoplasty for bullous keratopathy in eyes with an anterior chamber intraocular lens," *Journal of Cataract & Refractive Surgery*, vol. 39, no. 12, pp. 1835–1845, 2013.

[19] A. Matsuzawa, T. Hayashi, I. Oyakawa et al., "Use of four asymmetric marks to orient the donor graft during Descemet's membrane endothelial keratoplasty," *BMJ Open Ophthalmology*, vol. 1, no. 1, article e000080, 2017.

[20] T. Hayashi, K. Yuda, I. Oyakawa, and N. Kato, "Use of brilliant blue G in Descemet's membrane endothelial keratoplasty," *BioMed Research International*, vol. 2017, Article ID 9720389, 5 pages, 2017.

[21] T. Shimizu, T. Hayashi, K. Yuda et al., "Chandelier illumination for Descemet membrane endothelial keratoplasty," *Cornea*, vol. 36, no. 9, pp. 1155–1157, 2017.

[22] M. Dirisamer, K. van Dijk, I. Dapena et al., "Prevention and management of graft detachment in Descemet membrane endothelial keratoplasty," *Archives of Ophthalmology*, vol. 130, no. 3, pp. 280–291, 2012.

[23] E. Yoeruek, T. Bayyoud, J. Hofmann, and K.-U. Bartz-Schmidt, "Novel maneuver facilitating Descemet membrane unfolding in the anterior chamber," *Cornea*, vol. 32, no. 3, pp. 370–373, 2013.

[24] N. A. Afshari, M. S. Gorovoy, S. H. Yoo et al., "Dislocation of the donor graft to the posterior segment in Descemet stripping automated endothelial keratoplasty," *American Journal of Ophthalmology*, vol. 153, no. 4, pp. 638–642.e2, 2012.

[25] C. M. Mangione, R. S. Phillips, M. G. Lawrence, J. M. Seddon, E. J. Orav, and L. Goldman, "Improved visual function and attenuation of declines in health-related quality of life after cataract extraction," *Archives of Ophthalmology*, vol. 112, no. 11, pp. 1419–1425, 1994.

[26] P. Gogate, V. Vakil, R. Khandekar, M. Deshpande, and H. Limburg, "Monitoring and modernization to improve visual outcomes of cataract surgery in a community eyecare center in western India," *Journal of Cataract and Refractive Surgery*, vol. 37, no. 2, pp. 328–334, 2011.

[27] Y. Kim, E. S. Kim, S. Y. Yu, and H. W. Kwak, "Age-related clinical outcome after macular hole surgery," *Retina*, vol. 37, no. 1, pp. 80–87, 2017.

[28] T. Y. Wong, "Effect of increasing age on cataract surgery outcomes in very elderly patients," *BMJ*, vol. 322, no. 7294, pp. 1104–1106, 2001.

[29] V. Patel, M. R. Moster, L. Kishfy et al., "Sequential versus concomitant surgery of glaucoma drainage implant and Boston keratoprosthesis type 1," *European Journal of Ophthalmology*, vol. 26, no. 6, pp. 556–563, 2016.

[30] M. Vanathi, N. Sharma, R. Sinha, R. Tandon, J. S. Titiyal, and R. B. Vajpayee, "Indications and outcome of repeat penetrating keratoplasty in India," *BMC Ophthalmology*, vol. 5, no. 1, p. 26, 2005.

[31] E. Moisseiev, I. D. Fabian, J. Moisseiev, and A. Barak, "Outcomes of repeated pars plana vitrectomy for persistent macular holes," *Retina*, vol. 33, no. 6, pp. 1137–1143, 2013.

[32] W. E. Flanary, J. M. Vislisel, M. D. Wagoner et al., "Incidence of cystoid macular edema after Descemet membrane endothelial keratoplasty as a staged and solitary procedure," *Cornea*, vol. 35, no. 8, pp. 1040–1044, 2016.

[33] S. Heinzelmann, P. Maier, D. Böhringer, S. Hüther, P. Eberwein, and T. Reinhard, "Cystoid macular oedema following Descemet membrane endothelial keratoplasty," *British Journal of Ophthalmology*, vol. 99, no. 1, pp. 98–102, 2015.

14

Outcomes of Wound Dehiscence after Penetrating Keratoplasty and Lamellar Keratoplasty

Xin Wang,[1,2] Ting Liu,[3] Sai Zhang,[1,2] Xiaolin Qi,[2] Suxia Li,[2] Weiyun Shi,[2] and Hua Gao ⓘ[2]

[1]*Qingdao University, Qingdao 266071, China*
[2]*Shandong Eye Hospital, Shandong Eye Institute, Shandong Academy of Medical Sciences, Jinan 250021, China*
[3]*Qingdao Eye Hospital, Shandong Eye Institute, Shandong Academy of Medical Sciences, Qingdao 266071, China*

Correspondence should be addressed to Hua Gao; gaohua100@126.com

Academic Editor: Mehmet Borazan

Objective. To investigate the incidence, causes, occurrence time, and range of wound and outcomes of wound dehiscence in patients treated by penetrating keratoplasty (PK) or lamellar keratoplasty (LK). *Methods.* We retrospectively reviewed medical records of keratoplasty in Shandong Eye Hospital from January 2006 to June 2017. Thirty-one eyes of 30 patients had sustained wound dehiscence (WD) after surgical treatment. The surgical type, causes, occurrence time, extent of the wound, treatment, and outcomes were recorded. *Results.* The study population consisted of 26 men and 4 women. The mean age at the occurrence of WD was 44.6 years old (range: 12–78 years), and the mean time from keratoplasty to WD was 45.9 months (range: 1–204 months). WD occurred in 23 eyes (23/1385, 1.66%) after PK and 8 eyes (8/1632, 0.49%) after LK ($p < 0.05$). Twenty-seven eyes (27/31, 87.0%) had trauma-induced dehiscence. The mean range of dehiscence was 5.5 o'clock. The vision ranged from 20/50 to light perception after wound suture. The eyes receiving LK had fewer serious complications than PK. *Conclusions.* Compared with LK, PK seems to be more prone to result in wound dehiscence. The WD after LK may be less severe. The visual acuity after treatment of WD can be worse in the eyes with PK than LK.

1. Introduction

Corneal diseases represent the second leading cause of blindness globally. Keratoplasty is the major surgical procedure for visual restoration of corneal blindness. Corneal wound dehiscence (WD) is not an uncommon complication after keratoplasty. Although its incidence is relatively low, compared with other complications [1], WD may lead to delayed visual recovery, corneal graft edema, immune rejection, endophthalmitis, suprachoroidal hemorrhage, severe, and even irreversible damage to the vision function [2, 3]. In the recent decade, lamellar keratoplasty (LK) has an increasing trend. Due to retaining of the posterior corneal stroma, it theoretically has better biomechanical stability and might reduce the risk of postoperative WD. In the current study, we retrospectively reviewed medical records of keratoplasty in our hospital and analyzed the patient characteristics, causative factors, clinical features, and outcomes of WD in patients with penetrating keratoplasty (PK) or LK.

2. Methods

From January 2016 to June 2017, 3017 keratoplasties were performed in Shandong Eye Hospital, including 1385 PK surgeries, 1632 LK surgeries, and 75 endothelial transplantations. The patients were 1988 males and 1029 females. We retrospectively reviewed the medical records of these patients and recorded the characteristics, risk factors, and outcomes of corneal WD in patients with different surgical approaches. Data collected included patient age and gender, indication for keratoplasty, surgical procedures, duration between keratoplasty and WD, causative events for WD, size of dehiscence, treatment procedures, and vision outcomes after surgical repair.

All patients with WD were given eye shields or glasses to protect the eyes before treated with emergency corneal graft surgery. Patients who did not have eye content exposure or other serious complications underwent original corneal graft repair under topical anesthesia or general anesthesia. In the

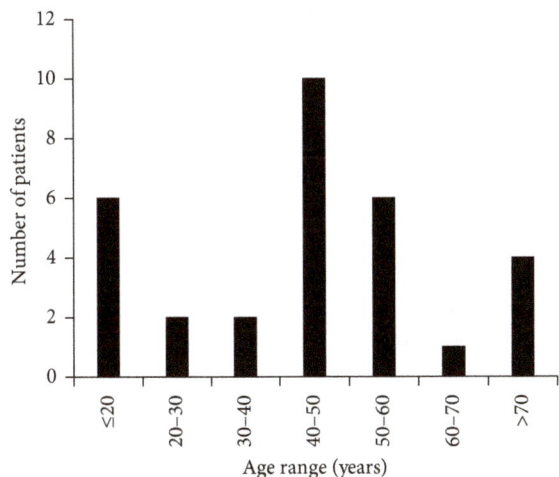

FIGURE 1: Age of patients with wound dehiscence.

eyes with iris or vitreous prolapse, corneal graft rejoint surgery was performed, and complicated fundus surgery was combined if needed. WD was sutured using 10-0 nylon sutures. Postoperatively, systemic and intravenous antibiotics were administered, as well as topical antirejection drugs. All data analyses were performed using SPSS statistical software (version 17.0, SPSS, Inc, Chicago, Illinois, USA). Quantitative data are presented as the mean ± standard deviation (range). A value of $p < 0.05$ was considered statistically significant.

3. Results

3.1. Patient Demography and Indications for Keratoplasty. Thirty-one eyes from 30 patients (1.0%) suffered WD after keratoplasty, including 26 males (86.7%) and 4 females (13.3%). The age span of the patients with WD was between 12 and 78 years old with the mean age being 44.6 ± 18.3 years old (Figure 1). The patients included 18 farmers, 4 students, two civil servants, one freelancer, one hobo, and 5 with unknown professions. The follow-up was 1–5 years.

The corneal graft WD occurred in 23 eyes (23/31, 74.2%) after PK and 8 eyes (8/31, 25.1%) after LK. The incidence of WD after PK and LK was 1.66% and 0.49%, respectively ($p = 0.01$). The major indications for PK among these patients were fungal keratitis (8 eyes, 34.8%), herpes simplex virus keratitis (5 eyes, 21.7%), keratoconus (3 eyes, 13.0%), and bullous keratopathy (3 eyes, 13.0%). The common indications for LK included keratoconus (4 eyes, 50.0%), fungal keratitis (2 eyes, 25.0%), interstitial keratitis (1 eye, 12.5%), and ocular chemical injury (1 eye, 12.5%) (Figure 2). The mean interval between the initial keratoplasty and occurrence of WD was 45.9 months, with 61.3% within 4 years; the mean interval between the initial PK procedure and WD was 45.0 ± 36.4 months, with 56.5% within 4 years (range, 1 to 126 months); and the mean interval between the initial LK and WD was 48.4 ± 66.2 months, with 75% within 3 years (range 5 to 204 months) (Figure 3).

3.2. Causes and Severity of Wound Dehiscence. As shown in Table 1, WD resulted from known trauma in 27 eyes (87.0%), was spontaneous in 4 eyes (13.0%), and had an unknown

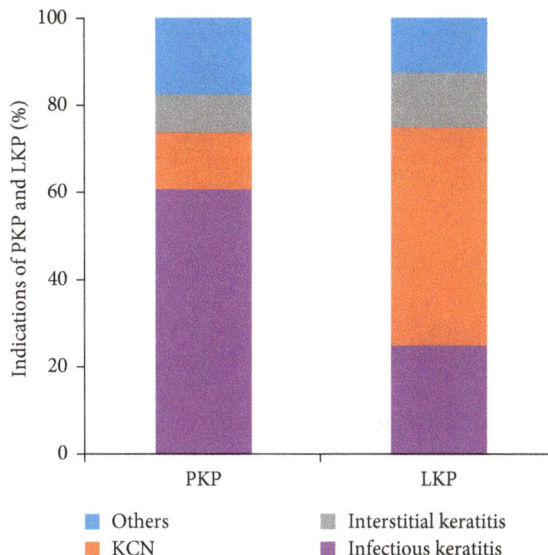

FIGURE 2: The indications of PK and LK.

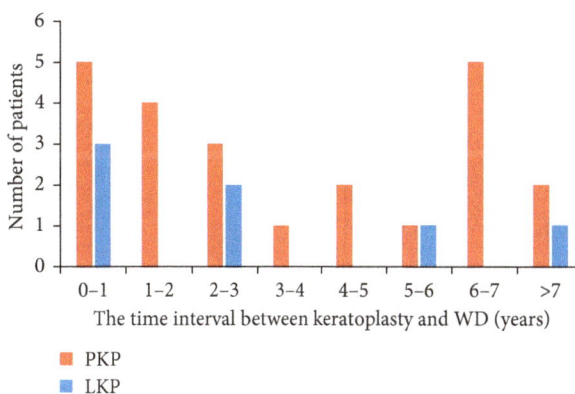

FIGURE 3: The time interval between keratoplasty and occurrence of WD.

predisposing cause in 6 eyes (19.4%). The specific trauma treated by PK included strike by obvious objects (41.9%), spontaneous injury (12.9%), strike by no obvious cause (19.4%), hurt by hand or elbow (22.6%), and accidental falling (3.2%). Twenty-two of the 30 patients purchased protective goggles, but none had worn protective goggles when they were injured.

Slit lamp examination showed that the corneal fissure was located in the corneal graft-host interface. Nearly one-third (10/31) of the eyes had sutures in place after trauma. 37.5% of the eyes with LK had sutures, while 30.4% of the eyes with PK had sutures in place. The suture technique used in the keratoplasty was interrupted suture. The mean range of dehiscence was 5.5 o'clock in the eyes with sutures, while 5.2 o'clock in the eyes without sutures. There is no significant difference in wound dehiscence ($p > 0.05$). And there is also no statistical significance ($p > 0.05$) in PK or LK. Two cases were excluded in that we did not know the location of WD. The mean range of dehiscence was 5.7 o'clock in all the eyes, 5.1 o'clock in the eyes with LK, and 5.9 o'clock in the eyes with PK. WD covered 1–3 clock hours in 6 eyes (20.7%), 4–6 clock hours in 11 eyes (37.9%), 7–9 clock hours in 11 eyes (37.9%), and 10–12 clock hours in one eye (3.5%).

TABLE 1: Characteristics of wound dehiscence following keratoplasty.

Case	Indication for keratoplasty	Type of keratoplasty	Age at the time of trauma (years)	Cause of trauma	Interval between trauma and keratoplasty (months)	Final visual acuity
1	PBK	PK	40	Unknown	6	FC/BE
2	HSK	PK	51	Struck by iron drill	13	FC/20 cm
3	KCN	PK	17	Finger poke	76	LP
4	FK	PK	58	Struck by own hand	2	20/400
5	HSK	PK	48	Spontaneous	1	20/1000
6	PBK	PK	75	Struck by wooden stick	29	20/167
7	Bacterial keratitis	PK	71	Struck by wooden stick	13	LP
8	HSK	PK	62	Unknown	99	HM/10 cm
9	Corneal endothelial decompensation	PK	42	Spontaneous	126	LP
10	PBK	PK	78	Spontaneous	52	20/500
11	FK	PK	48	Struck by desk	61	20/1000
12	FK	PK	54	Unknown	12	HM/BE
13	FK	PK	45	Struck by rebar	22	20/400
14	FK	PK	12	Struck by book	27	HM/50 cm
15	KCN	PK	19	Struck by phone	34	20/67
16	KCN	PK	23	Struck by basketball	21	20/200
17	FK	PK	49	Struck by shoes	1.5	20/133
18	HSK	PK	60	Struck by wooden stick	84	20/167
19	FK	PK	43	Struck by cabbage	48	FC/BE
20	FK	PK	29	Fall	56	HM/40 cm
21	Interstitial keratitis	PK	53	Punch	84	20/67
22	Corneal perforation	PK	50	Struck by door	84	20/133
23	Interstitial keratitis	PK	53	Punch	84	20/40
24	Ocular chemical injury	LK	46	Struck by cages	204	HM/BE
25	FK	LK	39	Punch	24	20/200
26	KCN	LK	16	Struck by elbow	28	Unknown
27	FK	LK	72	Struck by own hand	72	20/50
28	Interstitial keratitis	LK	47	Unknown	11	HM/30 cm
29	KCN	LK	48	Unknown	5	20/400
30	KCN	LK	16	Spontaneous	31	20/80
31	KCN	LK	20	Unknown	12	20/67

PBK, pseudophakic bullous keratopathy; HSK, herpes simplex virus; KCN, keratoconus; FK, fungal keratitis; PK, penetrating keratoplasty; LK, lamellar keratoplasty; HM, hand moving; FC, finger counting; BE, before eyes; LP, light perception.

Four patients after PK and 2 after LK had wound disruption of 1 to 3 clock hours. Seven after PK and 4 after LK had wound disruption of 4 to 6 clock hours. Nine after PK and 2 after LK had wound disruption of 7 to 9 clock hours. One after PK had disruption of 10–12 clock hours. The wound dehiscence encompassed the inferior temporal quadrant in 4 eyes (26.7%), inferior nasal quadrant in 6 eyes (40.0%), superior nasal quadrant in 9 eyes (60.0%), and superior temporal quadrant in 10 eyes (66.7%). The wound dehiscence with 180° or more occurred in 14 eyes (48.3%) with 12 eyes in PK and 2 eyes in LK. And the incidence of extensive wound dehiscence is not different between PK and LK ($p > 0.05$).

3.3. Accompanied Complications. With the increase in the range of corneal WD, the degree of eye prolapses increased. Accompanied complications included iris prolapse in 5 eyes (16.1%), lens expulsion or dislocation in 15 eyes (48.4%), and extrusion of vitreous in 11 eyes (35.5%). In the eyes treated by PK, the complications were iris prolapse in 4 eyes, lens

expulsion or dislocation in 15 eyes, and extrusion of vitreous in 10 eyes. In the eyes treated by LK, the complications were iris prolapse in 1 eye and extrusion of vitreous in 1 eye. The lens in one eye and the vitreous in the other eyes were not seen clearly. The extrusion of the lens and vitreous mainly occurred in the patients with an extent of wound disruption ≥ 6 o'clock hours (7/10, 70%).

3.4. Therapeutic Outcomes. The duration between the occurrence of corneal graft dehiscence and therapy was 2 to 72 hours. Among 31 eyes of 30 patients, 31 eyes, including 22 eyes after PK and 8 eyes after LK, just had the graft repaired, and only 1 eye after PK was treated with combined anterior chamber angioplasty surgery because of flat anterior chamber.

Final visual acuity was 20/200 or better in 12 eyes (40%), better than hand motions (HM) to 20/200 in 11 eyes (36.7%), HM to light perception (LP) in 7 eyes (23.3%), and unknown in one eye. In the follow-up period, BCVA was improved in 19 eyes (65.5%), including 16 eyes with PK and 3 eyes with

LK, unchanged in 9 eyes (31.0%), including 6 eyes with PK and 3 eyes with LK, and decreased in one eye with LK (3.5%). Patients after treatment of LK achieved better final visual acuity than those after PK, but the final visual acuity and the recovery of visual acuity were of no statistical significance ($p > 0.05$). In addition, patients with LK were less likely to suffer lens loss ($p < 0.05$). Although LK patients had less extrusion of the lens ($p > 0.05$) and vitreous ($p > 0.05$), there was no significant difference. Furthermore, there was no difference in the range of WD between PK and LK ($p > 0.05$).

4. Discussion

The cornea never regains the original tensile strength after keratoplasty [4], whether PK or LK. There is a risk of corneal WD in the postoperative cornea. The incidence of WD after corneal transplantation ranges from 0.6% to 5.8% [3, 5, 6], and one major reason is trauma reported to be 1.28%–2.53% [5–8]. In our study, the incidence of WD after keratoplasty was 1.0%, lower than the other reports. This may be because some patients were treated in the local medical units and were not referred to our hospital.

It was reported that the incidence of WD was related to age. Older people were found to be more likely to develop graft WD [5]. In contrast, some researchers believed that young patients with keratoconus were more liable to develop WD [9–11]. In our series, no significant age-related findings were found with 4 (12.9%) patients of less than 18 years old and 6 patients (19.4%) of more than 60 years old. Men were reported to be the majority of the injured patients [5]. Considering the working environment of our patients, farmers and students (61.3%) were easy to be hurt because their protective measures were poorer than other occupations. Wearing protective goggles was very necessary to avoid WD.

WD after keratoplasty has been divided into traumatic WD and spontaneous WD. In our study, the incidence of traumatic WD was 87.1%, but we also needed to notice that there were some cases with no obvious causes. Long-term using of topical corticosteroids could increase the risk of corneal WD after the removal of sutures [7]. The safety and side effects of postoperative glucocorticoid therapy should not be ignored. Since immunosuppressive agents could be partially replaced with topical corticosteroids, the amount of corticosteroids may be reduced and topical immunosuppressive eye drops are administered instead [7].

It was reported that corneal WD mostly occurred within two years. The mean interval between keratoplasty and WD was 45.9 months in our study, and dehiscence occurred during the first 4 years in 61.3% of the eyes. The longest duration between keratoplasty and WD occurrence in China was 9 years [12], and the longest in our survey was 17 years. According to Tran et al., the longest was 20 years [13]. All traumatic WDs were observed to occur in the corneal graft-host interface [3, 14], and our finding is consistent with it. This phenomenon indicated that the tensile strength of corneal graft-host junction after keratoplasty was weaker than original corneal tensile strength. It will never regain the same level of normal intact tissue even in many years. An experimental investigation disclosed that the junction after

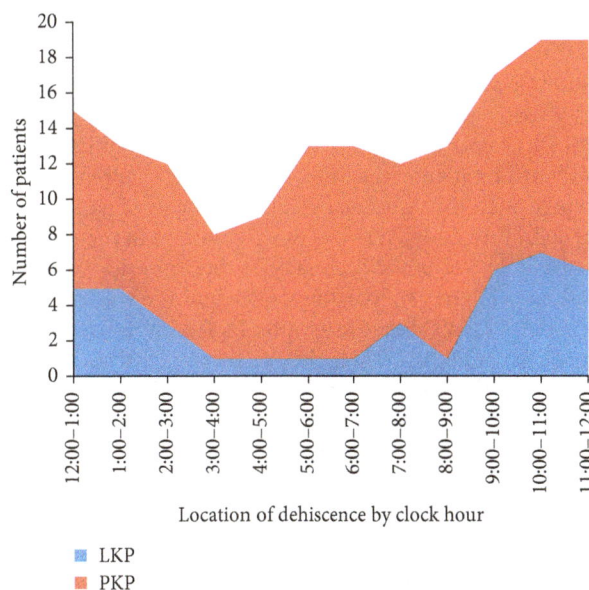

FIGURE 4: The location of wound dehiscence.

corneal transplantation could never return to normal intensity. In addition, increasing evidence indicated that WD was a lasting risk in all patients undergoing keratoplasty, regardless of their age, the type of operation, indication for surgery, and time to dehiscence after corneal transplantation [15]. Therefore, such patients should pay attention to take long-term protective measures such as wearing safety glasses.

In our hospital, the sutures were removed within 1.5 years. Therefore, the sutures were in place in the eyes in which WD happened within 1.5 years. To our surprise, we found that WD without sutures did not lead to more extensive WD compared with those with sutures. So we think that the remaining sutures did not affect WD. The extend of graft dehiscence attributed to the trauma after WD. This result was not consistent with other reports. We think the reason may be that our sample is too small. Meyer found that leaving sutures may maintain the integrity of the graft-host junction and dehiscence with sutures led to less dehiscence [16]. Even in the different type of operation, the remaining sutures did not help the eyes to have lower rate of WD. And the rate has no significant difference in LK or PK.

In the current study, the type of operation was found to be an important factor of the occurrence of WD. The incidence of WD was 1.66% after PK and 0.49% after LK ($p < 0.05$). We could get a primary conclusion that LK, compared with PK, was less liable to lead to WD. Retaining the posterior corneal stroma during LK can better recover vision and lower postoperative complications.

WD may result in many serious ocular complications including iris prolapse, crystalline or intraocular lens expulsion or dislocation, and extrusion of vitreous. As previously reported, lens expulsion or dislocation was associated with poor prognosis and the final visual acuity. We noticed that PK patients tended to suffer more severe complications from WD. The reason may be that the cornea still remained a part of the autologous corneal tissue after LK and was protected with the help of full thickness of the Descemet membrane [17, 18].

Once WD occurs, the degree of injury would directly affect the patient prognosis. It was reported that in patients with poor prognosis after injury, only 1/3 to 1/2 of patients had visual acuity of 20/200 [19]. In our patients with WD, only 9 had corrected visual acuity of 20/200, and the visual acuity of 11 patients was below FC. With the increase in the range of WD, the visual acuity and prognosis of patients got worse. In this study, WD was more common in the superior quadrant of the graft, especially in the superior temporal quadrant (Figure 4). We think this quarter was prone to occurrence of WD because temporal quadrant is without the help of the bone [18]. Then, the graft was directly faced with trauma. So the incidence of WD may be higher in the superior temporal quadrant. However, our opinion was not consistent with other reports. Farley and Petit reported that most of the eyes had dehiscence in the inferior quadrant because of lack of protection by the nose and eyelids [20]. And there was no quadrant that was prone to WD in previous observations [5, 21]. We also think that the specific trauma may decide the direction and location of the WD.

In conclusion, WD is a risk factor for patients undergoing corneal transplant. Compared with LK, PK seems to be more prone to result in wound dehiscence. The WD after LK may be less severe. The visual acuity after treatment of WD can be worse in the eyes with PK than LK. To reduce the incidence of WD after corneal transplantation, the patient's condition needs to be comprehensively analyzed before selecting appropriate surgical approaches, regular postoperative follow-up is important, and the protective awareness of the patient and family members should be improved.

Conflicts of Interest

The authors have no conflicts of interests to declare.

Acknowledgments

This work was supported by the National Natural Science Foundation of China (81370989, 81570821, and 81530027), Science and Technology Development Program of Shandong Province (2016GSF201182), Taishan Scholar Program (20081148), the Natural Science Foundation of Shandong Province (ZR2015YL026), and Innovation Project of Shandong Academy of Medical Sciences.

References

[1] M. Fiorentzis, B. Seitz, and A. Viestenz, "Traumatic keratoplasty rupture resulting from continuous positive airway pressure mask," *Cornea*, vol. 34, no. 6, pp. 717–719, 2015.

[2] A. Viestenz, W. Schrader, M. Küchle et al., "Management of a ruptured globe," *Der Ophthalmologe*, vol. 105, no. 12, pp. 1163–1174, 2008.

[3] M. Kawashima, T. Kawakita, S. Shimmura, K. Tsubota, and J. Shimazaki, "Characteristics of traumatic globe rupture after keratoplasty," *Ophthalmology*, vol. 116, no. 11, pp. 2072–2076, 2009.

[4] D. J. Pettinelli, C. E. Starr, and W. J. Stark, "Late traumatic corneal wound dehiscence after penetrating keratoplasty," *Archives in Ophthalmology*, vol. 123, no. 6, pp. 853–856, 2005.

[5] S. H. Tseng, S. C. Lin, and F. K. Chen, "Traumatic wound dehiscence after penetrating keratoplasty: clinical features and outcome in 21 cases," *Cornea*, vol. 18, no. 5, pp. 553–558, 1999.

[6] B. Kartal, B. Kandemir, T. Set et al., "Traumatic wound dehiscence after penetrating keratoplasty," *Turkish Journal of Trauma and Emergency Surgery*, vol. 20, no. 3, pp. 181–188, 2014.

[7] A. Foroutan, S. A. Tabatabaei, M. J. Behrouz, R. Zarei, and M. Soleimani, "Spontaneous wound dehiscence after penetrating keratoplasty," *International Journal of Ophthalmology*, vol. 7, no. 5, pp. 905–908, 2014.

[8] D. Pahor, "Characteristics of traumatic versus spontaneous wound dehiscence after penetrating keratoplasty," *Klinische Monatsblätter für Augenheilkunde*, vol. 230, no. 8, pp. 808–813, 2013.

[9] A. R. Foroutan, G. H. Gheibi, M. Joshaghani, A. Ahadian, and P. Foroutan, "Traumatic wound dehiscence and lens extrusion after penetrating keratoplasty," *Cornea*, vol. 28, no. 10, pp. 1097–1099, 2009.

[10] M. R. Jafarinasab, S. Feizi, H. Esfandiari, B. Kheiri, and M. Feizi, "Traumatic wound dehiscence following corneal transplantation," *Journal of Ophthalmic and Vision Research*, vol. 7, no. 3, pp. 214–218, 2012.

[11] U. Rehany and S. Rumelt, "Ocular trauma following penetrating keratoplasty: incidence, outcome, and postoperative recommendations," *Archives of Ophthalmology*, vol. 116, no. 10, pp. 1282–1286, 1998.

[12] T. Wang, W. Y. Shi, H. Gao, S. Fang, J. Zhao, and L. X. Xie, "Investigation of graft dehiscence after penetrating keratoplasty," *Zhongguo Shi Yong Yan ke Za Zhi*, vol. 24, no. 9, pp. 952–956, 2006.

[13] T. H. Tran, P. Ellies, F. Azan, E. Assaraf, and G. Renard, "Traumatic globe rupture following penetrating keratoplasty," *Graefe's Archive for Clinical and Experimental Ophthalmology*, vol. 243, no. 6, pp. 525–530, 2005.

[14] J. F. Ma, C. J. Rapuano, K. M. Hammersmith, P. K. Nagra, Y. Dai, and A. A. Azari, "Outcomes of wound dehiscence post-penetrating keratoplasty," *Cornea*, vol. 35, no. 6, pp. 778–783, 2016.

[15] P. F. Tzelikis, E. M. Fenelon, R. R. Yoshimoto, G. P. Rascop, R. L. Queiroz, and W. T. Hida, "Traumatic wound dehiscence after corneal keratoplasty," *Arquivos Brasileiros de Oftalmologia*, vol. 78, no. 5, pp. 310–312, 2015.

[16] J. J. Meyer and C. N. McGhee, "Incidence, severity and outcomes of traumatic wound dehiscence following penetrating and deep anterior lamellar keratoplasty," *British Journal of Ophthalmology*, vol. 100, no. 10, pp. 1412–1415, 2016.

[17] S. Zarei-Ghanavati, M. Zarei-Ghanavati, and S. Sheibani, "Traumatic wound dehiscence after deep anterior lamellar keratoplasty: protective role of intact descemet membrane after big-bubble technique," *Cornea*, vol. 29, no. 2, pp. 220-221, 2010.

[18] M. B. Goweida, H. A. Helaly, and A. A. Ghaith, "Traumatic wound dehiscence after keratoplasty: characteristics, risk factors, and visual outcome," *Journal of Ophthalmology*, vol. 2015, Article ID 631409, 5 pages, 2015.

[19] E. Abou-Jaoude, M. Brooks, D. G. Katz et al., "Spontaneous wound dehiscence after removal of single continuous penetrating keratoplasty suture," *Ophthalmology*, vol. 109, no. 7, pp. 1291–1296, 2002.

[20] M. K. Farley and T. H. Petit, "Traumatic wound dehiscence after penetrating keratoplasty," *American Journal of Ophthalmology*, vol. 104, pp. 44–49, 1987.

[21] M. A. Williams, S. D. Gawley, A. J. Jackson et al., "Traumatic graft dehiscence after penetrating keratoplasty," *Ophthalmology*, vol. 115, no. 2, pp. 276–278, 2008.

15

Characteristics of New Onset Herpes Simplex Keratitis after Keratoplasty

Xiaolin Qi ⓘD, Miaolin Wang ⓘD, Xiaofeng Li ⓘD, Yanni Jia ⓘD, Suxia Li ⓘD, Weiyun Shi ⓘD, and Hua Gao

Shandong Eye Hospital, Shandong Eye Institute, Shandong Academy of Medical Sciences, Jinan, China

Correspondence should be addressed to Hua Gao; gaohua100@126.com

Academic Editor: Nóra Szentmáry

Purpose. To observe clinical characteristics and treatment outcomes of new onset herpes simplex keratitis (HSK) after keratoplasty. *Methods.* Among 1,443 patients (1,443 eyes) who underwent keratoplasty (excluding cases of primary HSK) in Shandong Eye Hospital, 17 patients suffered postoperative HSK. The clinical manifestations, treatment regimens, and prognoses of the patients were evaluated. *Results.* The incidence of new onset HSK after keratoplasty was 1.18%. Epithelial HSK occurred in 10 eyes, with dendritic epithelial infiltration in 6 eyes and map-like epithelial defects in 4 eyes. Nine eyes had lesions at the junction of the graft and recipient. Stromal necrotic and endothelial HSK occurred in 7 eyes, presenting map-shaped ulcers in the entire corneal graft and recipient (two eyes) or at the graft-recipient junction (five eyes). Confocal microscopy revealed infiltration of a large number of dendritic cells at the junction of the lesion and transparent cornea. All 10 eyes with epithelial lesions and two eyes suffering stromal lesions of ≤1/3 corneal thickness healed after systematic and local antiviral treatment. Best-corrected visual acuity and corneal graft transparency were restored. For stromal HSK with an ulcer of >1/3 corneal thickness, amniotic membrane transplantation was performed, and visual acuity and graft transparency decreased significantly. *Conclusion.* New onset HSK after keratoplasty primarily resulted in epithelial and stromal lesion, involving both the graft and recipient. Effective treatments included antiviral medications and amniotic membrane transplantation. Delayed treatment may lead to aggravated graft opacification.

1. Introduction

It is possible that keratoplasty induces herpes simplex keratitis (HSK), resulting in epithelial defects or ulcers in the grafts, even if the patient has no history of viral keratitis [1–4]. The majority of related studies have just been case reports with no systematic reports of clinical characteristics, typing, and diagnosis or treatment. The diagnosis of HSK is usually difficult, and this viral infection is often confused with infectious ulcers or immunological rejection of the corneal graft, leading to inappropriate use of antiinfective drugs or glucocorticoids, thereby adversely affecting or even exacerbating the disease. To provide more information about the clinical diagnosis and management, we retrospectively analyzed clinical data from patients with new onset HSK after keratoplasty and evaluated the clinical characteristics, diagnoses, and treatment methods.

2. Materials and Methods

2.1. Patients. This study was approved by the Institutional Review Board of Shandong Eye Hospital and adhered to the tenets of the Declaration of Helsinki. Clinical data of 1,443 patients who underwent keratoplasty (excluding cases of primary HSK) from January 2013 to January 2017 in our hospital with a regular follow-up of more than 1 year were retrospectively analyzed. HSK was identified in 17 patients (17 eyes) during the postoperative follow-up. The diagnostic criteria of HSK included (1) subjective symptoms of the affected eye, including redness and swelling, paresthesia, photophobia, tearing, and decreased visual acuity; (2) typical eye signs like dendritic or map-like infiltration or ulcers, terminal expansion, positive fluorescein sodium staining, discoid edema of the stroma, and substantial keratic precipitates (KPs); (3) negative results of corneal scraping smear examination for bacteria and fungi and laser confocal microscopy for fungal hyphae and amoeba cysts; and (4) gradual improvement of the patient after systemic and local antiviral medications [5–7].

2.2. Outcome Measures. The medical history included symptoms associated with the patient's complaint, the time of HSK onset, medication, changes in disease condition, and recurrence. Best-corrected visual acuity (BCVA), intraocular pressure (IOP), typical eye signs, corneal graft transparency, and epithelial integrity were recorded. In vivo confocal microscopy (HRT3; Heidelberg Engineering, Dossenheim, Germany) was used to observe epithelial and stromal inflammatory changes of the corneal graft and the distribution of dendritic cells. RTVue optical coherence tomography (OCT; Optovue, Fremont, California, USA) was used to clarify the depth of corneal stromal lesions.

3. Results

The incidence of new onset HSK after keratoplasty was 1.18% during the follow-up period of 38 ± 14.7 months (range, 10–55 months). The patients were 10 males and 7 females, aged 4–67 years (mean, 51 ± 15.1 years). The primary lesions included bacterial corneal ulcers in 8 eyes, immune-related corneal ulcers in 4 eyes, corneal leucoma in 2 eyes, fungal corneal ulcers in 2 eyes, and keratoconus in 1 eye. The surgical treatment was penetrating keratoplasty for 10 eyes and anterior lamellar keratoplasty for 7 eyes. All donor corneal tissues were provided by Shandong Red Cross Eye Bank.

All 17 patients denied repeated symptoms of redness, photophobia, tearing, decreased vision, and other symptoms of HSK. The time interval between keratoplasty and HSK onset was 11.7 ± 9 months, with the earliest case occurring at 1 month postoperatively. The onset time was postoperative 1–3 months for 2 eyes, 3–6 months for 3 eyes, 6–12 months for 6 eyes, 12–18 months for 4 eyes, and 18–24 months for 2 eyes.

3.1. Clinical Manifestations. Sudden eye swelling, pain with rubbing, photophobia, tearing, decreased visual acuity, and other discomforts in the affected eye were noted by 15 patients. The average duration from the onset to seeking treatment was 5.4 ± 1.6 days (3.9 ± 1.3 days for epithelial lesions and 7.9 ± 2.6 days for stromal necrotic lesions).

The BCVA of the 17 eyes decreased after the onset of HSK by 2 lines in eight eyes, 3–4 lines in four eyes, and 5–6 lines in five eyes. The IOP was within the normal range in all eyes.

HSK in 10 eyes was epithelial type. Six eyes had dendritic epithelial infiltration, terminal expansion, and positive fluorescein sodium staining with no obvious edema of the graft (Figure 1). Among them, the lesion was located in the center of the graft in one eye and at the junction of the graft and recipient in five eyes. The other four eyes had mild edema in the corneal graft with map-like epithelial defects, terminal expansion, and positive fluorescein sodium staining (Figure 2). Defective areas were located at the junction of the graft and recipient between 4 and 6o'clock, with an area of

approximately $4 \times 6 \, \mathrm{mm}^2$. The endothelial cell layer had a relatively large amount of finely pigmented KPs.

Stromal necrotic and endothelial HSK was found in seven eyes, presenting with edema in the corneal graft and map-shaped ulcers. Five eyes had lesions located at the junction of the graft and recipient between 4 and 6o'clock, with an area of approximately $4 \times 8 \, \mathrm{mm}^2$; the endothelial cell layer had a relatively large amount of finely pigmented KPs (Figures 3 and 4). Two of them displayed ulcers covering the entire corneal graft and involving the whole transplant bed (Figure 5).

Moreover, anterior chamber reaction was graded as +1 flare and +1 cell. No HSK recurred after medical or surgical management.

3.2. In Vivo Confocal Microscopy. In the eyes with epithelial HSK, the epithelial cells in the lesions were swollen and necrotic. Few or no subbasal nerve plexuses were observed. A large number of dendritic cells and basal epithelial cells formed netting via long interdigitating dendrites. The anterior elastic layer was damaged. The polygonal cells of the stromal cells in the superficial stromal layer showed enhanced reflectivity and were arranged in a cross-hatched pattern, but most nuclei were not visible. Little KPs were observed in the endothelial cell layer (Figure 6).

For the stromal necrotic and endothelial type, scanning images of the stromal cells in the lesions were unclear, showing a large amount of inflammatory cell infiltration. At the junction of the lesion and transparent cornea, however, a large number of dendritic cells, basal epithelial cells, and subbasal nerve plexuses were observed to form netting via long interdigitating dendrites. Lots of KPs were present in the endothelial cell layer (Figure 7).

3.3. Rtvue OCT. Corneal OCT was mainly used to identify the depth of the stromal lesions. Among the 7 eyes with stromal necrosis, 2 eyes had an ulcer ≤1/3 corneal thickness and 5 eyes had an ulcer >1/3 corneal thickness. In the two eyes with the entire corneal graft affected, the ulcer depth was up to 1/2 corneal thickness.

3.4. Treatment and Outcomes. Systemic and local antiviral therapy was administered in all 17 patients. Acyclovir was given intravenously (5 mg/kg) every 8 hours for 7 days, and then Aciclovir Tablets ($3 \times 400 \, \mathrm{mg}$) were given orally for 3 months. Moreover, 0.1% acyclovir eye drops (Wuhan Wujing Pharmaceutical Co., Wuhan, China) were used every 2 hours. For cases of epithelial HSK, the use of glucocorticoids was prohibited. For cases of stromal and endothelial HSK, 0.1% fluorometholone eye drops (Santen, Osaka, Japan), tobramycin dexamethasone eye drops (Alcon, Puurs, Belgium), and tobramycin dexamethasone eye ointment (Alcon, Puurs, Belgium) were employed based on disease conditions.

In all eyes with epithelial type lesions, epithelial infiltration disappeared after systemic and local antiviral treatment and was resolved within an average of 3.2 ± 1.9

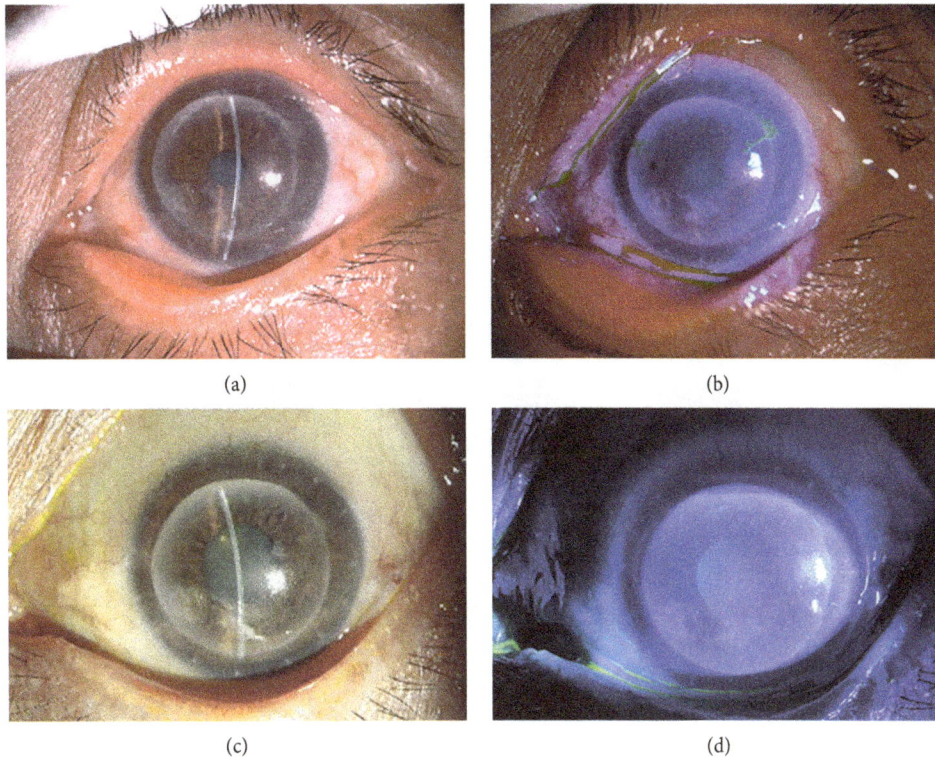

FIGURE 1: Slit lamp examination of patient 1 with epithelial HSK. (a) Two years after deep anterior lamellar keratoplasty for corneal leucoma. (b) Dendritic epithelial infiltration, terminal expansion, and positive fluorescein sodium staining at 2 and 10o'clock and the junction of the graft and recipient. (c) Epithelial infiltration disappearance after systemic and local antiviral treatment. (d) Negative fluorescein sodium staining.

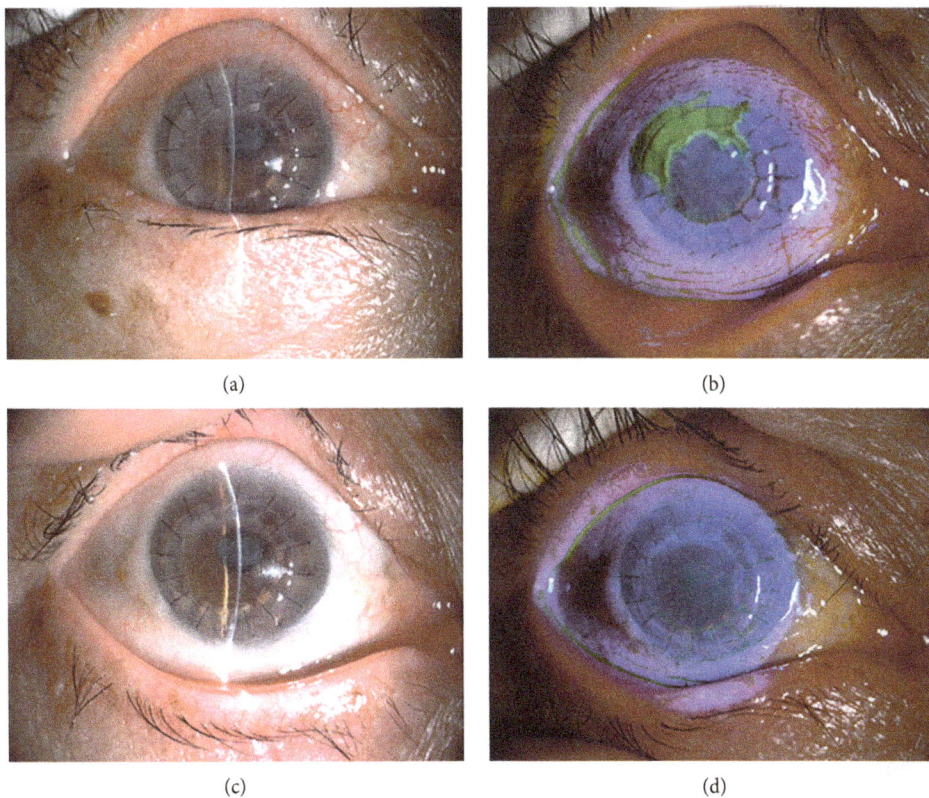

FIGURE 2: Slit lamp examination of patient 2 with epithelial HSK. (a) Two months after penetrating keratoplasty for bacterial corneal ulcers. (b) Map-shaped fluorescein sodium staining at the junction of the graft and recipient between 9 and 1o'clock. (c) The healed epithelium and clear cornea after systemic and local antiviral treatment. (d) Negative fluorescein sodium staining.

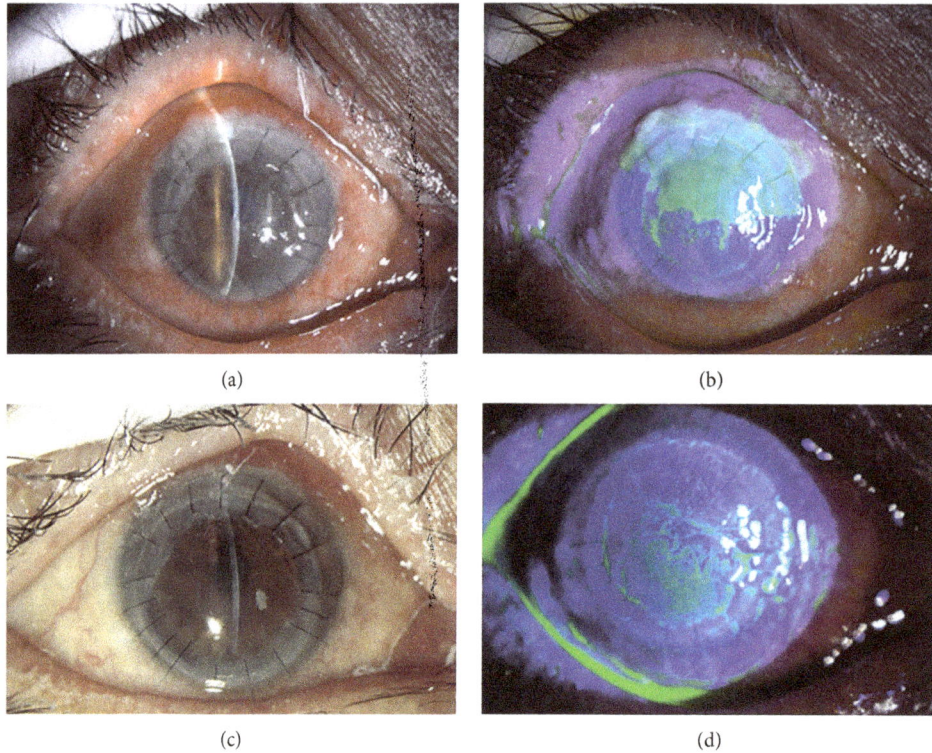

FIGURE 3: Slit lamp examination of patient 3 with stromal necrotic and endothelial HSK. (a) The edematous corneal graft at 6 months after penetrating keratoplasty for fungal corneal ulceration. (b) Map-shaped ulceration at the junction of the graft and recipient between 10 and 3o'clock. (c) The healed ulcer and clear cornea after systemic and local antiviral treatment. (d) Negative fluorescein sodium staining.

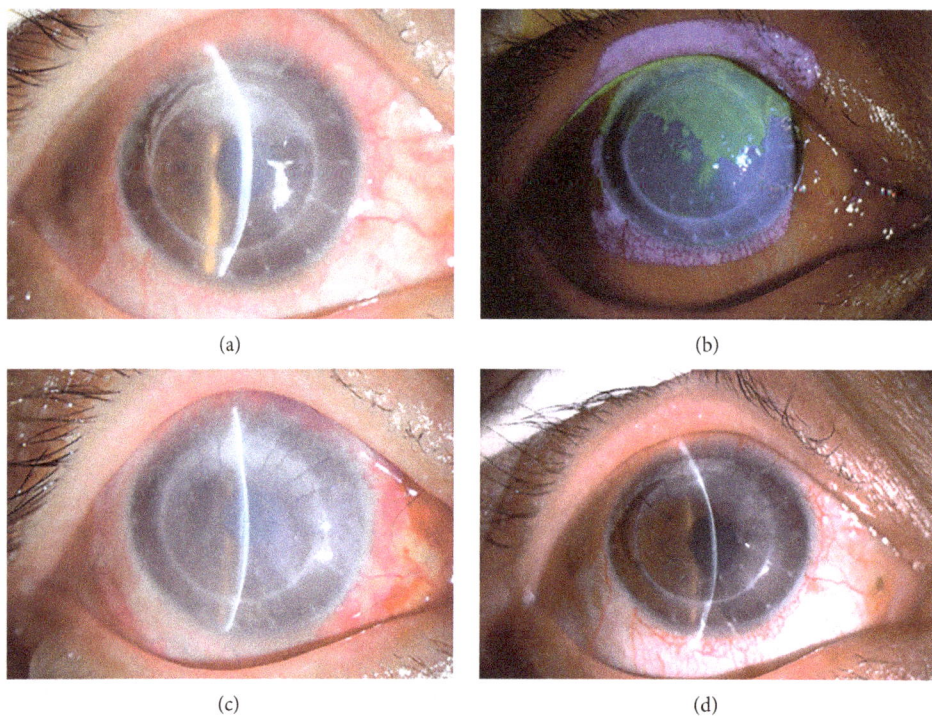

FIGURE 4: Slit lamp examination of patient 4 with stromal necrotic and endothelial HSK. (a) The edematous corneal graft at one and a half years after penetrating keratoplasty for bacterial corneal ulceration. (b) Map-shaped ulceration at the junction of the graft and recipient between 10 and 2o'clock. (c) The ulcer healing after amniotic membrane transplantation. (d) The corneal clarity was decreased.

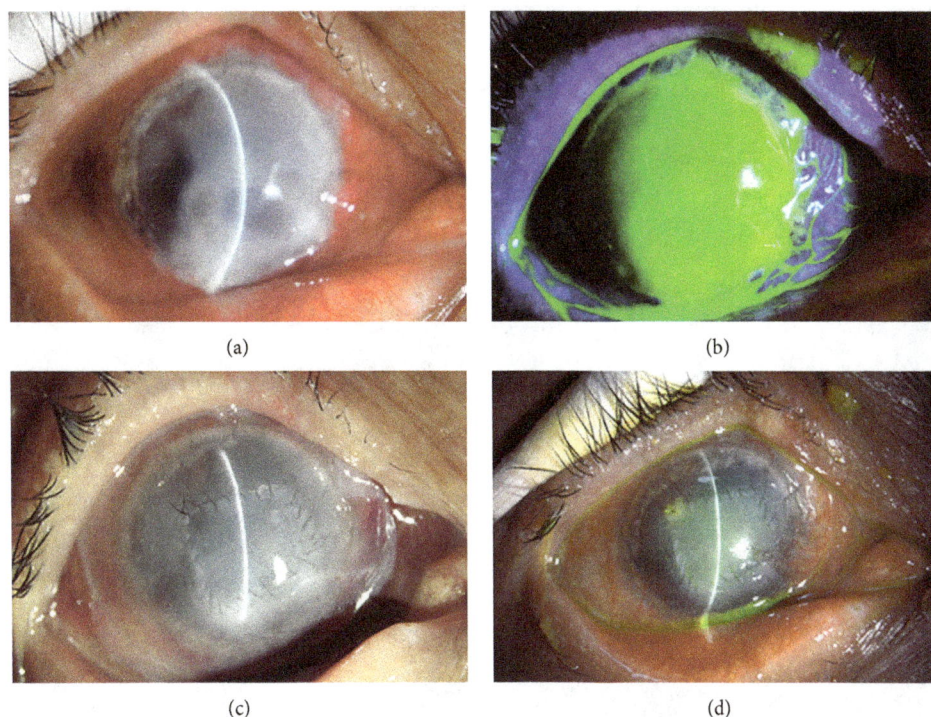

FIGURE 5: Slit lamp examination of patient 4 with stromal necrotic and endothelial HSK. (a) Corneal graft edema and opacity at one and a half years after penetrating keratoplasty for bacterial corneal ulceration. (b) Fluorescein sodium staining displaying ulceration of the entire corneal graft involving the whole transplant bed. (c) The ulcer healing after double amniotic membrane transplantation. (d) The residual amniotic membrane at the final follow-up. The corneal clarity was decreased significantly.

days (Figures 1 and 2). The BCVA was restored to the level before disease onset with a transparent corneal graft.

For patients with stromal necrotic lesions, the treatment options and the prognoses were closely related to the depth of the ulcers. The ulcers in two eyes with an ulcer ≤1/3 corneal thickness healed after systemic and local antiviral treatment, with an average healing time of 7.5 days, and the BCVA was restored to the level before HSK onset (Figure 3). In the five patients with an ulcer >1/3 corneal thickness, the ulcers did not heal after systemic and local antiviral treatment. Two patients with the entire corneal graft involved refused to undergo a second keratoplasty; therefore, double amniotic membrane transplantation was performed, and these ulcers healed after 18.5 days (Figure 5). The patients exhibited a BCVA of 3–4 lines less than that before disease onset, decreased transparency of the corneal grafts, and scars at the ulcer healing sites. The remaining 3 patients underwent amniotic membrane transplantation with an average healing time of 12.3 days (Figure 4). They exhibited a BCVA of 1–2 lines less than that before disease onset, decreased transparency of the corneal grafts, and scars at the ulcer healing sites.

4. Discussion

Recurrent herpetic keratitis is a leading cause of infectious blindness in the world [8, 9]. Ophthalmic surgery, especially keratoplasty, can induce the onset of HSK, even if the patient has never had symptoms of herpes simplex virus infection

prior to surgery [10–12]. Due to its low incidence, many physicians lack adequate understanding of the clinical manifestations of HSK. Misdiagnosis and inappropriate medical therapy may lead to treatment errors or delays so that the patient's vision and corneal graft transparency are affected. In this study, we evaluated the clinical characteristics and treatment outcomes of new onset HSK after keratoplasty in patients who had no prior HSK.

The lesion location of new onset HSK after keratoplasty was found to be mostly at the graft-recipient junction, and even at the entire corneal graft and surrounding transplant bed. This can be used to distinguish HSK from other corneal infections, because the other infectious graft ulcers, except for peripheral ulcers caused by loose sutures, are often located in the center of the graft and rarely involve the adjacent transplant bed. In the current study, most patients complained of decreased visual acuity within a short time, accompanied by conjunctival hyperemia and corneal edema, which made the physicians first suspect corneal graft rejection. The following 2 points may help to distinguish HSK from corneal graft rejection. First, in new onset HSK after keratoplasty, we observed typical dendritic or map-like epithelial infiltration, which may lead to stromal ulcers in severe cases and involve the adjacent transplant bed. Conversely, the immunological rejection of a corneal graft primarily manifests as edema of the corneal graft, an endothelial rejection line, neovascularization filling, and engorgement. Moreover, graft rejection is rarely associated with epithelial damage [13–15]. Second,

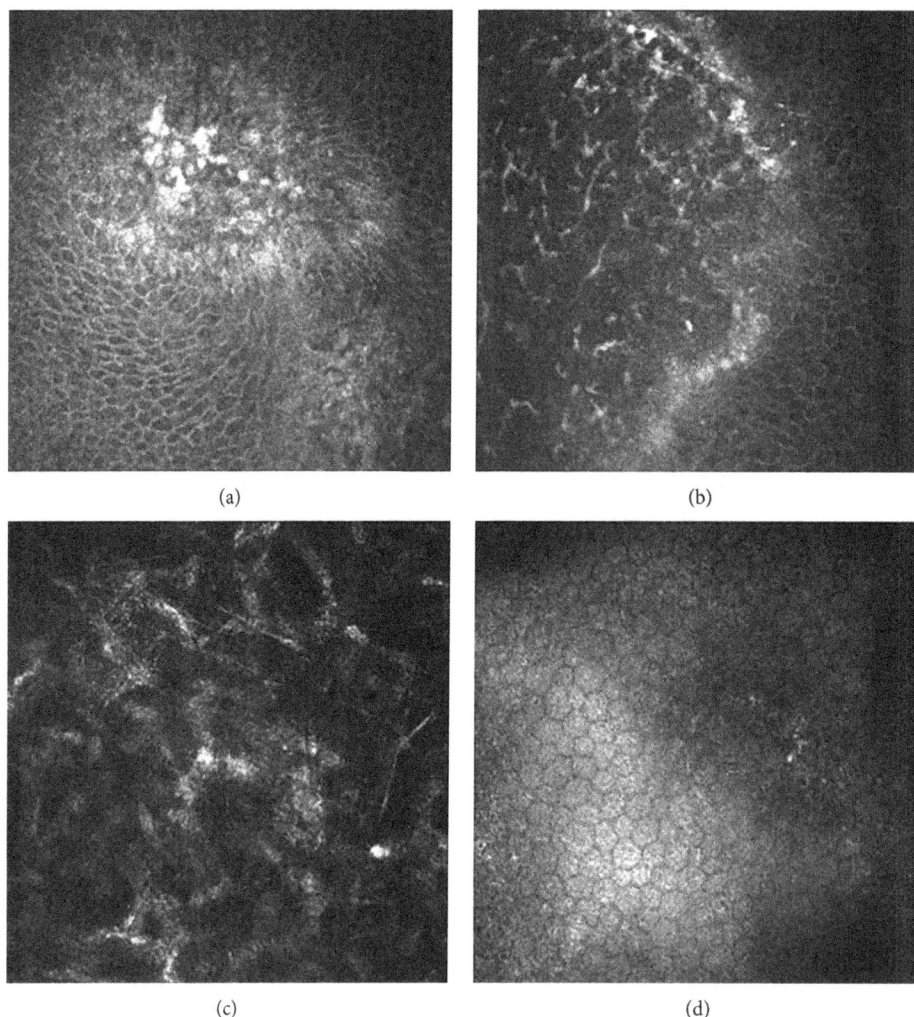

FIGURE 6: In vivo confocal microscopy examination of epithelial HSK. (a) The epithelial cells were swollen and necrotic. (b) A large number of dendritic cells were observed at the junction of the lesion and transparent cornea. (c) The polygonal cells of the stromal cells in the superficial stromal layer showed enhanced reflectivity and were arranged in a cross-hatched pattern. (d) Little KPs were observed in the endothelial cell layer.

in vivo confocal microscopy is a powerful tool that can assist in making a diagnosis [16–18]. The dendritic cells did not aggregate at the center of the corneal lesion but at the junction of the lesion area and transparent cornea in the new onset HSK cases [19]. In cases of corneal graft rejection, large numbers of dendritic cells and infiltration are only available in the area covering the epithelial or endothelial rejection line [20–22].

Fifteen of 17 patients complained of sudden discomfort with redness and decreased vision, but the degree of severity was related to whether they received treatment in time. The patients with timely treatment experienced mild, primarily epithelial type corneal lesions, with an average time of treatment of 3.9 ± 1.3 days; otherwise, the disease condition gradually worsened, leading to the formation of a map-like corneal ulcer after 7.9 ± 2.6 days, which can spread to the entire cornea. In all cases of epithelial lesions, epithelial infiltration disappeared quickly after antiviral treatment, with an average cure time of 3.2 ± 1.9 days, and corneal graft transparency was restored. The treatment option and prognoses of patients with stromal lesions were closely related to the depth of the ulcer. When the ulcer depth was ≤1/3 corneal thickness, the average healing time was 7.5 days after antiviral treatment, but corneal graft transparency and BCVA were not affected. Once the depth was >1/3 corneal thickness, the ulcers were not liable to heal after medication, and amniotic membrane transplantation or double amniotic membrane transplantation was required, with an average healing time extended to 18.5 days. After the surgical intervention, the patients exhibited scarring at the site of the healing ulcer, significantly decreasing corneal graft transparency and BCVA. Early diagnosis and standardized treatment may provide the greatest possible resolution of pathological changes; a lack of knowledge of the disease or delayed treatment can cause irreversible damage to vision and corneal graft transparency.

Herpes simplex virus-1 (HSV-1) can establish latent infections in the trigeminal ganglia [23]. HSV-1 DNA is also detected in the corneas of humans and animals with quiescent HSK, suggesting that the cornea might be

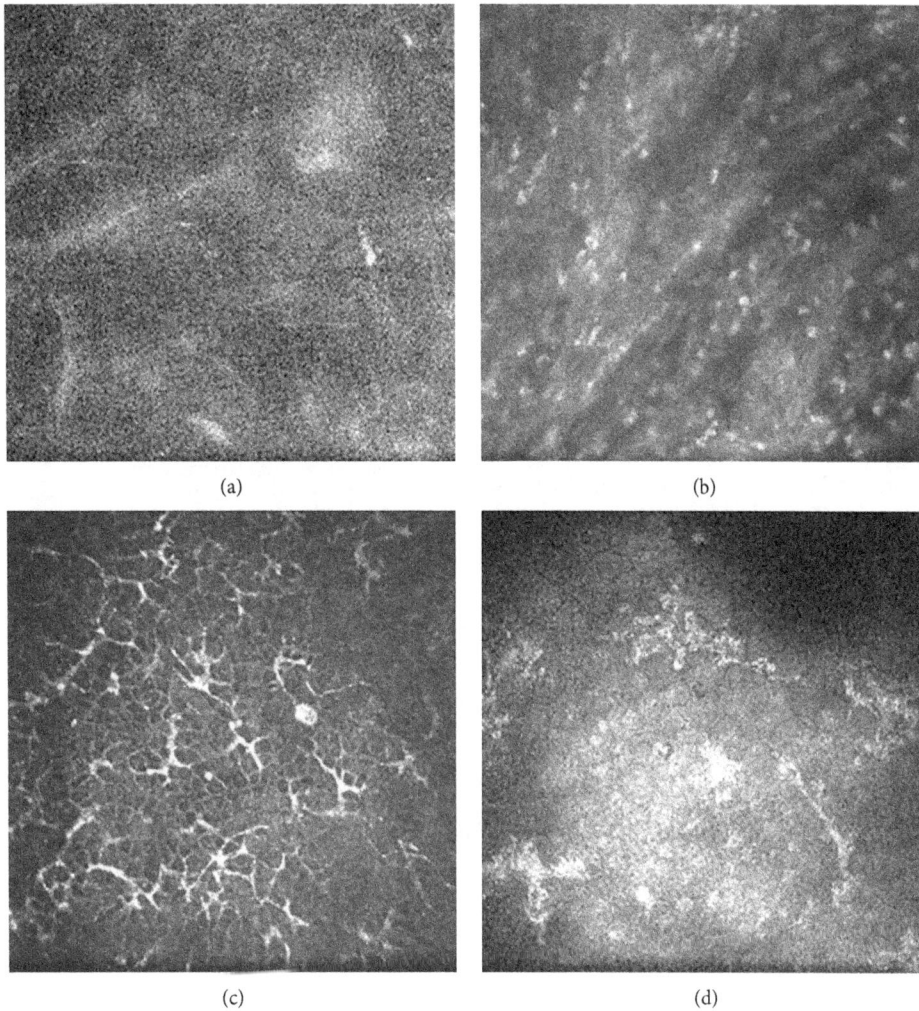

FIGURE 7: In vivo confocal microscopy examination of stromal necrotic and endothelial HSK. (a) Scanning images of the stromal cells were unclear. (b) A large amount of inflammatory cells were observed. (c) A large number of dendritic cells were observed, and wire netting was formed via long interdigitating dendrites at the junction of the lesion and transparent cornea. (d) Lots of KPs were observed in the endothelial cell layer.

another latency site of HSV-1 [24]. In patients without a clinical history of HSK, the emergence of HSV-1 DNA in corneas with primary graft failure suggested donor-recipient transmission through keratoplasty [25–27]. In our study, keratoplasty can induce the onset of HSK. The HSV infection may arise from any of three main mechanisms: intracorneal multiplication of virus after reactivation in sensitive ganglia, reactivation of latent-state virus in the residual cornea of the recipient, or through reactivation of a donor-recipient transmission virus [28]. But it is difficult to confirm the source of virus because donor corneas are not routinely screened for HSV-1 in our eye bank, which is the main limitation of this retrospective study. In addition, all 17 patients were considered as no episodes of HSK previously by means of limited medical records and their denial of repeated symptoms, with a lack of immunohistochemistry or polymerase chain reaction (PCR) assay, which is another limitation of this retrospective study. Improved detection methods and additional screening of donor corneas for HSV-1 may provide an improved understanding of corneal latency and its role in primary graft failure [29].

To conclude, the results of this study showed that HSK occurred in 1.18% of patients after keratoplasty. The diagnosis of HSK was mainly based on typical eye signs, such as dendritic epithelial infiltration and map-like epithelial lesions or ulcers, involving both the graft and adjacent recipient. Early stage lesions were primarily epithelial type, which could be cured quickly with antiviral treatment without affecting vision or corneal graft transparency. Delayed treatment may aggravate disease conditions and require amniotic membrane transplantation and even corneal transplantation, causing irreversible damage to vision and corneal graft transparency.

5. Conclusions

Keratoplasty can induce the onset of herpes simplex keratitis, resulting in epithelial defects or ulcers both in the graft and recipient. Effective treatments included antiviral medications and amniotic membrane transplantation. Delayed treatment causes irreversible damage to vision and corneal graft transparency.

Conflicts of Interest

The authors have no conflicts of interest in this article.

Acknowledgments

This study was supported by the National Natural Science Foundation of China (81370989, 81570821), Science & Technology Development Program of Shandong Province (2016GSF201182), Taishan Top Scholarship Program (grant number 20081148), Shandong Provincial Excellent Innovation Team Program, and the Young and Middle-Aged Scientists Research Awards Fund of Shandong Province (ZR2017BH004).

References

[1] M. J. Mannis, R. D. Plotnik, I. R. Schwab, and R. D. Newton, "Herpes simplex dendritic keratitis after keratoplasty," *American Journal of Ophthalmology*, vol. 111, no. 4, pp. 480–484, 1991.

[2] L. Remeijer, P. Doornenbal, A. J. Geerards, W. A. Rijneveld, and W. H. Beekhuis, "Newly acquired herpes simplex virus keratitis after penetrating keratoplasty," *Ophthalmology*, vol. 104, no. 4, pp. 648–652, 1997.

[3] R. A. Rezende, U. B. Uchoa, I. M. Raber, C. J. Rapuano, P. R. Laibson, and E. J. Cohen, "New onset of herpes simplex virus epithelial keratitis after penetrating keratoplasty," *American Journal of Ophthalmology*, vol. 137, no. 3, pp. 415–419, 2004.

[4] V. Jhanji, M. Ferdinands, H. Sheorey, N. Sharma, D. Jardine, and R. B. Vajpayee, "Unusual clinical presentations of new-onset herpetic eye disease after ocular surgery," *Acta Ophthalmologica*, vol. 90, no. 6, pp. 514–518, 2012.

[5] E. J. Holland and G. S. Schwartz, "Classification of herpes simplex virus keratitis," *Cornea*, vol. 18, no. 2, pp. 144–154, 1999.

[6] A. V. Farooq and D. Shukla, "Herpes simplex epithelial and stromal keratitis: an epidemiologic update," *Survey of Ophthalmology*, vol. 57, no. 5, pp. 448–462, 2012.

[7] T. N. Azher, X. T. Yin, D. Tajfirouz, A. J. Huang, and P. M. Stuart, "Herpes simplex keratitis: challenges in diagnosis and clinical management," *Clinical Ophthalmology*, vol. 11, pp. 185–191, 2017.

[8] K. J. Looker, A. S. Magaret, M. T. May et al., "Global and regional estimates of prevalent and incident herpes simplex virus type 1 Infections in 2012," *PLoS One*, vol. 10, no. 10, Article ID e0140765, 2015.

[9] T. J. Liesegang, "Herpes simplex virus epidemiology and ocular importance," *Cornea*, vol. 20, no. 1, pp. 1–13, 2001.

[10] H. D. Perry, S. J. Doshi, E. D. Donnenfeld, D. H. Levinson, and C. D. Cameron, "Herpes simplex reactivation following laser in situ keratomileusis and subsequent corneal perforation," *CLAO Journal: Official Publication of the Contact Lens Association of Ophthalmologists, Inc*, vol. 28, no. 2, pp. 69–71, 2002.

[11] G. D. Kymionis, D. M. Portaliou, D. I. Bouzoukis et al., "Herpetic keratitis with iritis after corneal crosslinking with riboflavin and ultraviolet A for keratoconus," *Journal of Cataract and Refractive Surgery*, vol. 33, no. 11, pp. 1982–1984, 2007.

[12] P. Prasher and O. Muftuoglu, "Herpetic keratitis after descemet stripping automated endothelial keratoplasty for failed graft," *Eye and Contact Lens: Science and Clinical Practice*, vol. 35, no. 1, pp. 41-42, 2009.

[13] A. Panda, M. Vanathi, A. Kumar, Y. Dash, and S. Priya, "Corneal graft rejection," *Survey of Ophthalmology*, vol. 52, no. 4, pp. 375–396, 2007.

[14] W. Shi, T. Wang, J. Zhang, J. Zhao, and L. Xie, "Clinical features of immune rejection after corneoscleral transplantation," *American Journal of Ophthalmology*, vol. 146, no. 5, pp. 707–713, 2008.

[15] I. Rahman, F. Carley, C. Hillarby, A. Brahma, and A. B. Tullo, "Penetrating keratoplasty: indications, outcomes, and complications," *Eye (Lond)*, vol. 23, no. 6, pp. 1288–1294, 2009.

[16] T. Hillenaar, C. Weenen, R. J. Wubbels, and L. Remeijer, "Endothelial involvement in herpes simplex virus keratitis: an in vivo confocal microscopy study," *Ophthalmology*, vol. 116, no. 11, pp. 2077–86.e1-2, 2009.

[17] T. Hillenaar, H. van Cleynenbreugel, G. M. Verjans, R. J. Wubbels, and L. Remeijer, "Monitoring the inflammatory process in herpetic stromal keratitis: the role of in vivo confocal microscopy," *Ophthalmology*, vol. 119, no. 6, pp. 1102–1110, 2012.

[18] M. C. Mocan, M. Irkec, D. G. Mikropoulos, B. Bozkurt, M. Orhan, and A. G. Konstas, "In vivo confocal microscopic evaluation of the inflammatory response in non-epithelial herpes simplex keratitis," *Current Eye Research*, vol. 37, no. 12, pp. 1099–1106, 2012.

[19] L. Mastropasqua, M. Nubile, M. Lanzini et al., "Epithelial dendritic cell distribution in normal and inflamed human cornea: in vivo confocal microscopy study," *American Journal of Ophthalmology*, vol. 142, pp. 736.e2–744.e2, 2006.

[20] R. L. Niederer, T. Sherwin, and C. N. McGhee, "In vivo confocal microscopy of subepithelial infiltrates in human corneal transplant rejection," *Cornea*, vol. 26, no. 4, pp. 501–504, 2007.

[21] W. J. Mayer, M. J. Mackert, N. Kranebitter et al., "Distribution of antigen presenting cells in the human cornea: correlation of in vivo confocal microscopy and immunohistochemistry in different pathologic entities," *Current Eye Research*, vol. 37, no. 11, pp. 1012–1018, 2012.

[22] D. Wang, P. Song, S. Wang et al., "Laser scanning in vivo confocal microscopy of clear grafts after penetrating keratoplasty," *BioMed Research International*, vol. 2016, Article ID 5159746, 6 pages, 2016.

[23] J. R. Baringer and P. Swoveland, "Recovery of herpes-simplex virus from human trigeminal ganglions," *New England Journal of Medicine*, vol. 288, no. 13, pp. 648–650, 1973.

[24] S. B. Kaye, C. Lynas, A. Patterson, J. M. Risk, K. McCarthy, and C. A. Hart, "Evidence for herpes simplex viral latency in the human cornea," *British Journal of Ophthalmology*, vol. 75, no. 4, pp. 195–200, 1991.

[25] G. C. Cockerham, A. E. Krafft, and I. W. McLean, "Herpes simplex virus in primary graft failure," *Archives of Ophthalmology*, vol. 115, no. 5, pp. 586–589, 1997.

[26] G. C. Cockerham, K. Bijwaard, Z. M. Sheng, A. A. Hidayat, R. L. Font, and I. W. McLean, "Primary graft failure:

a clinicopathologic and molecular analysis," *Ophthalmology*, vol. 107, no. 11, pp. 2083–2090, 2000.

[27] R. J. De Kesel, C. Koppen, M. Ieven, and T. Zeyen, "Primary graft failure caused by herpes simplex virus type 1," *Cornea*, vol. 20, no. 2, pp. 187–190, 2001.

[28] P. Y. Robert, J. P. Adenis, F. Denis, S. Alain, and S. Ranger-Rogez, "Herpes simplex virus DNA in corneal transplants: prospective study of 38 recipients," *Journal of Medical Virology*, vol. 71, no. 1, pp. 69–74, 2003.

[29] A. V. Farooq and D. Shukla, "Corneal latency and transmission of herpes simplex virus-1," *Future Virology*, vol. 6, no. 1, pp. 101–108, 2011.

16

A Comparative Study of Vitrectomy Combined with Internal Limiting Membrane Peeling for the Treatment of Idiopathic Macular Hole with Air or C3F8 Intraocular Tamponade

Xiang Chen ⓘ, Yi Yao, Xiaolu Hao, Xiaocui Liu, and Tiecheng Liu

Department of Ophthalmology, The Chinese PLA General Hospital, No. 28 Fuxing Road, Haidian District, Beijing 100853, China

Correspondence should be addressed to Xiang Chen; chenxianghoo@163.com

Academic Editor: Dirk Sandner

Purpose. The treatment of idiopathic macular holes has been basically modeled, and vitreoretinal surgery is recognized as an effective treatment. However, the postoperative tamponade of gas will still make the patient uncomfortable and may have related complications. The purpose of this study is to investigate whether air as an intraocular tamponade is equivalent to gas and what advantages may exist. *Methods.* A retrospective study was performed in one hundred and ninety-eight patients from 2013 to 2017; 112 received gas tamponade and 86 received air tamponade. After receiving retinal surgery, the outcomes of best corrected visual acuity, intraocular pressure, slit lamp examination, fundus examination, and imaging of the macula by spectral-domain optical coherence tomography were analyzed. *Results.* Before operation, there was no statistically significant difference in age, sex, macular hole diameter, or visual acuity between groups. The median follow-up period for the C3F8 group was 26 months, and the median follow-up for the air group was 25 months. After the operation, the best corrected visual acuity and macular hole closure rate were not significantly different between the two groups. The face-down time after the operation, the incidence of lens opacity on the third postoperative day, the intraocular pressure on the third postoperative day, and the operation time were significantly different between the two groups. *Conclusions.* In idiopathic macular hole surgery, the effect of air as an intraocular tamponade material can be similar to that of C3F8 but has fewer complications. In particular, it is a better choice for patients for whom the face-down position is not suitable.

1. Introduction

Most macular holes are idiopathic macular holes (IMH), but MH can also be seen in high myopia, trauma, and other situations. The prevalence of IMH is approximately 4/1000 [1] in people over 40 years of age. Among them, 60 to 80 years old is the age with the highest incidence, and it is more commonly seen in women [2, 3]. Although the etiology of IMH is varied and the exact mechanism of the development of IMH remains to be further explored, the consensus has not changed that the principle treatment for MH is vitreoretinal surgery. Currently, the classic procedure for treating IMH is pars plana vitrectomy with peeling of the internal limiting membrane and intraocular gas tamponade, followed by a face-down position for several days [4, 5]. Because of gas tamponade, the face-down position after the IMH surgery can cause much discomfort. It can also cause complicated cataracts, elevated intraocular pressure, secondary glaucoma, and other postoperative complications [6].

Compared to gas, air as an intraocular tamponade has a shorter absorption time in the eye, which means a shorter postoperative face-down time, more comfort for the patient, a lower probability of increased intraocular pressure, and a reduced possibility of concurrent cataracts. However, there are few reports about the use of air for intraocular tamponade: the number of studies is few, and the observed indexes are not comprehensive. It has been reported in the literature that air tamponade is equivalent to long-effect gas filling [7–10] and that the air tamponade effectiveness is poor [11].

Therefore, this study retrospectively analyzed the data of patients undergoing vitrectomy for idiopathic macular hole to investigate whether air as an intraocular tamponade is equivalent to gas and what advantages exist.

2. Patients and Methods

2.1. Study Design and Patients. Patients were included who consulted the Chinese PLA General Hospital between January 2013 and May 2017, underwent transconjunctival 25-gauge pars plana vitrectomy for the treatment of an idiopathic macular hole, and were followed up for 6 months or longer. All patients gave their written informed consent before participating in the study. No agreement from the ethical committee was needed as only standard procedures were performed.

This study consists of a retrospective evaluation of anatomical and functional results of idiopathic macular hole patients. A total of 198 eyes (46 male and 152 female) from 198 patients (46 men and 152 women) aged 38–80 years (average age of 60 years) were identified.

The inclusion criteria were IMH receiving vitrectomy combined with internal limiting membrane peeling. The exclusion criteria were ocular trauma, high myopia (>6 diopters), optic neuropathy, previous vitreoretinal surgery, and other diseases that may affect visual function.

2.2. Surgical Method. All surgeries were carried out under retrobulbar anesthesia. All patients underwent 25-gauge pars plana vitrectomy by a single surgeon. The surgery consisted of a standard 3-port transconjunctival 25-gauge pars plana vitrectomy with triamcinolone-assisted induction of posterior hyaloid separation, and core vitrectomy was performed. Phacoemulsification with intraocular lens implantation was performed simultaneously in 21 of 22 eyes (95.5%). After visualization using indocyanine green, peeling of the inner limiting membrane (ILM) was performed. Finally, a fluid-air exchange was performed. Intraocular tamponade with air or 15% C3F8 was employed at the end of the intervention.

2.3. Main Outcome Measures. All patients underwent preoperative and postoperative ophthalmic examinations. Best corrected visual acuity (BCVA) was measured and converted to the logarithm of the minimum angle of resolution (logMAR) scale. Measurements of intraocular tension were carried out using applanation tonometry, evaluation of the anterior segment was by slit-lamp, and examination of the posterior pole was by indirect ophthalmoscopy. The structure of the macular region was evaluated by spectral-domain optical coherence tomography (SD-OCT).

2.4. Statistical Analysis. The BCVA results were converted to logMAR equivalents. Statistical analysis was performed using Fisher's exact test or unpaired *t*-test. A *P* value ≤ 0.05 was considered statistically significant. The statistical analyses were performed with SPSS statistics, software version 23.0 (SPSS Inc., Chicago, IL).

TABLE 1: Patient characteristics.

	Air group	C3F8 group	P
Age (SD)	62.05 (5.788)	57.88 (7.289)	0.4013
Sex, M/F	20/66	26/86	0.8706
Minimum diameter of MH, μm (SD)	333.8 (148.041)	403.625 (148.041)	0.4263
Basal diameter of MH, μm (SD)	665.4 (437.950)	873.111 (488.687)	0.4458
Preoperative mean logMAR VA (SD)	0.86 (0.241)	0.963 (0.451)	0.6516
Preoperative IOP, mmHg	14.8 (3.701)	15.286 (2.138)	0.7783

M, male; F, female; MH, macular hole; logMAR, logarithm of minimal angle resolution; VA, visual acuity; IOP, intraocular pressure.

TABLE 2: The choice of intraocular tamponade material (classification by the diameter of MH).

Diameter of MH, μm	Air group	C3F8 group	P
<250	16/86	25/112	0.5223
250–400	40/86	46/112	0.4440
>400	30/86	41/112	0.8021

MH, macular hole.

3. Results

A total of 198 patients were included in the study. The air tamponade group had 86 patients, and the C3F8 group had 112 patients. The average age of the air group was 62.05 years, and the average age of the C3F8 group was 57.88 years, $P = 0.4013$. The gender ratios (male/female) were 20/66 and 26/86, $P = 0.8706$. Mean macular hole diameters were 333.800 and 403.625, $P = 0.4263$, and mean macular hole basal diameters were 665.40 and 873.11 microns, $P = 0.4448$. Preoperative mean logMAR visual acuity scores were 0.86 and 0.96, $P = 0.6516$, and mean preoperative intraocular pressures were 14.80 and 15.28 mmHg, $P = 0.7783$ (Table 1).

All patients were classified according to the diameter of macular hole and divided into 3 groups: <250 microns, 250–400 microns, and >400 microns. The constituent ratios of these three groups were not significantly different, and the P values were 0.5223, 0.4440, and 0.8021 (Table 2).

The postoperative follow-up times for the two groups were 25.22 months and 26.37 months, $P = 0.3722$, and postoperative logMAR visual acuity scores were 0.520 and 0.387, $P = 0.5678$. The face-down times were 6.05 days and 17.98 days, $P = 0.001$. On the third day after the operation, the incidence of lens opacity was 17/86 and 58/112, $P = 0.001$, intraocular pressures on the third postoperative day were 12.6 and 22.64, $P = 0.0375$, and the operation times were 35.07 and 41.63, $P = 0.0006$ (Table 3).

The structure of the macular area was examined by OCT before and after operation. The results suggest that the macular hole closure rates were 91.8% and 91.0%, with no significant difference between the two groups ($P = 0.8443$). The outer segment layer reconstruction rates at final postoperative follow-up time were 50/86 and 71/112, $P = 0.7704$,

TABLE 3: Clinical details of patients after surgery.

	Air group	C3F8 group	P
Follow-up time, months (SD)	25.219 (9.085)	26.326 (8.437)	0.3772
Prone posturing period, days (SD)	6.05 (0.912)	17.98 (3.320)	0.0005
Opacity of the lens, third day after operation	17/86	58/112	0.0003
Postoperative logMAR visual acuity (SD)	0.520 (0.497)	0.387 (0.340)	0.5678
Operation time, minutes (SD)	35.07 (9.21)	41.63 (10.32)	0.0006
Intraocular pressure, third day after operation, mmHg (SD)	12.6 (2.88)	22.635 (10.78)	0.0375

LogMAR, logarithm of minimal angle resolution.

TABLE 4: Postoperative OCT results.

	Air group	C3F8 group	P
Macular hole closure rate (%)	91.8%	91.0%	0.8443
Ellipsoid zone defect diameter, μm (SD)	1306.5 (960.958)	335.750 (325.696)	0.1146
Ellipsoid zone restructuring rate (%)	58.1%	63.4%	0.7704

with no significant difference between the two groups (Table 4, Figures 1 and 2).

4. Discussion

Before 1991, scholars thought that IMH was incurable. With a deep understanding of the pathogenesis of idiopathic macular holes, vitreomacular traction is considered to be the most important factor. In 1991, Kelly and Wendel first reported vitreoretinal surgery for IMH [12]. At present, the standard treatment for idiopathic macular hole is vitrectomy combined with ILM peeling, gas filling, and postoperative face down positioning. For a long time, the industry focused on whether the IMH surgery required stripping of the ILM and, during the procedure of stripping the ILM, whether there is a need for the use of stains due to their toxicity. After improving our understanding of macular interface disease, the treatment of IMH has become increasingly more precise.

For an aperture size of less than 250 microns in IMH, intravitreal injection of ocriplasmin may prevent some patients from requiring surgical treatment [13]. For large IMH, the ILM flap reversal technique is often used [14]. The face-down position after the IMH surgery may contribute to patients' discomfort. Lange et al. conducted a randomized controlled study of 30 patients with IMH with a diameter of <400 microns and suggested that the face-down position is not necessary [15]. Of course, the reliability of single-center research is not enough, and a multicenter, large sample study of the face-down position is needed.

Sulfur hexafluoride (SF6), octafluoropropane (C3F8), air, and silicone oil are the most common intraocular tamponade materials. The most widely used tamponade materials is gas, which means SF6 or C3F8. There were some reports of exploratory research on tamponade materials after MH surgery. There are several reports describing using air as the tamponade material after MH surgery, and the conclusion is somewhat controversial. Some doctors reported that air filling is equivalent to gas filling [7–10], but Gesser has reported that the effectiveness of air filling is poor [11].

Compared to the patients who underwent MH surgery with gas, the time in the prone position with air tamponade was shorter, and the patient was more comfortable. The volume of air does not expand, so the probability of elevated intraocular pressure decreases, and the possibility of concurrent cataracts can be reduced. Air filling has many advantages. Therefore, we carried out a study about whether air is a good intraocular tamponade material.

Previous studies have suggested that the stage of MH, duration of symptoms, preoperative visual acuity, size of the MH, and OCT image are predictive factors relevant to postoperative outcome. The most sensitive index for evaluating the recovery of visual function after macular hole surgery is the diameter of the hole before the operation [16, 17]. There were no statistically significant differences between the two groups we chose in terms of patient age, sex, or macular hole diameter, which was an important factor in ensuring the reliability of the study.

The closure of the macular hole requires two important elements. The first is the movement of the traction of the vitreoretinal interface, and the second is the dry environment of the macular interface, which can be achieved by gas or air filling [18, 19]. The blocking effect of the bubble on the hole breaks the fluid from the vitreous cavity into the subretinal space and restricts the cell composition and growth factor from entering the subretinal space.

According to the study by He et al., most of the macular holes of air tamponade eyes can be seen as closed by OCT images 48–72 h after surgery. In addition, the closure time of the macular hole was less than 24 h in SF6 tamponade eyes [10]. Our study showed that most macular holes were closed by the third day after surgery, and the closure rate of air group was 91.8%, while the closure rate of C3F8 group was 91.0%. There was no difference in the closure rate between the two groups, indicating that air tamponade was equivalent to gas tamponade.

There are few articles comparing the effects of air and gas on idiopathic macular hole surgery. Researchers [8] reported that the use of air tamponade for idiopathic macular hole surgery had an equal effect compared with the SF6 group, the postoperative best corrected visual acuity and macular hole closure rate were not significantly different, and the air tamponade group had a shorter face-down time after the operation. Usui et al. [9] reported that the air and SF6 groups had the same macular hole closure rate, postoperative face-down time was different, and the IS/OS layer restructuring rate was not significantly different, which was confirmed by

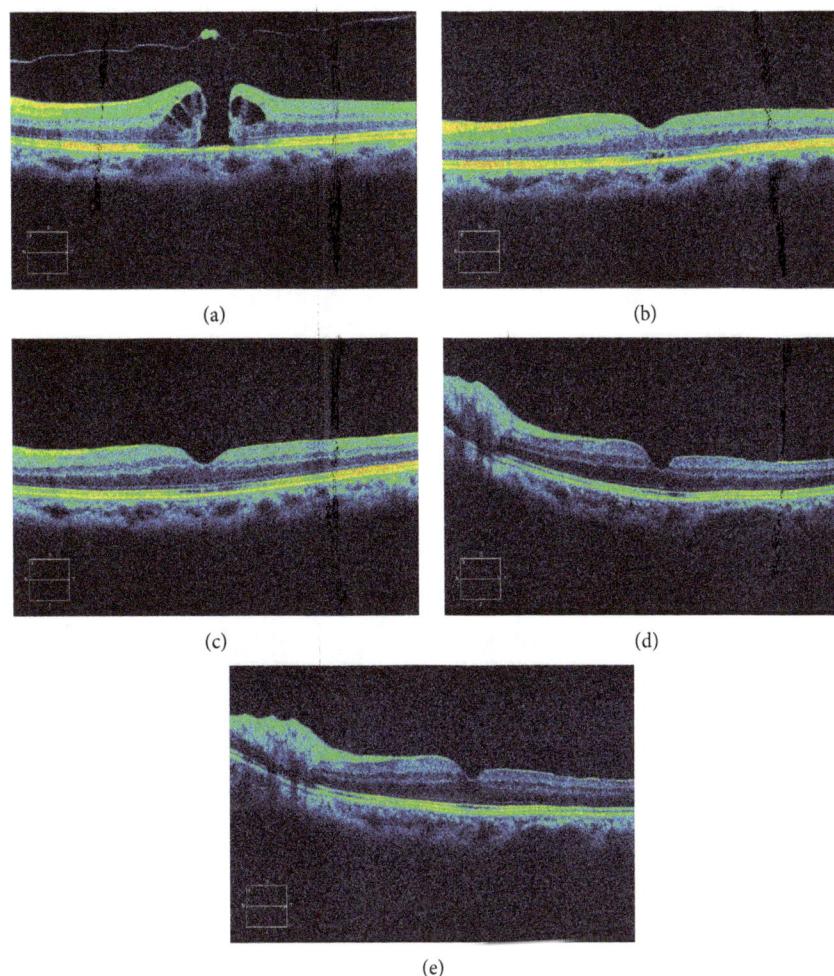

FIGURE 1: Images from SD-OCT of a 58-year-old woman with a 333 μm diameter MH and a photoreceptor layer defect of 1433 μm in the air group. MH was repaired 3 days after the operation. The ellipsoid zone was restructured at month 3. (a) Preoperative; (b) 3 days after surgery; (c) 1 month after surgery; (d) 3 months after surgery; (e) 6 months after surgery.

OCT examination. They drew the same conclusion we found here. We observed that there was no difference between the two groups in best corrected visual acuity or macular hole closure rate. The best corrected visual acuity was 0.520 and 0.387, respectively, and the rate of hiatus closure was as previously mentioned. The junction between the IS/OS of the photoreceptors seems to play an important role in the final BCVA. Preoperative reorganization of the IS/OS line is probably achieved by gradual migration of the photoreceptor cells from the surrounding healthy area. There was no significant difference in the length or defect rate of the photoreceptor outer layer between the two groups after the surgery on the photoreceptor outer layer.

The postoperative face-down time in the air tamponade group was 6.05 ± 0.912 days, and the postoperative face-down time in the C3F8 tamponade group was 17.98 ± 3.320 days. The difference between the two groups was statistically significant, and the patients with air tamponade had a shorter face-down time and were more comfortable. We found that on the third day after surgery, there was a higher rate of transient lens opacity in the C3F8 group, which reached 58/112, while the air group was significantly lower,

only 17/86. This difference between the two groups was statistically significant. The intraocular pressure (IOP) after the operation was also recorded. On the third day after the operation, the IOP of the C3F8 tamponade group was 22.635 ± 10.78 mmHg, which was significantly higher than that of the air tamponade group at 12.6 ± 2.88 mmHg. Moreover, the operation time for the air tamponade group was shorter than that of the gas tamponade group, and there was a statistically significant difference between the two groups.

The reason for lens opacification may be due to contact and the compression effect of intraocular gas in the posterior capsule of the lens and gas that blocks the metabolic pathway of the lens. We observed that with intravitreal gas absorption, the lens turns transparent again and only a few lenses cannot be restored to transparent; the pathogenesis for this state of permanent opacity needs further study [20]. The causes of ocular hypertension after vitrectomy are varied [21]. It may contribute to laser photocoagulation, combined cataract surgery, severity of postoperative vitreous hemorrhage, and use of expanding gas tamponade. The reason for transient high intraocular pressure after the operation may be the

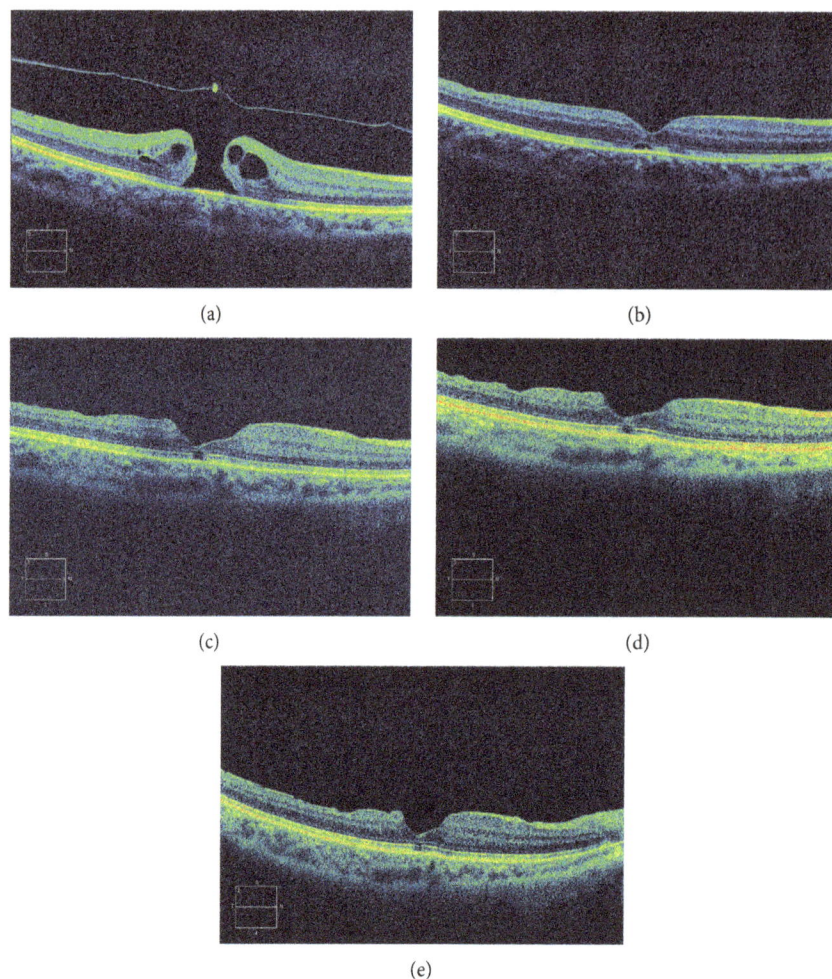

FIGURE 2: Images from SD-OCT of a 60-year-old woman with a 371 μm diameter MH and a photoreceptor layer defect of 692 μm in the C3F8 group. MH was repaired 3 days after the operation. The ellipsoid zone was not restructured at month 6 with a defect of 606 μm. (a) Preoperative; (b) 3 days after surgery; (c) 1 month after surgery; (d) 3 months after surgery; (e) 6 months after surgery.

relation to the expansion of C3F8 in our results, because maximal expansion of C3F8 occurred 48–72 hours postoperatively. This time, the interval overlapped with the time of postoperative intraocular hypertension.

Fewer surgical procedures and shorter operation time will reduce the probability of postoperative complications [22]. The main reason for the shorter operation time is the omission of intraocular long-acting gas injection, as the completion of gas fluid exchange is sufficient [23].

In conclusion, the present study revealed air filling has the same therapeutic effect as C3F8 filling, and there is no difference between the macular hole closure rate and the recovery of vision. Additionally, the face-down time is shorter after the operation. Furthermore, we reported that the probability of opacification of the lens and the IOP after the operation was reduced in the air group, and the operation time was shorter. These advantages can make the patient more comfortable.

Conflicts of Interest

The authors declare that there are no conflicts of interest regarding the publication of this paper.

References

[1] S. M. Meuer, C. E. Myers, B. E. Klein et al., "The epidemiology of vitreoretinal interface abnormalities as detected by spectral-domain optical coherence tomography: the beaver dam eye study," *Ophthalmology*, vol. 122, no. 4, pp. 787–795, 2015.

[2] L. A. Casuso, I. U. Scott, H. W. Flynn Jr. et al., "Long-term follow-up of unoperated macular holes," *Ophthalmology*, vol. 108, no. 6, pp. 1150–1155, 2001.

[3] J. W. Kim, W. R. Freeman, W. el-Haig, A. M. Maguire, J. F. Arevalo, and S. P. Azen, "Baseline characteristics, natural history, and risk factors to progression in eyes with stage 2 macular holes. Results from a prospective randomized clinical trial. Vitrectomy for Macular Hole Study Group," *Ophthalmology*, vol. 102, no. 12, pp. 1818–1828, 1995.

[4] M. Parravano, F. Giansanti, C. M. Eandi, Y. C. Yap, S. Rizzo, and G. Virgili, "Vitrectomy for idiopathic macular hole," *Cochrane Database of Systematic Reviews*, vol. 5, p. CD009080, 2015.

[5] S. Thinda, R. J. Shah, and S. J. Kim, "Two-year anatomical and functional outcomes after macular hole surgery: a prospective, controlled study," *Ophthalmic Surgery, Lasers & Imaging Retina*, vol. 46, no. 9, pp. 926–934, 2015.

[6] Y. Hasegawa, F. Okamoto, Y. Sugiura, Y. Okamoto, T. Hiraoka, and T. Oshika, "Intraocular pressure elevation after vitrectomy

for various vitreoretinal disorders," *European Journal of Ophthalmology*, vol. 24, no. 2, pp. 235–241, 2014.

[7] L. Hejsek, A. Stepanov, J. Dusova et al., "Microincision 25G pars plana vitrectomy with peeling of the inner limiting membrane and air tamponade in idiopathic macular hole," *European Journal of Ophthalmology*, vol. 27, no. 1, pp. 93–97, 2017.

[8] Y. Hasegawa, Y. Hata, Y. Mochizuki et al., "Equivalent tamponade by room air as compared with SF(6) after macular hole surgery," *Graefe's Archive for Clinical and Experimental Ophthalmology*, vol. 247, no. 11, pp. 1455–1459, 2009.

[9] H. Usui, T. Yasukawa, Y. Hirano, H. Morita, M. Yoshida, and Y. Ogura, "Comparative study of the effects of room air and sulfur hexafluoride gas tamponade on functional and morphological recovery after macular hole surgery: a retrospective study," *Ophthalmic Research*, vol. 50, no. 4, pp. 227–230, 2013.

[10] F. He, F. Dong, W. Yu, and R. Dai, "Recovery of photoreceptor layer on spectral-domain optical coherence tomography after vitreous surgery combined with air tamponade in chronic idiopathic macular hole," *Ophthalmic Surgery, Lasers & Imaging Retina*, vol. 46, no. 1, pp. 44–48, 2015.

[11] C. Gesser, T. Eckert, U. Eckardt, U. Porkert, and C. Eckardt, "Macular hole surgery with air tamponade. Does air suffice for short-term tamponade?," *Der Ophthalmologe: Zeitschrift der Deutschen Ophthalmologischen Gesellschaft*, vol. 107, no. 11, pp. 1043–1050, 2010.

[12] N. E. Kelly and R. T. Wendel, "Vitreous surgery for idiopathic macular holes: results of a pilot study," *Archives of Ophthalmology*, vol. 109, no. 5, pp. 654–659, 1991.

[13] B. Lescrauwaet, L. Duchateau, T. Verstraeten, and T. L. Jackson, "Visual function response to ocriplasmin for the treatment of vitreomacular traction and macular hole: the OASIS study," *Investigative Ophthalmology & Visual Science*, vol. 58, no. 13, pp. 5842–5848, 2017.

[14] J. S. Duker, P. K. Kaiser, S. Binder et al., "The International Vitreomacular Traction Study Group classification of vitreomacular adhesion, traction, and macular hole," *Ophthalmology*, vol. 120, no. 12, pp. 2611–2619, 2013.

[15] C. A. Lange, L. Membrey, N. Ahmad et al., "Pilot randomised controlled trial of face-down positioning following macular hole surgery," *Eye*, vol. 26, no. 2, pp. 272–277, 2012.

[16] E. Beausencourt, A. E. Elsner, M. E. Hartnett, and C. L. Trempe, "Quantitative analysis of macular holes with scanning laser tomography," *Ophthalmology*, vol. 104, no. 12, pp. 2018–2029, 1997.

[17] E. Byhr and B. Lindblom, "Preoperative measurements of macular hole with scanning laser ophthalmoscopy. Correlation with functional outcome," *Acta Ophthalmologica Scandinavica*, vol. 76, no. 5, pp. 579–583, 1998.

[18] Y. Shiode, Y. Morizane, R. Matoba et al., "The role of inverted internal limiting membrane flap in macular hole closure," *Investigative Ophthalmology & Visual Science*, vol. 58, no. 11, pp. 4847–4855, 2017.

[19] K. Boninska, J. Nawrocki, and Z. Michalewska, "Mechanism of "flap closure" after the inverted internal limiting membrane flap technique," *Retina*, 2017.

[20] H. Schaefer, R. Al Dwairi, P. Singh, C. Ohrloff, T. Kohnen, and F. Koch, "Can postoperative accelerated lens opacification be limited by lying in "face-down position" after vitrectomy with gas as tamponade?," *Klinische Monatsblatter fur Augenheilkunde*, vol. 232, no. 8, pp. 966–975, 2015.

[21] A. Miele, A. Govetto, C. Fumagalli et al., "Ocular hypertension and glaucoma following vitrectomy: a systematic review," *Retina*, vol. 38, no. 5, pp. 883–890, 2017.

[22] S. Naruse, H. Shimada, and R. Mori, "27-gauge and 25-gauge vitrectomy day surgery for idiopathic epiretinal membrane," *BMC Ophthalmology*, vol. 17, no. 1, p. 188, 2017.

[23] L. Cheng, S. P. Azen, M. H. El-Bradey et al., "Duration of vitrectomy and postoperative cataract in the vitrectomy for macular hole study," *American Journal of Ophthalmology*, vol. 132, no. 6, pp. 881–887, 2001.

Visual Outcomes of Ultrathin-Descemet Stripping Endothelial Keratoplasty versus Descemet Stripping Endothelial Keratoplasty

Konstantinos Droutsas [1,2] Myrsini Petrelli [1] Dimitrios Miltsakakis,[3]
Konstantinos Andreanos,[1] Anastasia Karagianni,[3] Apostolos Lazaridis [1,2]
Chrysanthi Koutsandrea,[1] and George Kymionis[1,4]

[1]*First Department of Ophthalmology, National and Kapodistrian University of Athens, General Hospital "G. Gennimatas",*
 Athens, Greece
[2]*Department of Ophthalmology, Philipps University, Marburg, Germany*
[3]*State Ophthalmology Clinic, General Hospital "G. Gennimatas", Athens, Greece*
[4]*Jules Gonin Eye Hospital, Faculty of Biology and Medicine, University of Lausanne, Lausanne, Switzerland*

Correspondence should be addressed to Konstantinos Droutsas; konstantinos_droutsas@yahoo.gr

Academic Editor: Florence Cabot

Purpose. To examine the impact of graft thickness (GT) on postoperative visual acuity and endothelial cell density after ultrathin-Descemet stripping automated endothelial keratoplasty (UT-DSAEK) versus conventional DSAEK. *Methods.* The medical records of all patients who underwent DSAEK at our institute during a 2-year period were reviewed. After excluding subjects with low visual potential, 34 eyes were divided into two groups based on the postoperative GT as measured with anterior segment optical coherence tomography (AS-OCT): an UT-DSAEK group (GT ≤ 100 μm, $n = 13$ eyes) and a DSAEK group (GT > 100 μm, $n = 21$ eyes). The groups were compared with regard to best-corrected visual acuity (BCVA), subjective refraction, central corneal thickness (CCT), GT, and endothelial cell density (ECD). *Results.* Preoperative BCVA (logMAR) was 1.035 ± 0.514 and 0.772 ± 0.428 for UT-DSAEK and DSAEK, respectively ($P = 0.072$). At 6 months postoperatively, BCVA was 0.088 ± 0.150 following UT-DSAEK and 0.285 ± 0.158 following DSAEK ($P = 0.001$). *Conclusion.* DSAEK grafts with a thickness under 100 μm offered better visual outcomes during the early postoperative period.

1. Introduction

Over the past decade, Descemet stripping automated endothelial keratoplasty (DSAEK) has surpassed penetrating keratoplasty (PK) as the preferred treatment method for patients with corneal endothelial dysfunction [1]. The numerous advantages of DSAEK over PK include the avoidance of an open sky procedure, absence of suture-related complications, better tectonic and refractive stability, and faster visual rehabilitation [2, 3].

In contrast to PK, where all layers of the host cornea are replaced, DSAEK represents an additive procedure, where a graft consisting of a layer of posterior donor stroma of variable thickness and a layer of healthy corneal endothelium is placed on the posterior surface of the host cornea. This increased corneal thickness may limit the visual outcome after DSAEK [4]. Thus, a trend has emerged [5–7] favouring thinner grafts (i.e., thin and UT-DSAEK) and even alternative surgical procedures, such as Descemet membrane endothelial keratoplasty (DMEK) and pre-Descemet's endothelial keratoplasty (PDEK).

To date, the evidence for differences in visual outcomes depending on GT remains controversial. A number of studies have demonstrated a positive correlation between GT and postoperative visual acuity after DSAEK [8–10], whereas others have not provided supporting data for this hypothesis [11–13]. Thus, the aim of this study was to further elucidate the possible impact of GT on postoperative visual acuity by comparing visual outcomes of UT-DSAEK to those of DSAEK.

2. Materials and Methods

The medical records of all patients who had undergone DSAEK surgery between October 2015 and August 2017 at a tertiary referral centre (General Hospital "G. Gennimatas," Athens, Greece) were reviewed. Cases with low visual potential (e.g., glaucoma, retinal macular disease, corneal scars, amblyopia) or concurrent ocular surgery (e.g., phacoemulsification) were excluded. Failed or complicated procedures requiring reinterventions such as rebubbling or repeat DSAEK were also excluded. In bilateral cases, only the right was included in the study. All procedures were performed by 3 surgeons (K.D., D.M., and G.K.) with the same surgical technique [14] using precut grafts acquired from an eye bank network that uses a single-pass donor DSAEK graft preparation technique (https://www.sightlife.org/Resources/prepared-corneal-tissue). Notably, the surgeons did not request grafts of a specific thickness range; therefore, the grafts used were of random thickness.

All patients underwent laser iridotomy prior to surgery. The DSAEK procedure was performed under subtenon's block and involved placement of a 4.5 mm limbal incision (temporally in left eyes and nasally in right eyes), followed by three side ports at 1.00, 6.00, and 9.00. After filling the anterior chamber with air, stripping of the recipient's Descemet membrane was performed using a reverse Sinskey hook. Following removal of the anterior cap of the precut donor tissue, the posterior lamella was mounted on a silicon bank (Geuder AG, Heidelberg, Germany) with the endothelium facing up. The donor lenticule was trephined with an 8.0 to 8.5 mm punch (Katena, U.S.A.), based on the corneal diameter of the recipient. The graft was then loaded onto a Busin glide (Moria SA, Germany), and a fine intraocular forceps (Moria SA) was used to pull the graft through the limbal incision. Incision wounds were sutured using 10-0 nylon. Following this, the anterior was filled completely with 100% air. After 60 to 120 minutes, the patient was examined at the slit lamp and some air was released by gently pressing on a side port in the case of pupillary block.

Preoperative and postoperative best-corrected visual acuity (BCVA), subjective refraction, central corneal thickness (CCT), GT, and endothelial cell density (ECD) were recorded.

CCT and GT were measured using swept-source anterior segment optical coherence tomography (AS-OCT) (DRI-OCT Triton, Topcon, Japan). More specifically, the average thickness of 5 points was recorded—measured at the vertex and at 1 mm located superiorly, inferiorly, temporally, and nasally to the vertex (Figure 1). In addition, four peripheral graft thickness measurements were taken, at two perpendicular axes within 3 mm from the centre, and the mean value of the latter measurements was calculated (P). Following this, the ratio of central to peripheral graft thickness (C:P) was calculated. Patients were divided into two groups based on postoperative GT: UT-DSAEK (GT $\leq 100\,\mu$m) and DSAEK (GT $> 100\,\mu$m). Donor ECD was extracted from the

donor information form, provided by the supplying eye bank. Postoperative ECD was measured with a noncontact specular microscope (EM-3000, Tomey, USA). BCVA was measured in Snellen and converted to a logarithm of the minimum angle of resolution (logMAR) in order to facilitate statistical analysis.

All data were collected with Excel software (version 14, Microsoft Corp.), analyzed with SPSS software (version 17.0, SPSS, Inc.,) and reported as central tendency and dispersion. Differences of means between the groups were assessed by the Mann–Whitney U test for independent samples. A P value less than 0.05 was considered statistically significant.

3. Results

The study enrolled 43 eyes of 43 patients. Thirteen eyes ($n = 13$) fell within the UT-DSAEK group and 30 eyes ($n = 30$) within the DSAEK group (Table 1). Postoperative GT was $87 \pm 13\,\mu$m and $145 \pm 21\,\mu$m following UT-DSAEK and DSAEK, respectively ($P < 0.001$). No significant difference between groups with respect to age and preoperative BCVA was observed ($P \geq 0.072$, Mann–Whitney U test). The mean corneal donor lenticule C:P ratio in the UT-DSAEK group was 0.65 ± 0.12 ($n = 12$) and 0.86 ± 0.17 in the DSAEK group ($n = 6$) ($P = 0.027$). In the ultrathin group, mean logMAR improved from 1.035 (range 0.521 to 1.549) at baseline to 0.088 (range −0.062 to 0.238) at 6 months after surgery. In the DSAEK group, mean logMAR improved from 0.772 (range 0.344 to 1.2) at baseline to 0.285 (range −0.127 to 0.443) at 6 months. Postoperative logMAR was significantly better following UT-DSAEK ($P = 0.001$).

A statistically significant moderate positive relationship between postoperative GT and logMAR values ($r^2 = 0.423$, $P = 0.006$, linear regression analysis) was found in the total group.

Donor ECD was significantly higher in the UT-DSAEK group ($P = 0.029$). Postoperative ECD was 1403 ± 473 cells/mm^2 and 1407 ± 411 cells/mm^2 ($P = 0.715$).

4. Discussion

DSAEK has replaced PK as the treatment of choice for corneal endothelial dysfunction. Thus, considering the increasing popularity of DSAEK, elucidating the contribution of various factors that influence the final visual outcome is highly significant. A number of factors, including donor-recipient interface, tissue irregularities, anterior corneal scarring, and high-order aberrations, have been suggested as influencing the visual outcome following DSAEK [15–17]. Moreover, a more regular posterior corneal surface has been shown to be achieved with thinner grafts, which, in turn, results in fewer, high-order aberrations. This reduction could explain the faster and better visual recovery observed with thinner DSAEK grafts [10, 18].

The aim of this retrospective study was to examine if GT less than $100\,\mu$m is associated with better postoperative visual acuity, as this could provide guidance for optimizing DSAEK graft thickness. Therefore, we assessed the impact of GT on BCVA following UT-DSAEK versus conventional

(a)

(b)

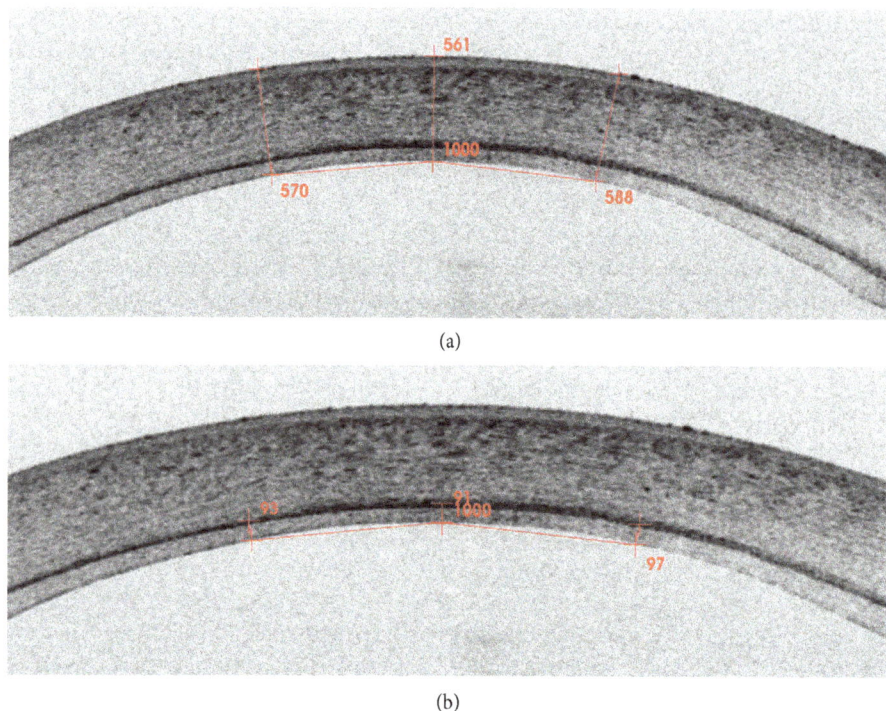

FIGURE 1: Thickness of a DSAEK graft as measured on an AS-OCT image. Both total (a) and graft (b) corneal thickness were measured at 5 points (at the point of intersection of the measurement's reference axis and the graft and at 1 mm distance in the superior, inferior, nasal, and temporal meridian). Here are depicted three horizontal points: at the point of intersection of the measurement's reference axis and the graft, and at 1 mm distance on both sides nasally and temporally to the centre.

TABLE 1: Baseline and 6-month postoperative characteristics.

	Ultrathin DSAEK (GT $\leq$ 100 μm)		DSAEK (GT > 100 μm)		MWU test
	Mean ± SD	n	Mean ± SD	n	P value
Age (years)	72.7 ± 8.8	13	71.4 ± 7.3	30	0.701
Follow-up (months)	9.3 ± 4.6	13	7.4 ± 4.4	30	0.274
logMARpre	1.035 ± 0.514	13	0.772 ± 0.428	30	0.072
logMARpost	0.088 ± 0.150	13	0.285 ± 0.158	27	0.001*
SEpost (D)	0.11 ± 0.54	13	0.31 ± 1.24	26	0.227
REFcylpost (D)	1.173 ± 0.874	13	1.154 ± 0.863	26	0.641
CCTpost (μm)	579 ± 45	12	621 ± 56	16	0.039*
Gtpost (μm)	87 ± 13	13	145 ± 21	30	0.000*
ECDpre (cells/mm^2)	2698 ± 401	13	2457 ± 249	30	0.029*
ECDpost (cells/mm^2)	1403 ± 473	13	1407 ± 411	19	0.715
ECL (%)	47 ± 19	9	44 ± 16	19	0.418

*Statistically significant; CCT: central corneal thickness; D: diopters; ECD: endothelial cell density; GT: graft thickness; logMAR: decadic logarithm of the minimal angle of resolution; mo: months; MWU: Mann–Whitney U test; post: postoperatively; pre: preoperatively; REFcyl: refractive cylinder; SE: spherical equivalent.

DSAEK and found significantly better BCVA after UT-DSAEK at 6 months after surgery, as well as a moderate positive correlation of GT with BCVA.

Our results are consistent with the findings of previous studies. Neff et al. conducted a retrospective study (n = 33) and concluded that grafts that postoperatively were 131 μm or thinner had a higher percentage of 20/25 and 20/20 final visual acuity results compared to grafts with a postoperative central GT greater than 131 μm [9]. Pogorelov et al. correlated postoperative GT and BCVA 6 months after DSAEK

and found a statistically significant relationship (n = 15) [8]. Dickman et al. confirmed these results in a larger cohort of eyes without significant comorbidity (n = 79) [10]. Acar et al. reported that thinner DSAEK grafts (GT < 150 μm) are associated with better visual rehabilitation and less endothelial loss (n = 37) [19]. The findings of a recent randomized multicenter clinical trial indicated that UT-DSAEK, compared to DSAEK, promotes faster and better visual acuity results with a similar endothelial cell loss at 1 year postoperatively (n = 66) [20]. Finally, results from a relatively recent review of the literature and meta-analysis suggest a weak relationship between GT and BCVA following DSAEK [21].

Nevertheless, several other studies have not provided evidence supporting a clear association between GT and visual acuity following DSAEK [11–13, 22–24].

To our knowledge, there is currently no consensus on the basis upon which the categorization of GT should be done. The exact thickness defining UT, as opposed to conventional DSAEK, is not uniform in the literature and has been described variously as sub-130 μm or sub-100 μm [25, 26]. Moreover, some studies refer to the GT measurement immediately after graft preparation [13, 23, 27], while others use the measurement after surgery *in vivo* [10, 22, 24]. Here, we have used the definition of UT-DSAEK based on postoperative GT measurement as previously reported by others [4].

In order to assess donor corneal lenticule morphology, we calculated the C:P ratio of the DSAEK graft, an index that represents the ratio of the central graft thickness to the peripheral as formerly described [28]. Interestingly, the C:P ratio was found to be higher in the DSAEK group.

Different endothelial keratoplasty techniques have not shown significantly different ECL up to date. The slightly higher but not significant ECL in the UT-DSAEK group (47% versus 44% following UT-DSAEK and DSAEK, respectively) agrees with previous observations [20].

Limitations of this study include its retrospective nature and the small number of the studied eyes. Randomized, prospective studies with larger sample size are required in order to examine the relationship between both preoperative and postoperative donor thickness and postoperative vision and to confirm the theory that better visual outcomes can be achieved with the use of ultrathin DSAEK grafts.

Conflicts of Interest

The authors declare that there are no conflicts of interest regarding the publication of this article.

References

[1] M. O. Price and F. W. Price Jr., "Endothelial keratoplasty—a review," *Clinical & Experimental Ophthalmology*, vol. 38, no. 2, pp. 128–140, 2010.

[2] M. A. Terry, N. Shamie, E. S. Chen, K. L. Hoar, and D. J. Friend, "Endothelial keratoplasty a simplified technique to minimize graft dislocation, iatrogenic graft failure, and pupillary block," *Ophthalmology*, vol. 115, no. 7, pp. 1179–1186, 2008.

[3] E. S. Chen, M. A. Terry, N. Shamie, K. L. Hoar, and D. J. Friend, "Descemet-stripping automated endothelial keratoplasty," *Cornea*, vol. 27, no. 5, pp. 514–520, 2008.

[4] A. M. J. Turnbull, M. Tsatsos, P. N. Hossain, and D. F. Anderson, "Determinants of visual quality after endothelial keratoplasty," *Survey of Ophthalmology*, vol. 61, no. 3, pp. 257–271, 2016.

[5] M. Busin, S. Madi, P. Santorum, V. Scorcia, and J. Beltz, "Ultrathin descemet's stripping automated endothelial keratoplasty with the microkeratome double-pass technique," *Ophthalmology*, vol. 120, no. 6, pp. 1186–1194, 2013.

[6] G. R. J. Melles, T. S. Ong, B. Ververs, and J. van der Wees, "Descemet membrane endothelial keratoplasty (DMEK)," *Cornea*, vol. 25, no. 8, pp. 987–990, 2006.

[7] A. Agarwal, H. S. Dua, P. Narang et al., "Pre-Descemet's Endothelial Keratoplasty (PDEK)," *British Journal of Ophthalmology*, vol. 98, no. 9, pp. 1181–1185, 2014.

[8] P. Pogorelov, C. Cursiefen, B. O. Bachmann, and F. E. Kruse, "Changes in donor corneal lenticule thickness after Descemet's Stripping Automated Endothelial Keratoplasty (DSAEK) with organ-cultured corneas," *British Journal of Ophthalmology*, vol. 93, no. 6, pp. 825–829, 2009.

[9] K. D. Neff, J. M. Biber, and E. J. Holland, "Comparison of central corneal graft thickness to visual acuity outcomes in endothelial keratoplasty," *Cornea*, vol. 30, no. 4, pp. 388–391, 2011.

[10] M. M. Dickman, Y. Y. Y. Cheng, T. T. J. M. Berendschot, F. J. H. M. van den Biggelaar, and R. M. M. A. Nuijts, "Effects of graft thickness and asymmetry on visual gain and aberrations after Descemet Stripping Automated Endothelial Keratoplasty," *JAMA Ophthalmology*, vol. 131, no. 6, p. 737, 2013.

[11] M. O. Price and F. W. Price, "Descemet's stripping with endothelial keratoplasty," *Ophthalmology*, vol. 113, no. 11, pp. 1936–1942, 2006.

[12] K. A. Ahmed, J. W. McLaren, K. H. Baratz, L. J. Maguire, K. M. Kittleson, and S. V. Patel, "Host and graft thickness after Descemet stripping endothelial keratoplasty for fuchs endothelial dystrophy," *American Journal of Ophthalmology*, vol. 150, no. 4, pp. 490–497.e2, 2010.

[13] H. Van Cleynenbreugel, L. Remeijer, and T. Hillenaar, "Descemet stripping automated endothelial keratoplasty: effect of intraoperative lenticule thickness on visual outcome and endothelial cell density," *Cornea*, vol. 30, no. 11, pp. 1195–1200, 2011.

[14] M. Busin, P. R. Bhatt, and V. Scorcia, "A modified technique for Descemet membrane stripping automated endothelial keratoplasty to minimize endothelial cell loss," *Archives of Ophthalmology*, vol. 126, no. 8, p. 1133, 2008.

[15] S. V. Patel, K. H. Baratz, D. O. Hodge, L. J. Maguire, and J. W. McLaren, "The effect of corneal light scatter on vision after Descemet stripping with endothelial keratoplasty," *Archives of Ophthalmology*, vol. 127, no. 2, p. 153, 2009.

[16] M. Rudolph, K. Laaser, B. O. Bachmann, C. Cursiefen, D. Epstein, and F. E. Kruse, "Corneal higher-order aberrations after descemet's membrane endothelial keratoplasty," *Ophthalmology*, vol. 119, no. 3, pp. 528–535, 2012.

[17] M. Dirisamer, J. Parker, M. Naveiras et al., "Identifying causes for poor visual outcome after DSEK/DSAEK following secondary DMEK in the same eye," *Acta Ophthalmologica*, vol. 91, no. 2, pp. 131–139, 2013.

[18] M. Busin and E. Albé, "Does thickness matter," *Current Opinion in Ophthalmology*, vol. 25, no. 4, pp. 312–318, 2014.

[19] B. T. Acar, M. O. Akdemir, and S. Acar, "Visual acuity and endothelial cell density with respect to the graft thickness in Descemet's stripping automated endothelial keratoplasty: one year results," *International Journal of Ophthalmology Press*, vol. 7, no. 6, pp. 974–979, 2014.

[20] M. M. Dickman, P. J. Kruit, L. Remeijer et al., "A randomized multicenter clinical trial of ultrathin Descemet Stripping Automated Endothelial Keratoplasty (DSAEK) versus DSAEK," *Ophthalmology*, vol. 123, no. 11, pp. 2276–2284, 2016.

[21] K. Wacker, W. M. Bourne, and S. V. Patel, "Effect of graft thickness on visual acuity after Descemet stripping endothelial keratoplasty: a systematic review and meta-analysis," *American Journal of Ophthalmology*, vol. 163, pp. 18–28, 2016.

[22] A. J. Shinton, M. Tsatsos, A. Konstantopoulos et al., "Impact of graft thickness on visual acuity after Descemet's stripping endothelial keratoplasty," *British Journal of Ophthalmology*, vol. 96, no. 2, pp. 246–249, 2012 Feb.

[23] M. A. Terry, M. D. Straiko, J. M. Goshe, J. Y. Li, and D. Davis-Boozer, "Descemet's stripping automated endothelial keratoplasty: the tenuous relationship between donor thickness and postoperative vision," *Ophthalmology*, vol. 119, no. 10, pp. 1988–1996, 2012.

[24] M. A. Woodward, D. Raoof-Daneshvar, S. Mian, and R. M. Shtein, "Relationship of visual acuity and lamellar thickness in Descemet stripping automated endothelial keratoplasty," *Cornea*, vol. 32, no. 5, pp. e69–e73, 2013.

[25] M. Busin, A. K. Patel, V. Scorcia, and D. Ponzin, "Microkeratome-assisted preparation of ultrathin grafts for Descemet stripping automated endothelial keratoplasty," *Investigative Opthalmology & Visual Science*, vol. 53, no. 1, p. 521, 2012.

[26] M. Hsu, W. L. Hereth, and M. Moshirfar, "Double-pass microkeratome technique for ultra-thin graft preparation in Descemet's stripping automated endothelial keratoplasty," *Clinical Ophthalmology Dove Press*, vol. 6, pp. 425–432, 2012.

[27] P. M. Phillips, L. J. Phillips, and C. M. Maloney, "Preoperative graft thickness measurements do not influence final BSCVA or speed of vision recovery after Descemet stripping automated endothelial keratoplasty," *Cornea*, vol. 32, no. 11, pp. 1423–1427, 2013.

[28] S. H. Yoo, G. D. Kymionis, A. A. Deobhakta et al., "One-year results and anterior segment optical coherence tomography findings of Descemet stripping automated endothelial keratoplasty combined with phacoemulsification," *Archives of Ophthalmology American Medical Association*, vol. 126, no. 8, p. 1052, 2008.

18

Graft Survival after Penetrating Keratoplasty in Cases of Trabeculectomy versus Ahmed Valve Implant

Abdelhamid Elhofi ⓘ **and Hany Ahmed Helaly** ⓘ

Ophthalmology Department, Faculty of Medicine, Alexandria University, Egypt

Correspondence should be addressed to Hany Ahmed Helaly; hany209209@yahoo.com

Academic Editor: Edward Manche

Purpose. To compare the corneal graft survival rates after penetrating keratoplasty (PKP) in cases of post-PKP glaucoma managed by either trabeculectomy with mitomycin C or Ahmed glaucoma valve (AGV). *Methods.* This study was a retrospective interventional comparative study that included 40 eyes of 40 patients. The included patients had undergone previous PKP for anterior segment reconstruction after microbial or fungal keratitis, chemical burns, trauma, or perforated corneal ulcer. Post-PKP glaucoma was managed surgically by either trabeculectomy with mitomycin C (group 1) or Ahmed glaucoma valve (group 2). *Results.* The first group ($n = 20$) had undergone trabeculectomy with MMC, and the second group ($n = 20$) had undergone AGV implantation. Regarding BCVA, there was no statistically significant difference between the 2 groups. Mean IOP was significantly lower in the AGV group at 6 months, 12 months, and 24 months ($p = 0.001$). Mean IOP at 24 months dropped significantly from preglaucoma surgery levels in both groups ($p = 0.001$). Rejection episodes occurred in 2 eyes (10%) of the trabeculectomy group versus 8 eyes (40%) in the AGV group ($p = 0.028$). In the trabeculectomy group, corneal graft failure occurred in 1 (5%), 3 (15%), and 6 (30%) eyes at 6 months, 12 months, and 24 months, respectively. In the AGV group, corneal graft failure occurred in 2 (10%), 5 (25%), and 10 (50%) eyes at 6 months, 12 months, and 24 months, respectively. The mean time to failure in the trabeculectomy group was 12.33 ± 5.60 months versus 11.90 ± 5.70 months in the AGV group ($p = 0.027$). *Conclusion.* Managing postpenetrating keratoplasty glaucoma could be bothersome especially in complex cases. Ahmed glaucoma valve implant controls the intraocular pressure more effectively than trabeculectomy with mitomycin C. However, Ahmed glaucoma valve can result in higher rates of corneal graft failure in a shorter duration of time. This trial is registered with PACTR201712002861391 on 21 Dec 2017.

1. Introduction

Penetrating keratoplasty (PKP) is a common procedure for anterior segment reconstruction in cases of damaged corneas such as chemical burns, microbial keratitis, and perforated corneal ulcers [1, 2]. Lamellar keratoplasty in such conditions is of no use as it does not replace the damaged endothelium. In cases of preserved corneal endothelium, deep anterior lamellar keratoplasty may be successful for treating infectious keratitis or ocular burns. However, PKP carries higher risk of rejection and longer postoperative rehabilitation time than lamellar keratoplasty [3–5].

The reported incidence of raised intraocular pressure (IOP) and/or glaucoma after penetrating keratoplasty is variable according to the previous state of the eye before PKP. It was reported as low as 0–12% in PKP done for keratoconus and up to 75% in PKP done for infectious keratitis [6–9]. The pathogenesis of post-PKP glaucoma is multifactorial and may be due to postoperative inflammatory response, the formation of peripheral anterior synechiae (PAS), distortion of the trabecular meshwork, and previously undiagnosed glaucoma [6, 10].

The management of post-PKP glaucoma can be done using topical antiglaucoma medications, trabeculectomy with mitomycin C (MMC), deep sclerectomy, or glaucoma drainage device (GDD) [11–14]. Deep sclerectomy is valuable when the angle is not closed by synechiae and is associated with higher graft survival compared with trabeculectomy with MMC. The GDD may be valved, for example, Ahmed glaucoma valve, or nonvalved, for example, Molteno implant and Baerveldt implant [15–18].

An advantage of a valved implant such as Ahmed glaucoma valve is the low frequency of hypotony besides the easy insertion [19, 20]. However, it has higher rate of increased IOP in the first few months that may require needling and 5-fluorouracil injection [21].

The aim of the current study was to compare the corneal graft survival rates after penetrating keratoplasty (PKP) in cases of post-PKP glaucoma managed by either trabeculectomy with mitomycin C or Ahmed glaucoma valve.

2. Subjects and Methods

This study was a retrospective interventional comparative study that included 40 eyes of 40 patients. The included patients had undergone previous PKP for anterior segment reconstruction after microbial or fungal keratitis, chemical burns, trauma, or perforated corneal ulcer. Those patients developed uncontrolled IOP despite maximal medical therapy (i.e., 3 topical antiglaucoma medications), did not tolerate the medical therapy, or were not compliant. Post-PKP glaucoma was managed surgically by either trabeculectomy with mitomycin C (group 1) or Ahmed glaucoma valve (group 2). Included patients had a clear corneal graft before the glaucoma surgery, were >18 years of age, and had complete records of at least two years follow-up after glaucoma surgery. Data of the patients were recorded including best-corrected visual acuity (BCVA), IOP, clarity of the corneal graft, indication of the original PKP, corneal graft endothelial cell count, and any complications. Patients were recalled for a final follow-up visit. Snellen's BCVA was transformed into logMAR units. Counting fingers was considered as 2.1 logMAR, and hand motions was considered as 2.4 logMAR [22, 23].

The current study was approved by the local ethics committee of the faculty medicine, Alexandria University, Egypt. Tenets of the Declaration of Helsinki were followed. All patients signed an informed consent at the final follow-up visit.

3. Surgical Technique

Penetrating keratoplasty was performed under general anesthesia. Trephination was done using Hessburg–Barron trephines (Katena, Denville, USA). The donor graft was oversized by 0.25 mm larger than the recipient bed. Partial trephination of the recipient cornea was done using suction trephine size 7.5, 7.75, or 8 mm centered on the geometric center of the cornea, and cutting of the recipient cornea was completed by corneal scissors after full thickness trephination. For all patients, 10-0 nylon sutures (Alcon Laboratories, Fort Worth, Texas, USA) were applied. The donor cornea was initially secured in the recipient bed with four cardinal sutures at the 12, 6, 3, and 9 o'clock positions. Then the patients received 16 interrupted sutures. Any adhesions in the anterior segment were dissected, and cataract removal was done when applicable with or without intraocular lens implantation. Patients received topical gatifloxacin (Zymar, Allergan, Irvine, California, USA) every 6 hours for 30 days and topical prednisolone (Pred Forte, Allergan, Irvine, California, USA)

every 6 hours tapered over 2 to 3 months and then replaced by topical fluorometholone (Flucon, Alcon Laboratories, Fort Worth, Texas, USA).

Trabeculectomy was performed under general anesthesia. Limbal-based conjunctival flap was dissected followed by dissection of a partial thickness triangular scleral flap. Application of a soaked sponge with 0.02% mitomycin C for 2 minutes above and under the scleral flap was done followed by a thorough wash with balanced salt solution. A paracentesis was done to test for aqueous drainage and to form the anterior chamber if needed. Then a corneoscleral block was excised and a peripheral iridectomy was performed. Closure of the scleral flap with interrupted 10-0 nylon sutures was done. The conjunctiva was closed with 10-0 running nylon sutures to form the filtration bleb. All surgeries were performed by the same surgeon (A.E.) with a reproducible technique.

Ahmed glaucoma valve (AGV) was performed under general anesthesia. Priming of the AGV using 26-gauge needle was done with injection of balanced salt solution to ensure functionality. A superior-temporal fornix based conjunctival flap was dissected between the 2 recti muscles. Tenon's capsule is dissected from the episclera. The body of AGV is placed 8–10 mm from the limbus and sutured with 10-0 nylon sutures to the sclera. The tube is then cut to allow 2–3 mm inside the anterior chamber and beveled up with an angle of 30°. Using 23-gauge needle, a tract is formed entering the anterior chamber parallel to the iris plane starting 1–3 mm posterior to the limbus. The beveled tube was then inserted through this tract avoiding contact with the iris or the corneal endothelium. All surgeries were performed by the same surgeon (A.E.) with a reproducible technique.

Graft failure was defined as corneal edema for 1 month or more despite the use of intense steroid therapy or irreversible corneal graft opacity as a result of scarring or neovascularization. Time to failure was defined as the time interval between the glaucoma surgery and the diagnosis of graft failure according to the previous criteria. Glaucoma surgery was considered successful if the IOP was ≤21 mmHg with (qualified success) or without (complete success) topical medications and/or needling with subconjunctival 5-fluorouracil.

Data analysis was performed using the software SPSS for Windows version 20.0 (SPSS Inc., Chicago, USA). Quantitative data were described using range, mean, and standard deviation. The Mann–Whitney test was used to compare means of independent samples. Wilcoxon rank-sum test was used for comparisons between means of the preoperative and postoperative data. The Kruskal–Wallis test was used to compare means of two or more groups. Kaplan–Meier was used for survival analysis. The chi-square test was used to compare between different percentages and ratios. Differences were considered statistically significant when the associated p-value was less than 0.05.

4. Results

Forty post-PKP glaucoma patients were included and divided into two equal groups. The first group ($n = 20$) had undergone trabeculectomy with MMC, and the second group (n = 20) had undergone AGV implantation. Table 1 summarizes the characteristics of the included eyes of both groups. Microbial or fungal keratitis was the main indication for PKP in both groups. Using Mann–Whitney and chi-square tests, there were no statistically significant differences between the 2 groups regarding different parameters. Before the glaucoma surgery, the eyes of the Ahmed glaucoma valve group had higher mean IOP and lower post-PKP endothelial cell count (ECC), but this was not statistically significant. Gonioscopy was done to evaluate the degree of PAS. Total PAS more than 270° was found in 11 versus 13 eyes in groups 1 and 2, respectively. Partial PAS less than 180° was found in 6 versus 5 eyes in groups 1 and 2, respectively. None of the included cases had a history of previous glaucoma.

Table 2 shows the characteristics of the included eyes of both groups after the glaucoma surgery. Regarding BCVA, there was no statistically significant difference between the 2 groups. Also, there is no statistically significant difference between the preoperative mean BCVA and 24-month postoperative mean BCVA in both groups (p = 0.511 and 0.532 in groups 1 and 2, respectively). Two patients from each group have lost 2 lines of BCVA after the glaucoma surgery. Mean IOP was significantly lower in the AGV group at 6 months, 12 months, and 24 months (p = 0.001). Mean IOP at 24 months dropped significantly from preglaucoma surgery levels in both groups (p = 0.001). Regarding mean number of antiglaucoma medications used, there is a significant decrease after the glaucoma surgery from preoperative levels. It was significantly lower in the AGV group at 24 months (p = 0.034) but not at 6 and 12 months (p = 0.157, 0.102, respectively). At 24 months, six patients of the trabeculectomy group received one topical antiglaucoma medication, and 4 patients received 2 medications. While in the AGV group, six patients received 1 medication, and 1 patient received 2 medications.

The needling procedure with subconjunctival 5-fluorouracil injection was needed in a total of 14 eyes (70%) of the trabeculectomy group versus 6 eyes (30%) in the AGV group (p = 0.011) at 24 months. The total success rate (complete and qualified) was higher in the AGV group than the trabeculectomy group. This difference was statistically significant at 12 and 24 months (p = 0.048 and 0.001, respectively) but not at 6 months (p = 0.179).

Regarding postoperative complications, two cases had vitreous hemorrhage in the trabeculectomy group, and none developed hypotony or choroidal effusion. Cases with aphakia needed anterior vitrectomy to prevent vitreous clogging. In the AGV group, one case developed vitreous hemorrhage in the early postoperative period that persisted after pars plana vitrectomy with failed 3 times needling and subconjunctival 5-fluorouracil to control IOP. Cyclo-cryodestruction was needed to control IOP in this case. Two other cases developed vitreous hemorrhage that resolved spontaneously with no further intervention. One case had early tube obstruction due to a vitreous strand and required anterior vitrectomy. Three cases had tube-related complications. One case had a small conjunctival hole that was managed conservatively using topical tetracycline ointment. Another case developed larger exposure of the implant

TABLE 1: Characteristics of the included patients of trabeculectomy and Ahmed glaucoma valve groups before the glaucoma surgery.

	Trabeculectomy group (n = 20)	Ahmed valve group (n = 20)	p value*
Age (years)	37.3 ± 9.6 (19–60)	35.7 ± 11.2 (20–61)	0.521
Sex (male : female)	11 : 9	10 : 10	0.752
Diabetes mellitus	2 (10%)	2 (10%)	1.000
Hypertension	5 (25%)	4 (20%)	0.705
Indication of keratoplasty			0.739
Microbial or fungal keratitis	9 (45%)	8 (40%)	
Chemical burn	5 (25%)	7 (35%)	
Trauma	4 (20%)	2 (10%)	
Others	2 (10%)	3 (15%)	
Pre-op BCVA (logMAR)	1.40 ± 0.55 (0.9–2.4)	1.30 ± 0.50 (0.8–2.1)	0.655
Pre-op IOP (mmHg)	31.22 ± 4.91 (26–40)	33.54 ± 4.59 (29–42)	0.375
Pre-op number of medications	2.11 ± 0.55	2.34 ± 0.61	0.410
Pre-op endothelial count (cells/mm²)	2812 ± 270 (2400–3210)	2776 ± 291 (2450–3120)	0.288
Pre-op lens status			0.881
Phakic	4	3	
Pseudophakic	12	12	
Aphakic	4	5	
Time interval from PKP to glaucoma surgery (months)	9.41 ± 7.22 (2–30)	8.66 ± 6.51 (2–28)	0.321

*Using the Mann–Whitney test or the chi-square test where appropriate.

which required a scleral patch graft. Another case had tube extrusion from the anterior chamber and required a tube extensor with a scleral patch graft. By the end of 2nd year of follow-up, seven cases of the trabeculectomy group required another glaucoma surgery in the form of Ahmed glaucoma valve implantation versus three cases in the AGV group.

Rejection episodes occurred in 2 eyes (10%) of the trabeculectomy group versus 8 eyes (40%) in the AGV group (p = 0.028). Among the 8 eyes of the AGV group, one eye had 3 rejection episodes, four eyes had 2 rejection episodes, and three eyes had 1 rejection episode. In the trabeculectomy group, corneal graft failure occurred in 1 (5%), 3 (15%), and 6 (30%) eyes at 6 months, 12 months, and 24 months, respectively. In the AGV group, corneal graft failure occurred in 2 (10%), 5 (25%), and 10 (50%) eyes at 6 months, 12 months, and 24 months, respectively. However, this difference was not statistically significant (p = 0.902). Figure 1 shows Kaplan–Meier survival analysis graph for the cumulative corneal graft survival in both groups. The mean time to failure in the trabeculectomy group was 12.33 ± 5.60 months (range 4–18 months). The mean time to failure in the AGV group was 11.90 ± 5.70 months (range 3–18 months). There was a statistically significant difference between the two groups (p = 0.027). Cases with graft failure required another PKP. One case in the AGV group required two PKP surgeries.

TABLE 2: Characteristics of the included patients of trabeculectomy and Ahmed glaucoma valve groups after the glaucoma surgery.

	Trabeculectomy group ($n = 20$)	Ahmed valve group ($n = 20$)	p value*
Post-op BCVA (logMAR)			
6 months	1.21 ± 0.65 (0.7–2.4)	1.27 ± 0.56 (0.8–2.1)	0.491
12 months	1.29 ± 0.67 (0.8–2.1)	1.33 ± 0.60 (0.9–2.1)	0.544
24 months	1.35 ± 0.59 (0.8–2.1)	1.36 ± 0.64 0.9–2.1)	0.697
Post-op IOP (mmHg)			
6 months	13.20 ± 4.51 (8–21)	11.20 ± 3.32 (5–20)	0.001#
12 months	13.50 ± 4.76 (8–25)	11.88 ± 3.55 (7–22)	0.001#
24 months	13.98 ± 3.44 (10–26)	12.28 ± 3.71 (8–23)	0.001#
Post-op number of medications			
6 months	0.25 ± 0.44	0.15 ± 0.37	0.157
12 months	0.50 ± 0.76	0.25 ± 0.44	0.102
24 months	0.70 ± 0.80	0.40 ± 0.60	0.034#
Eyes required needling + 5-fluorouracil			
6 months	5 (25%)	2 (10%)	0.212
12 months	10 (50%)	4 (20%)	0.047#
24 months	14 (70%)	6 (30%)	0.011#
Total success rate			
6 months	90%	95%	0.179
12 months	80%	90%	0.048#
24 months	55%	80%	0.001#

*Using the Mann–Whitney test or the chi-square test where appropriate.
#Significant.

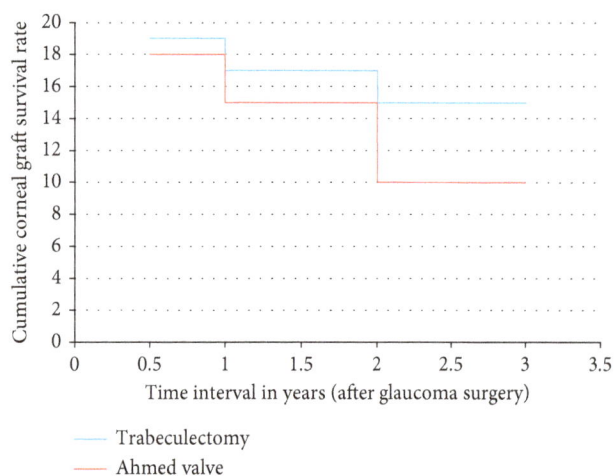

FIGURE 1: Kaplan–Meier survival analysis for corneal graft survival among trabeculectomy and Ahmed valve groups.

5. Discussion

Postpenetrating keratoplasty glaucoma is not uncommon. It is the second leading cause for corneal graft failure.

Post-PKP glaucoma is a problematic issue because of difficulties met in diagnosis and management. The increase in IOP may have damaging effect on the corneal endothelial cells and therefore the corneal graft failure. Early diagnosis of post-PKP rise of IOP is essential in preserving the integrity of optic nerve head and corneal graft clarity [24, 25].

In the current study, the incidence of post-PKP glaucoma was high (more than 50%). This is due to the complex nature of the indication for PKP of the included patients. About half of the cases had microbial or fungal keratitis, and one quarter had chemical burns. Many of those patients developed PAS. Other possible mechanisms may be due to postoperative steroid medications used, trabecular meshwork damage either due to the original disease or due to anterior chamber collapse, or postoperative inflammatory response [6, 10]. As stated above, the incidence of post-PKP glaucoma varies according to the indication of PKP. Yildirim et al. [26] reviewed 122 eyes of PKP. Post-PKP glaucoma occurred in 42 eyes which represented 34% of the cases during the first 4 years of follow-up. They reported a mean time interval from PKP to the diagnosis of post-PKP glaucoma of 24 weeks. The difference in incidence rate from our study may be related to the different indications for PKP. The longer the duration of follow-up, it is expected to have higher incidence of post-PKP glaucoma.

In the current study, all cases of trabeculectomy surgery included the application of 0.02% of mitomycin C for 2 minutes in the subconjunctival and subscleral spaces. Mitomycin C application significantly improved the success rates of trabeculectomy for managing post-PKP glaucoma. Mitomycin C should be thoroughly washed before the entry of the anterior chamber to avoid endothelial cell damage. The reported success rates of IOP control in such patients vary from 67 to 90% [26, 27]. In the current study, the success rate for the trabeculectomy group was 90% at 6 months postoperative which dropped to 55% at the end of the second year. It is important during the surgery to take care to prevent collapse or shallowing of the anterior chamber to decrease the damage to the endothelial cells. The use of 5-fluorouracil for subconjunctival injection may be of benefit with needling procedure, but it is associated with corneal epithelial toxicity. The incidence of corneal graft failure in the current study was 5% at 6 months postoperative and reached 30% at the end of 2 years follow-up. Some studies reported the rate of graft failure after trabeculectomy for post-PKP glaucoma to be 12–18% [26–30].

The success rate of IOP control in the Ahmed glaucoma valve group was 95% at 6 months and 80% at 2 years. This was significantly higher than the trabeculectomy group. Rejection episodes occurred at a higher incidence with the AGV group. Corneal graft rejection occurred in 10% at 6 months and in 50% at 2 years. However, this difference failed to show statistical significance despite of the clinical significance. It may be resorted to the smaller number of the included patients due to the search for more complicated cases to be included in the study. The mean time to failure was significantly shorter in the AGV group. Kirkness [31] was the first one to report the use of a glaucoma drainage device for the management of post-PKP glaucoma in the late 80's. Ahmed glaucoma valve has an advantage over the nonvalved devices being easy to insert and having a lower incidence of postoperative hypotony. On the opposite, it is associated with higher incidence of postoperative rise of intraocular pressure that might indicate the use of needling and subconjunctival 5-fluorouracil [32, 33]. After 2 years follow-up, the included AGV group in the current study needed less postoperative needling than the trabeculectomy group (30% versus 70%). Ahmed glaucoma valve and other glaucoma drainage devices in general control IOL in a high percentage of the reported population (average of 84%) [32–35] which is comparable with the results of our study despite the complex nature of the included patients. However, they appear to have a higher incidence of corneal graft failure (average of 36%) [32–34]. Again, the incidence of graft failure in our AGV study group was higher due to the complex nature of the included cases and also due to the higher damage to the graft endothelium induced by the AGV compared with trabeculectomy. Helmy et al. [35] reported a graft survival rate of 94% at 4 years follow-up in their series of 38 eyes of post-PKP glaucoma managed by Ahmed valve. The cause of increased incidence of corneal graft failure after glaucoma drainage device may be related to the retrograde passage of inflammatory cells into the anterior chamber, postoperative inflammation that breaks down the blood aqueous barrier, formation of peripheral anterior synechiae, and shallow anterior chamber with iris or tube endothelial touch.

The advantages of the current study are the comparative nature of two study groups with two different surgeries, relatively moderate follow-up period of 2 years, and focusing on selecting complex cases requiring anterior segment reconstruction with extensive PAS. The limitations of the current study included the need for larger number of included patients. However, the complex cases are not available in larger number. Also, it might have been useful to include a longer duration of follow-up to record the long-term effects.

In conclusion, managing postpenetrating keratoplasty glaucoma could be bothersome especially in complex cases. Ahmed glaucoma valve implant controls the intraocular pressure more effectively than trabeculectomy with mitomycin C. However, Ahmed glaucoma valve can result in higher rates of corneal graft failure in a shorter duration of time.

Abbreviations

PKP: Penetrating keratoplasty
IOP: Intraocular pressure
PAS: Peripheral anterior synechia
MMC: Mitomycin C
BCVA: Best-corrected visual acuity
AGV: Ahmed glaucoma valve.

Conflicts of Interest

The authors declare that they have no conflicts of interest.

Authors' Contributions

Dr. Abdelhamid Elhofi conceived the idea and concept of the study and shared in writing the manuscript and collection of data. Dr. Hany Helaly shared in the idea of the study, writing the manuscript, and analysis of the data. All authors contributed equally to the drafting, critical revision, and final approval of the manuscript.

References

[1] M. O. Price, P. Calhoun, C. Kollman, F. W. Price, and J. H. Lass, "Descemet stripping endothelial keratoplasty: ten-year endothelial cell loss compared with penetrating keratoplasty," *Ophthalmology*, vol. 123, no. 7, pp. 1421–1427, 2016.

[2] D. J. Coster, M. T. Lowe, M. C. Keane, K. A. Williams, and A. C. Contributors, "A comparison of lamellar and penetrating keratoplasty outcomes: a registry study," *Ophthalmology*, vol. 121, no. 5, pp. 979–987, 2014.

[3] V. Romano, A. Iovieno, G. Parente, A. M. Soldani, and L. Fontana, "Long-term clinical outcomes of deep anterior lamellar keratoplasty in patients with keratoconus," *American Journal of Ophthalmology*, vol. 159, no. 3, pp. 505–511, 2015.

[4] R. MacIntyre, S. P. Chow, E. Chan, and A. Poon, "Long-term outcomes of deep anterior lamellar keratoplasty versus penetrating keratoplasty in Australian keratoconus patients," *Cornea*, vol. 33, no. 1, pp. 6–9, 2014.

[5] P. Steven, S. Siebelmann, D. Hos, F. Bucher, and C. Cursiefen, "Immune reactions and dry eye after Posterior Lamellar keratoplasty," in *Proceedings of Current Treatment Options for Fuchs Endothelial Dystrophy*, pp. 227–235, Springer International Publishing, Basel, Switzerland, 2017.

[6] F. Oruçoglu, E. Z. Blumenthal, J. Frucht-Pery, and A. Solomon, "Risk factors and incidence of ocular hypertension after penetrating keratoplasty," *Journal of Glaucoma*, vol. 23, no. 9, pp. 599–605, 2014.

[7] V. M. Borderie, P. Loriaut, N. Bouheraoua, and J. P. Nordmann, "Incidence of intraocular pressure elevation and glaucoma after lamellar versus full-thickness penetrating keratoplasty," *Ophthalmology*, vol. 123, no. 7, pp. 1428–1434, 2016.

[8] D. T. Quek, C. W. Wong, T. T. Wong et al., "Graft failure and intraocular pressure control after keratoplasty in iridocorneal endothelial syndrome," *American Journal of Ophthalmology*, vol. 160, no. 3, pp. 422.e1–429.e1, 2015.

[9] H. C. Chen, C. Y. Lee, H. Y. Lin et al., "Shifting trends in microbial keratitis following penetrating keratoplasty in Taiwan," *Medicine*, vol. 96, no. 5, article e5864, 2017.

[10] T. Dada, A. Aggarwal, K. B. Minudath et al., "Post-penetrating keratoplasty glaucoma," *Indian Journal of Ophthalmology*, vol. 56, no. 4, p. 269, 2008.

[11] J. W. Doyle and M. F. Smith, "Glaucoma after penetrating keratoplasty," *Seminars in Ophthalmology*, vol. 9, no. 4, pp. 254–257, 1994.

[12] I. Beiran, D. S. Rootman, G. E. Trope, and Y. M. Buys, "Long-term results of transscleral Nd: YAG cyclophotocoagulation for refractory glaucoma postpenetrating keratoplasty," *Journal of Glaucoma*, vol. 9, no. 3, pp. 268–272, 2000.

[13] M. Banitt and R. K. Lee, "Management of patients with combined glaucoma and corneal transplant surgery," *Eye*, vol. 23, no. 10, pp. 1972–1979, 2009.

[14] A. Panda, V. J. Prakash, T. Dada, A. K. Gupta, S. Khokhar, and M. Vanathi, "Ahmed glaucoma valve in post-penetrating-keratoplasty glaucoma: a critically evaluated prospective clinical study," *Indian Journal of Ophthalmology*, vol. 59, no. 3, p. 185, 2011.

[15] R. K. Lee and F. Fantes, "Surgical management of patients with combined glaucoma and corneal transplant surgery," *Current Opinion in Ophthalmology*, vol. 14, no. 2, pp. 95–99, 2003.

[16] J. D. Levinson, A. L. Giangiacomo, A. D. Beck et al., "Glaucoma drainage devices: risk of exposure and infection," *American Journal of Ophthalmology*, vol. 160, no. 3, pp. 516–521.e2, 2015.

[17] K. W. Muir, A. Lim, S. Stinnett, A. Kuo, H. Tseng, and M. M. Walsh, "Risk factors for exposure of glaucoma drainage devices: a retrospective observational study," *BMJ Open*, vol. 4, no. 5, article e004560, 2014.

[18] A. Chen, F. Yu, S. K. Law, J. A. Giaconi, A. L. Coleman, and J. Caprioli, "Valved glaucoma drainage devices in pediatric glaucoma: retrospective long-term outcomes," *JAMA Ophthalmology*, vol. 133, no. 9, pp. 1030–1035, 2015.

[19] Z. Li, M. Zhou, W. Wang et al., "A prospective comparative study on neovascular glaucoma and non-neovascular refractory glaucoma following Ahmed glaucoma valve implantation," *Chinese Medical Journal*, vol. 127, no. 8, pp. 1417–1422, 2014.

[20] J. Jiménez-Román, F. Gil-Carrasco, V. P. Costa et al., "Intraocular pressure control after the implantation of a second Ahmed glaucoma valve," *International Ophthalmology*, vol. 36, no. 3, pp. 347–353, 2016.

[21] A. M. Al-Omairi, A. H. Al Ameri, S. Al-Shahwan et al., "Outcomes of Ahmed glaucoma valve revision in pediatric glaucoma," *American Journal of Ophthalmology*, vol. 183, pp. 141–146, 2017.

[22] T. L. Jackson, P. H. Donachie, J. M. Sparrow, and R. L. Johnston, "United Kingdom National Ophthalmology Database study of vitreoretinal surgery: report 1; case mix, complications, and cataract," *Eye*, vol. 27, no. 5, pp. 644–651, 2013.

[23] T. L. Jackson, P. H. Donachie, A. Sallam, J. M. Sparrow, and R. L. Johnston, "United Kingdom National Ophthalmology Database study of vitreoretinal surgery: report 3, retinal detachment," *Ophthalmology*, vol. 121, no. 3, pp. 643–648, 2014.

[24] S. E. Wilson and H. E. Kaufman, "Graft failure after penetrating keratoplasty," *Survey of Ophthalmology*, vol. 34, no. 5, pp. 325–356, 1990.

[25] D. B. Goldberg, D. J. Schanzlin, and S. I. Brown, "Incidence of increased intraocular pressure after keratolasty," *American Journal of Ophthalmology*, vol. 92, no. 3, pp. 372–377, 1981.

[26] N. Yildirim, H. Gursoy, A. Sahin, A. Ozer, and E. Colak, "Glaucoma after penetrating keratoplasty: incidence, risk factors, and management," *Journal of ophthalmology*, vol. 30, pp. 1–6, 2011.

[27] I. Chowers and U. Ticho, "Mitomycin-C in combined or two stage procedure trabeculectomy followed by penetrating keratoplasty," *Journal of Glaucoma*, vol. 8, pp. 184–187, 1999.

[28] R. S. Ayyala, L. Pieroth, and A. F. Vinals, "Comparison of mitomycin C trabeculectomy, glaucoma drainage device implantation and laser neodymium YAG cyclophotocoagulation in the management of intractable glaucoma after penetrating keratoplasty," *Ophthalmology*, vol. 105, no. 8, pp. 1550–1556, 1998.

[29] A. Raj, R. Dhasmana, and H. Bahadur, "Comparative evaluation of trabeculectomy with releasable suture versus subconjunctival mitomycin C in post keratoplasty glaucoma," *Sudanese Journal of Ophthalmology*, vol. 9, no. 1, p. 16, 2017.

[30] S. M. Iverson, O. Spierer, G. C. Papachristou et al., "Comparison of primary graft survival following penetrating keratoplasty and descemet's stripping endothelial keratoplasty in eyes with prior trabeculectomy," *British Journal of Ophthalmology*, vol. 99, no. 11, pp. 1477–1482, 2015.

[31] C. M. Kirkness, "Penetrating keratoplasty, glaucoma and silicon drainage tubing," *Developments in Ophthalmology*, vol. 14, pp. 161–165, 1987.

[32] J. K. Parihar, V. K. Jain, J. Kaushik, and A. Mishra, "Pars plana-modified versus conventional Ahmed glaucoma valve in patients undergoing penetrating keratoplasty: a prospective comparative randomized study," *Current Eye Research*, vol. 42, no. 3, pp. 436–442, 2017.

[33] R. S. Ayyala, D. Zurakowski, and J. A. Smith, "A clinical study of Ahmed valve implant in advanced glaucoma," *Ophthalmology*, vol. 105, no. 10, pp. 1968–1976, 1998.

[34] A. Tandon, L. Espandar, D. Cupp, S. Ho, V. Johnson, and R. S. Ayyala, "Surgical management for postkeratoplasty glaucoma: a meta-analysis," *Journal of Glaucoma*, vol. 23, no. 7, pp. 424–429, 2014.

[35] H. Helmy, O. Hashem, S. Abouelkhir, and M. M. Murad, "Ahmed valve implantation in post-penetrating keratoplasty glaucoma: four-years follow up," *Cataract and Cornea: Journal of the Egyptian Society of Cataract and Corneal Diseases*, vol. 22, pp. 41–46, 2016.

19

A Review of Surgical Outcomes and Advances for Macular Holes

Peng-peng Zhao ⓘ,[1] Shuang Wang,[2] Nan Liu,[1] Zhi-min Shu,[1] and Jin-song Zhao ⓘ[1]

[1]Department of Ophthalmology, The Second Hospital of Jilin University, Changchun, China
[2]Department of Ophthalmology, The Third People's Hospital of Chengdu, Chengdu, China

Correspondence should be addressed to Jin-song Zhao; jinsongzhao2003@163.com

Academic Editor: Toshihide Kurihara

The surgical outcomes of macular holes (MHs) have improved greatly in recent years. The closure rate is as high as 90–100%, but the outcomes of some special types of MHs remain unsatisfactory. Internal limiting membrane (ILM) peeling dramatically improves the anatomic success rate, but recent studies have found that it could also cause mechanical and subclinical traumatic changes to the retina. Dyes are widely used, and apart from indocyanine green (ICG), the toxicities of other dyes require further research. Face-down posturing is necessary for MHs larger than $400\,\mu m$, and the duration of this posture is determined by the type of tamponade and the case. The ellipsoid zone has been shown to be highly correlated with visual outcome and recovery. New surgical methods include the inverted ILM flap technique and the ILM abrasion technique. However, they require further research to determine their effectiveness.

1. Introduction

A macular hole (MH) is a full-thickness or partial-thickness defect in the macular region, and its pathogenesis can be idiopathic or result from myopia, trauma, or other causes [1, 2]. Before the application of vitrectomy, there was no specific treatment for MH [3], although some MHs were known to close spontaneously [4]. Surgery for MH has undergone great developments since Kelly and Wendel [5] first applied vitrectomy to treat MH. Both closure rate and visual recovery have improved dramatically; internal limiting membrane (ILM) peeling in particular has significantly improved the closure rate. The use of dyes and the development of microincision surgery have reduced both the duration of surgery and the risk of damage from surgery. Furthermore, a recent postoperative posturing study reported pain relief for patients, and new surgical methods may soon offer novel solutions to the remaining problems. This article reviews the outcomes of and advances in MH surgery.

2. The Surgical Outcomes

2.1. Visual Outcomes. Kelly and Wendel [5] reported that 73% patients who underwent vitrectomy resulting in successful macular reattachment experienced an improvement in visual acuity of two lines or better. With the continuous improvement in surgical techniques, the closure rate is improved and the rate of visual acuity recovery has been improved.

However, visual acuity outcomes differ by the MH type. Compared with the idiopathic MH, the postoperative visual outcomes for high myopic MH are limited. For idiopathic MHs, Tewari et al. [6] reported a final visual acuity of 20/50 following ILM peeling. Wu and Kung [4] reported that the mean logMAR visual acuity improved in a group with high myopia from 0.92 to 0.63, while a group without high myopia showed an improvement from 1.02 to 0.48. Thus, visual outcomes were less successful in highly myopic eyes. Due to the relatively less favorable outcomes of ILM peeling techniques for myopic eyes and for large and refractory MHs, the inverted flap technique was proposed in 2010. Guber et al. [7] reported that most patients with large MHs (diameter > 400 μm) showed best-corrected visual acuity (BCVA) improvements of 1 to 2 lines following surgery using the inverted flap technique. Khodani et al. [8] reported that visual acuity was improved in patients with very large MHs (diameter > 1000 μm), from a baseline visual acuity of 20/120 to a final visual acuity of 20/80 following surgery using the inverted flap technique.

Visual acuity improvements are known to differ depending on the stage of MH and the type of stain used in ILM peeling. Mean visual acuity has been reported to improve to 20/50 for stage 2 holes, 20/110 for stage 3 holes, and 20/145 for stage 4 holes [9]. Further, better visual outcomes following ILM peeling have been reported with brilliant blue (BB) compared to indocyanine green (ICG). Williamson and Lee [9] reported that postoperative visual acuity was 20/100 for patients who underwent surgery where ICG was used, while the postoperative visual acuity was 20/70 for patients who underwent surgery with BB.

2.2. Closure Rate. Before the introduction of vitrectomy to treat MH, the spontaneous closure rate for Gass stage 3 and 4 MHs was merely 4%, while that for stage 2 MHs was 11.4% [4]. Following the introduction of vitrectomy by Kelly and Wendel [5], the closure rate increased to 58%. As surgical techniques and instrumentation have improved, the closure rate has increased to as high as 90% [10].

However, as with visual outcomes, surgical outcomes differ by the MH type. Idiopathic MHs have the best outcomes, with reported closure rates ranging from 90 to 100% [6, 11–20]. Vitrectomy can reduce tangential traction at the prefoveal vitreous cortex and/or the epiretinal membranes (ERMs) as well as anteroposterior traction at the vitreoretinal interface. Compared with idiopathic MHs, the postoperative closure rates for myopic, traumatic, and large MHs are limited and these MHs require a second surgery [4, 21–29]. Traumatic MH is hypothesized to result from axial compression of the globe, which can suddenly reduce the globe's anterior-posterior diameter and cause the eyeball to expand in the equatorial direction to compensate. This change can lead to splitting of the retinal layers at the fovea [21]. The postoperative closure rate for a traumatic MH has been reported to range from approximately 83% to 92.3% [21, 30]. For a myopic MH, the closure rate has been reported to range from 63% to 90% [4, 22–25]. Although the reasons for these less favorable outcomes are not fully understood, some authors speculated that a long axial length (>30 mm) and posterior staphyloma, which can exert additional traction on the retinal surface and impede hole closure, are the two main causes for the low closure rates and limited visual recovery [4, 26].

Additionally, MH diameter is also an important issue in hole closure [28, 29, 31–35]. One study in particular indicated that when the MHs with diameters less than 400 μm, the closure rate is approximately 92–97%, while MHs with diameters greater than 500 μm show a closure rate of just 50% [31]. This difference in closure rates is caused by both hole diameter and the associated Gass stage. Indeed, other studies have shown that closure rate differs by stage in

idiopathic MH, with lower rates being observed in stage 3 and 4 MHs compared to stage 2 MHs [9, 36–38]. Williamson and Lee [9] reported that among 351 cases, the stage 2, 3, and 4 closure rates were 95.8%, 73.0%, and 56.3%, respectively, and this difference was significant.

2.3. Microstructural Changes. Using histology results, postoperative MH can be divided into four types: U-shaped closures, V-shaped closures, irregular closures, and flat/open closures [39, 40]. Michalewska et al. [39] described a U-shaped closure as a normal foveal contour that results in the best visual outcomes and is present in about 45% of all patients. A V-shaped closure, described as a steep foveal contour, has been reported to be present in about 26% of cases and is associated with less favorable visual outcomes compared to U-shaped closures. Irregular closures show an irregular foveal contours and are reported to be present in about 8.8% of cases. Flat/open closures are observed in approximately 19% of cases and show foveal defects of the neurosensory retina with a flattened cuff of fluid around the hole. Visual recovery for flat/open closures is limited.

Before the advent of spectral-domain optical coherence tomography (SD-OCT), authors using time-domain OCT (TD-OCT) found that photoreceptor defects were correlated with postoperative BCVA. However, they could not determine the causing mechanisms and could only describe the foveal contour as irregular or regular due to the limited resolution of TD-OCT [41–43]. SD-OCT has a higher resolution and can enhance the intraretinal architectural morphology, especially that of the photoreceptor layer [41]. There are four distinct hyperreflective lines that can be viewed by SD-OCT: the photoreceptor inner segment/outer segment (IS/OS) junction, the external limiting membrane (ELM), the cone outer segment tips (COST), and the retinal pigment epithelium (RPE) [44]. The International Nomenclature OCT Consensus refers to the IS/OS junction as the ellipsoid zone and the COST as the interdigitation zone [45], and thus we use this nomenclature in the remainder of this review. Studies have reported that defects in the ellipsoid zone are a major reason for unsatisfactory visual recovery, and the length of the ellipsoid zone defect is negatively correlated with visual recovery. Further, as the ellipsoid zone is restored, visual acuity is expected to improve [46–51]. Other studies have found that the ELM and the interdigitation zone are also associated with visual recovery [49]. The ELM has further been shown to be correlated with the ellipsoid zone: a disrupted ELM has been reported to always be accompanied by a disrupted ellipsoid zone, but a restored or intact ELM is not always associated with an intact ellipsoid zone [50]. It has also been demonstrated that the integrity of the ELM and ellipsoid zone is the most important factor related to postoperative visual acuity [44].

A less common mechanism of MH formation is by ERM traction, usually on a lamellar macular hole (LMH) [52]. Recently, a study proposed by Pang and associates [53] found that the lamellar hole-associated epiretinal proliferation (LHEP) appears on SD-OCT images as a substantial material of homogenous medium reflectivity located on the epiretinal surface, which is a unique feature in LMH or LMH-induced full-thickness macular hole (FTMH). In addition, unlike the common configuration observed with MH, SD-OCT images show ERM-induced MHs as narrow base with wider separation in the inner retina [52].

3. The Surgical Techniques

3.1. ILM Peeling and New Surgical Methods. Several meta-analyses have indicated that ILM peeling can significantly improve initial postoperative closure rate and visual recovery and reduce the chance of a second operation [54–56]. Several studies have reported that there is no difference between peeling and nonpeeling for stage 1 and 2 MHs but there is a significant difference for stages 3 and 4 between peeling and nonpeeling, regarding the closure rate. ILM peeling releases traction caused by glial cells, which then migrate on the surface of the ILM, as it acts as a scaffold for cellular proliferation [20, 57, 58]. ILM peeling is now a standard procedure in MH surgery.

Although ILM peeling can result in improvements in MH treatment, recent research has found that it can cause mechanical and subclinical traumatic changes to the retinal nerve fiber layer (RNFL) [59, 60]. The earliest change is swelling of the arcuate retinal nerve fiber layer (SANFL) [61]. Indeed, Clark et al. [61] found that patients who underwent vitrectomy and ILM peeling presented with hypoautofluorescent arcuate striae in the macular region on infrared and autofluorescence imaging with corresponding hyperreflectantive swelling demonstrated on spectral-domain optical coherence tomography (SD-OCT). The SANFL does not appear to impact the final BCVA and can be expected to disappear in about 3 months [59]. There are two hypotheses regarding the cause of SANFL [61]. The first hypothesis is that surgical forceps cause direct damage to the retina when grasping the ILM while the second is that ILM peeling causes damage to the Müller cell endplates that are attached to the ILM.

The dissociated optic nerve fiber layer (DONFL), which is similar to the SANFL [10, 58, 59, 62], is observed as small, spindle-shaped splitting adjacent nerve fiber bundles on SD-OCT. Not all patients who undergo ILM peeling will present with the DONFL postoperatively, and there have been no significant differences observed between eyes with and those without the DONFL with respect to BCVA or macular sensitivity. The reason for DONFL presentation is also unclear, although some authors speculated that the DONFL is caused by irregularly distributed Müller cells following ILM peeling in regions that show a higher density of nerve fiber bundles in the RNFL.

Although ILM peeling is generally used for MH surgery, several surgical technique modifications have been studied in recent years. Bae et al. [20] demonstrated that the extent of ILM peeling affects the degree of postoperative metamorphopsia. They divided the radius of ILM removal into two groups of 0.75 and 1.5 disc diameter (DD) and found that a larger extent of ILM removal was related to significantly better postoperative metamorphopsia improvement. There have also been developments of new surgical methods for MHs that are associated with unsatisfactory anatomic

outcomes and visual recovery, including large MHs, highly myopic MHs, and traumatic MHs. Ho et al. [63] performed the foveola nonpeeling surgery in early-stage 2 MHs. They peeled off a donut-shaped ILM, leaving a 400 μm diameter ILM over the foveola. And in this way, they successfully prevented inner retinal damages, maintained the integrity of the foveolar structure, and led to better final visual acuity. In 2010, Michalewska et al. [27] first adopted the inverted ILM flap technique to treat large MHs. The authors of this study did not grasp the ILM completely but left it attached at the edges of the MH. Next, they rolled the ILM to cover the hole and left the ILM's retinal face adjacent to the vitreous cavity. This new method was shown to significantly improve the closure rates of large MHs (>400 μm) and to change the flat/open closures into U-shaped or V-shaped closures. Later, the authors applied this method to highly myopic, traumatic, and other refractory MHs and were again able to achieve higher closure rates and improved visual outcomes [7, 8, 25, 28, 64–71]. However, the mechanism of the ILM flap technique is not yet clear. The results of a study by Kase et al. [70] suggest that glial cells placed on the hole may produce intermediate filaments and provoke tissue remodeling within the MH. Further, Shiode et al. [72] proposed that the ILM functions as a scaffold for the proliferation and migration of Müller cells, allowing the neurotrophic factors and basic fibroblast growth factors that are produced by the Müller cells to contribute to MH closure.

Recent studies have improved on the inverted ILM flap technique: a rolled segment of the peeled ILM into a single-layered ILM. A single-layered ILM can now be rolled and used to fill the MH [73–75]. Song et al. [73] developed a vitrectomy combined with a Viscoat- (Alcon Laboratories, Fort Worth, TX, USA) assisted single-layered inverted ILM flap technique. The use of Viscoat effectively prevents retroversion of the ILM flap during the fluid-air exchange and minimizes the toxic effect of ICG staining on the RPE. Morizane et al. [64] further developed an autologous transplantation of the ILM for refractory MHs in which the surgeon grasps the ILM flap from the ungrasped area to cover the hole for patients who undergo ILM peeling. Michalewska et al. [76] reported that the temporal inverted ILM flap technique, which involves grasping the ILM from the temporal area, reduced the incidence of the DONFL and SANFL. Chen and Yang [77] reported a technique that uses the autologous anterior or posterior lens capsule flap as a scaffold to plug the MH. Finally, Grewal and Mahmoud [78] introduced a new technique involving the use of the autologous neurosensory retinal free flap for closure of refractory myopic MHs.

Mahajan et al. [79] reported a new ILM abrasion technique for postvitrectomy in which a diamond-dusted membrane scraper is brushed over the macula in the 1 DD area surrounding the MH. This technique achieves similar results as ILM peeling (total, 94% closure) and achieves a rate of 93.5% (58/62) closure for Gass stage 3 and 4 holes [79]. They also found that this method would not penetrate the RNFL [80]. Therefore, they believe that the ILM abrasion technique is another option for MH surgery. More studies are required to determine the effectiveness of both the inverted ILM flap technique and the ILM abrasion technique.

3.2. Dyes and Adjuvants. Even for experienced surgeons, it is difficult to visualize the ILM during MH surgery. The application of dyes and adjuvants can make MH surgeries safer, reduce the duration of surgery, and decrease the risk of mechanical trauma to the retina.

Commonly used dyes include indocyanine green (ICG), trypan blue (TB), brilliant blue G (BBG), and acid violet 17 [58]. Adjuvants include triamcinolone acetonide (TA) and blood [58, 81].

Among these dyes, the earliest and most widely used is ICG [10], but studies have demonstrated that ICG can cause toxicity. ICG has an impact on the retinal ganglion cells (RGCs), glial cells, and RPE cells [82, 83]. Two meta-analyses have reported that eyes treated with ICG have poorer visual acuity and field outcomes than those treated with other dyes [84, 85]. Additionally, the visual field defect present after ILM removal has been shown to further progress after surgery when ICG is used [86]. TB is another widely used dye [10, 81, 87–89], but several *in vitro* experiments have shown that it causes dose- and time-dependent neurotoxicity on RGCs. However, the RGC toxicity observed for TB has been less than that observed for ICG [58, 90, 91].

Authors have also reported RPE atrophy following TB-assisted ILM peeling [92, 93]. TA has been shown to be safe and effective compared with ICG, and its usage has thus become common [81, 94–97]. The main side effect of TA is high postoperative intraocular pressure, and one *in vitro* study has reported that TA is toxic to RPE cells when applied at a normal dose [98]. However, a pig study failed to observe the same RPE atrophy 6 weeks after surgery [95]. Blood can also be used for staining [58], and one report has demonstrated that the use of whole blood before staining the ILM with BBG causes earlier and better visual postoperative rehabilitation [99]. BBG is another safe dye used in ophthalmological surgery [100]. Although ICG and TB injections have both been shown to cause retinal cell degeneration, subretinal injection of BBG had no such effect in a study using a rat model [101]. One *in vitro* experiment used ICG, TB, TA, and BBG in a rat model and reported that only ICG caused retinal cell dysfunction and structural damage [102]. Further, one electroretinogram and histopathology study used ICG, TA, and BBG in a pig eye model and reported that the cytotoxicity of ICG is significantly higher than that of TA or BBG [95]. Another experiment found that neither BBG nor TA use had a significant effect on postoperative mfERG (multifocal electroretinogram) responses or histology in pig eye [95, 103]. A meta-analysis further showed that there is no significant difference in the rate of hole closure following MH surgery using BBG versus other dyes, but significantly better recovery of postoperative visual function was present when BBG was used compared to ICG or other dyes [104]. Acid violet 17 is a dye that has been recently introduced for use in MH surgery and is specific to the ILM. This dye allows clear intraoperative visualization and provides a greater contrast than BBG. Although its safety has been confirmed at concentrations of 0.25 g/L and 0.5 g/L, further studies are required to confirm its long-term safety [58].

Indeed, further study is required to determine the toxicities of each dye, with the exception of ICG, during MH surgery.

3.3. Postoperative Posturing and Tamponade. When Kelly and Wendel [5] first introduced vitrectomy for MH treatment, they used room air to fill the vitreous cavity and required that the patients stay face-down for one week. Face-down posturing has thus become a standard of MH treatment.

However, face-down posturing is accompanied by great inconvenience, and some patients, especially children and the elderly, cannot tolerate it. Therefore, there is still debate about the necessity and duration of face-down posturing [105, 106]. A meta-analysis by Hu and colleagues [107] found that patients who stay face-down show better anatomic outcomes than those who do not. However, when the MH diameter was <400 μm, face-down posturing showed no significant difference in anatomic success, while face-down posturing was associated with a higher success rate when the MH diameter was >400 μm [108]. Thus, face-down posturing currently seems to be necessary, especially for large MHs.

The duration of face-down posturing is strongly related to the type of tamponade that is used in MH surgery. Two kinds of tamponades can be used in the vitreous cavity: gas and silicone oil. Gas plays a very important role in MH surgery because air not only can provide scaffolds for cellular proliferation but also can cause the extrusion of subretinal fluid from surface tension [109]. Although room air was originally used for MH surgery, long-lasting gas can also be applied [105]. Then, long-lasting gas became widely used to improve the effect of the gas, and the duration was extended to 1 month. Recently, some researchers have found that room air can have similar outcomes to a long-lasting gas, but the hole diameters in their cases were small, so the conclusions that can be drawn are limited [110, 111]. Commonly used long-lasting gases include sulfur hexafluoride (SF_6) and perfluoropropane (C_3F_8) [112], and no significant differences in anatomic success or visual outcomes have been reported between these [108, 112–114]. When long-lasting gas became widely used as an improved tamponade, the duration was extended to 1 month. Recently, two studies have reported that room air can have similar outcomes to long-lasting gas, but the conclusions that can be drawn from these studies are limited because they only included holes with small diameters [110, 111]. The degree of gas fill also affects MH closure, as a gas fill above at least 65% on postoperative day 4 has been shown to reduce the risk of poor gas-macula contact and surgical failure [106]. Kannan et al. [115] reported that a smaller volume of SF_6 can be used for a longer duration in order to achieve good surgical outcomes at a decreased cost.

Silicone oil, which is also used as a tamponade, is available in heavy and light varieties [116]. There is no consensus about which of these is better with respect to closure rate [117], but one report found that high intraocular pressure is more common following the use of heavy silicone oil

[118]. Heavy silicone oil can also cause complications such as intraocular inflammation reaction, media opacification, and secondary glaucoma [119, 120]. Face-down posturing is not strictly necessary when using silicone oil [83, 116], and heavy silicone oil only requires that the patient be lied flat [116]. Silicone oil is mainly used for patients who cannot tolerate face-down posturing (e.g., children) [121], for large MHs [21], for MHs that remain open after the first operation [122], for highly myopic MHs with retinal detachment, and for cases involving posterior staphyloma [117]. Studies have demonstrated that initial closure rates and visual outcomes are lower with silicone oil than with gas [111, 123–126], mainly because of silicone oil's lower buoyant force [124], toxic effect on photoreceptor cells, and the cases that are chosen for silicone oil use [21, 83, 124]. In addition, the use of silicone oil requires another operation to remove it. Finally, a recent study has indicated that the use of ILM flap repositioning and autologous gluconated blood clumps as a macular plug is effective in achieving satisfactory hole closure with statically significant functional improvements and in reducing the occurrence of cataract and high intraocular pressure after surgery [127].

Apart from the tamponade type, the duration of face-down posturing is also dependent on the MH itself. One study indicated that most MHs close during the first postoperative day [128]. Research using short-lasting gases and shorter durations has shown similar outcomes [83, 109, 129–131]. Tatham and Banerjee's meta-analysis found that a duration of 24 h versus 5–10 days resulted in no significant differences in the closure rate [132]. Iezzi and Kapoor [133] reported that MH surgery using broad ILM peeling, 20% SF_6 gas, and no face-down positioning is highly effective for idiopathic MH. More studies are needed to investigate short durations of face-down posturing.

4. Conclusion

There is no doubt that MH surgery has made huge progress leading to better accuracy and convenience and less damage. The continual development of new instruments helps surgeons to better assess microstructural changes, while new surgical methods provide a promising direction for treatment. However, these new advances are still being explored, and more research is needed in order to develop more definitive conclusions.

Conflicts of Interest

The authors declare that there is no conflict of interest regarding the publication of this article.

Acknowledgments

This study was supported by "Binding activity of sugar glycosaminoglycans and RPE mediated by CD44 receptor" (NO20160101094JC) and "The project of emergency treatment for ocular trauma" (3D5172173429).

References

[1] M. Landolfi, M. A. Zarbin, and N. Bhagat, "Macular holes," *Ophthalmology Clinics of North America*, vol. 15, no. 4, pp. 565–572, 2002.

[2] M. la Cour and J. Friis, "Macular holes: classification, epidemiology, natural history and treatment," *Acta Ophthalmologica*, vol. 80, no. 6, pp. 579–587, 2002.

[3] A. R. Margherio, "Macular hole surgery in 2000," *Current Opinion in Ophthalmology*, vol. 11, no. 3, pp. 186–190, 2000.

[4] T. T. Wu and Y. H. Kung, "Comparison of anatomical and visual outcomes of macular hole surgery in patients with high myopia vs. non-high myopia: a case-control study using optical coherence tomography," *Graefe's Archive for Clinical and Experimental Ophthalmology*, vol. 250, no. 3, pp. 327–331, 2012.

[5] N. E. Kelly and R. T. Wendel, "Vitreous surgery for idiopathic macular holes. Results of a pilot study," *Archives of Ophthalmology*, vol. 109, no. 5, pp. 654–659, 1991.

[6] A. Tewari, A. Almony, and G. K. Shah, "Macular hole closure with triamcinolone-assisted internal limiting membrane peeling," *Retina*, vol. 28, no. 9, pp. 1276–1279, 2008.

[7] J. Guber, C. Lang, and C. Valmaggia, "Internal limiting membrane flap techniques for the repair of large macular holes: a short-term follow-up of anatomical and functional outcomes," *Klinische Monatsblätter für Augenheilkunde*, vol. 234, no. 4, pp. 493–496, 2017.

[8] M. Khodani, P. Bansal, R. Narayanan, and J. Chhablani, "Inverted internal limiting membrane flap technique for very large macular hole," *International journal of Ophthalmology*, vol. 9, no. 8, pp. 1230–1232, 2016.

[9] T. H. Williamson and E. Lee, "Idiopathic macular hole: analysis of visual outcomes and the use of indocyanine green or brilliant blue for internal limiting membrane peel," *Graefes Archive for Clinical and Experimental Ophthalmology*, vol. 252, no. 3, pp. 395–400, 2014.

[10] E. K. Chin, D. R. P. Almeida, and E. H. Sohn, "Structural and functional changes after macular hole surgery: a review," *International Ophthalmology Clinics*, vol. 54, no. 2, pp. 17–27, 2014.

[11] L. Jančo, R. Vida, M. Bartoš, and K. Villémová, "Surgical treatment of the idiopatic macular hole - our experience," *Ceska A Slovenska Oftalmologie Casopis Ceske Oftalmologicke Spolecnosti A Slovenske Oftalmologicke Spolecnosti*, vol. 69, no. 3, pp. 102–105, 2013.

[12] F. Jordan, S. Jentsch, R. Augsten, J. Strobel, and J. Dawczynski, "Study on the time course of macular pigment density measurement in patients with a macular hole – clinical course and impact of surgery," *Klinische Monatsbltter Für Augenheilkunde*, vol. 229, no. 11, pp. 1124–1129, 2012.

[13] T. Baba, S. Yamamoto, R. Kimoto, T. Oshitari, and E. Sato, "Reduction of thickness of ganglion cell complex after internal limiting membrane peeling during vitrectomy for idiopathic macular hole," *Eye*, vol. 26, no. 9, pp. 1173–1180, 2012.

[14] H. Sakaguchi, M. Ohji, Y. Oshima et al., "Long-term follow-up after vitrectomy to treat idiopathic full-thickness macular holes: visual acuity and macular complications," *Clinical Ophthalmology*, vol. 6, pp. 1281–1286, 2012.

[15] D. R. P. Almeida, J. Wong, M. Belliveau, J. Rayat, and J. Gale, "Anatomical and visual outcomes of macular hole surgery with short-duration 3-day face-down positioning," *Retina*, vol. 32, no. 3, pp. 506–510, 2012.

[16] K. Yamamoto and S. Hori, "Long-term outcome of vitrectomy combined with internal limiting membrane peeling for idiopathic macular holes," *Nippon Ganka Gakkai Zasshi*, vol. 115, no. 1, pp. 20–26, 2011.

[17] H. Nomoto, F. Shiraga, H. Yamaji et al., "Macular hole surgery with triamcinolone acetonide–assisted internal limiting membrane peeling: one-year results," *Retina*, vol. 28, no. 3, pp. 427–432, 2008.

[18] T. Hikichi, Y. Furukawa, H. Ohtsuka et al., "Improvement of visual acuity one-year after vitreous surgery in eyes with residual triamcinolone acetonide at the macular hole," *American Journal of Ophthalmology*, vol. 145, no. 2, pp. 267–272.e1, 2008.

[19] K. Kumagai, M. Furukawa, N. Ogino, E. Larson, and A. Uemura, "Long-term outcomes of macular hole surgery with triamcinolone acetonide–assisted internal limiting membrane peeling," *Retina*, vol. 27, no. 9, pp. 1249–1254, 2007.

[20] K. Bae, S. W. Kang, J. H. Kim, S. J. Kim, J. M. Kim, and J. M. Yoon, "Extent of internal limiting membrane peeling and its impact on macular hole surgery outcomes: a randomized trial," *American Journal of Ophthalmology*, vol. 169, pp. 179–188, 2016.

[21] J. B. Miller, Y. Yonekawa, D. Eliott, and D. G. Vavvas, "A review of traumatic macular hole: diagnosis and treatment," *International Ophthalmology Clinics*, vol. 53, no. 4, pp. 59–67, 2013.

[22] M. Alkabes, L. Padilla, C. Salinas et al., "Assessment of OCT measurements as prognostic factors in myopic macular hole surgery without foveoschisis," *Graefe's Archive for Clinical and Experimental Ophthalmology*, vol. 251, no. 11, pp. 2521–2527, 2013.

[23] K. Suda, M. Hangai, and N. Yoshimura, "Axial length and outcomes of macular hole surgery assessed by spectral-domain optical coherence tomography," *American Journal of Ophthalmology*, vol. 151, no. 1, pp. 118–127.e1, 2011.

[24] J. Qu, M. Zhao, Y. Jiang, and X. Li, "Vitrectomy outcomes in eyes with high myopic macular hole without retinal detachment," *Retina*, vol. 32, no. 2, pp. 275–280, 2012.

[25] S. Kuriyama, H. Hayashi, Y. Jingami, N. Kuramoto, J. Akita, and M. Matsumoto, "Efficacy of inverted internal limiting membrane flap technique for the treatment of macular hole in high myopia," *American Journal of Ophthalmology*, vol. 156, no. 1, pp. 125–131.e1, 2013.

[26] M. Alkabes, F. Pichi, P. Nucci et al., "Anatomical and visual outcomes in high myopic macular hole (HM-MH) without retinal detachment: a review," *Graefe's Archive for Clinical and Experimental Ophthalmology*, vol. 252, no. 2, pp. 191–199, 2014.

[27] Z. Michalewska, J. Michalewski, R. A. Adelman, and J. Nawrocki, "Inverted internal limiting membrane flap technique for large macular holes," *Ophthalmology*, vol. 117, no. 10, pp. 2018–2025, 2010.

[28] P. Mahalingam and K. Sambhav, "Surgical outcomes of inverted internal limiting membrane flap technique for large macular hole," *Indian Journal of Ophthalmology*, vol. 61, no. 10, pp. 601–603, 2013.

[29] S. Ullrich, C. Haritoglou, C. Gass, M. Schaumberger, M. W. Ulbig, and A. Kampik, "Macular hole size as a prognostic factor in macular hole surgery," *British Journal of Ophthalmology*, vol. 86, no. 4, pp. 390–393, 2002.

[30] N. Brennan, I. Reekie, A. P. Khawaja, N. Georgakarakos, and E. Ezra, "Vitrectomy, inner limiting membrane peel, and gas tamponade in the management of traumatic paediatric macular holes: a case series of 13 patients," *Ophthalmologica*, vol. 238, no. 3, pp. 119–123, 2017.

[31] A. Susini and P. Gastaud, "Macular holes that should not be operated," *Journal Français d'Ophtalmologie*, vol. 31, no. 2, pp. 214–220, 2008.

[32] R. Reis, N. Ferreira, and A. Meireles, "Management of stage IV macular holes: when standard surgery fails," *Case Reports in Ophthalmology*, vol. 3, no. 2, pp. 240–250, 2012.

[33] Z. Michalewska, J. Michalewski, and J. Nawrocki, "Long-term decrease of retinal pigment epithelium defects in large stage IV macular holes with borders mechanically joined during surgery," *Case Reports in Ophthalmology*, vol. 2, no. 2, pp. 215–221, 2011.

[34] T. Brockmann, C. Steger, M. Weger, A. Wedrich, and A. Haas, "Risk assessment of idiopathic macular holes undergoing vitrectomy with dye-assisted internal limiting membrane peeling," *Retina*, vol. 33, no. 6, pp. 1132–1136, 2013.

[35] T. M. Jenisch, F. Zeman, M. Koller, D. A. Märker, H. Helbig, and W. A. Herrmann, "Macular hole surgery: an analysis of risk factors for the anatomical and functional outcomes with a special emphasis on the experience of the surgeon," *Clinical Ophthalmology*, vol. 11, pp. 1127–1134, 2017.

[36] A. K. Kwok, T. Y. Lai, W. Man-Chan, and D. C. Woo, "Indocyanine green assisted retinal internal limiting membrane removal in stage 3 or 4 macular hole surgery," *British Journal of Ophthalmology*, vol. 87, no. 1, pp. 71–74, 2003.

[37] S. Foulquier, A. Glacet-Bernard, M. Sterkers, G. Soubrane, and G. Coscas, "Study of internal limiting membrane peeling in stage-3 and -4 idiopathic macular hole surgery," *Journal Français d'Ophtalmologie*, vol. 25, no. 10, pp. 1026–1031, 2002.

[38] S. W. Kang, K. Ahn, and D. I. Ham, "Types of macular hole closure and their clinical implications," *British Journal of Ophthalmology*, vol. 87, no. 8, pp. 1015–1019, 2003.

[39] Z. Michalewska, J. Michalewski, S. Cisiecki, R. Adelman, and J. Nawrocki, "Correlation between foveal structure and visual outcome following macular hole surgery: a spectral optical coherence tomography study," *Graefe's Archive for Clinical and Experimental Ophthalmology*, vol. 246, no. 6, pp. 823–830, 2008.

[40] M. Imai, H. Iijima, T. Gotoh, and S. Tsukahara, "Optical coherence tomography of successfully repaired idiopathic macular holes," *American Journal of Ophthalmology*, vol. 128, no. 5, pp. 621–627, 1999.

[41] M. Inoue, Y. Watanabe, A. Arakawa, S. Sato, S. Kobayashi, and K. Kadonosono, "Spectral-domain optical coherence tomography images of inner/outer segment junctions and macular hole surgery outcomes," *Graefes Archive for Clinical and Experimental Ophthalmology*, vol. 247, no. 3, pp. 325–330, 2009.

[42] T. Baba, S. Yamamoto, M. Arai et al., "Correlation of visual recovery and presence of photoreceptor inner/outer segment junction in optical coherence images after successful macular hole repair," *Retina*, vol. 28, no. 3, pp. 453–458, 2008.

[43] C. Haritoglou, A. S. Neubauer, I. W. Reiniger, S. G. Priglinger, C. A. Gass, and A. Kampik, "Long-term functional outcome of macular hole surgery correlated to optical coherence tomography measurements," *Clinical & Experimental Ophthalmology*, vol. 35, no. 3, pp. 208–213, 2007.

[44] G. Landa, R. C. Gentile, P. M. T. Garcia, T. O. Muldoon, and R. B. Rosen, "External limiting membrane and visual outcome in macular hole repair: spectral domain OCT analysis," *Eye*, vol. 26, no. 1, pp. 61–69, 2012.

[45] G. Staurenghi, S. Sadda, U. Chakravarthy, R. F. Spaide, and International Nomenclature for Optical Coherence Tomography (IN•OCT) Panel, "Proposed lexicon for anatomic landmarks in normal posterior segment spectral-domain optical coherence tomography: the IN•OCT consensus," *Ophthalmology*, vol. 121, no. 8, pp. 1572–1578, 2014.

[46] M. Sano, Y. Shimoda, H. Hashimoto, and S. Kishi, "Restored photoreceptor outer segment and visual recovery after macular hole closure," *American Journal of Ophthalmology*, vol. 147, no. 2, pp. 313–318, 2009.

[47] M. Shimozono, A. Oishi, M. Hata, and Y. Kurimoto, "Restoration of the photoreceptor outer segment and visual outcomes after macular hole closure: spectral-domain optical coherence tomography analysis," *Graefe's Archive for Clinical and Experimental Ophthalmology*, vol. 249, no. 10, pp. 1469–1476, 2011.

[48] J. Oh, W. E. Smiddy, H. W. Flynn Jr, G. Gregori, and B. Lujan, "Photoreceptor inner/outer segment defect imaging by spectral domain OCT and visual prognosis after macular hole surgery," *Investigative Ophthalmology & Visual Science*, vol. 51, no. 3, pp. 1651–1658, 2010.

[49] J. M. Ruiz-Moreno, F. Lugo, J. A. Montero, and D. P. Piñero, "Restoration of macular structure as the determining factor for macular hole surgery outcome," *Graefe's Archive for Clinical and Experimental Ophthalmology*, vol. 250, no. 10, pp. 1409–1414, 2012.

[50] Y. Mitamura, S. Mitamura-Aizawa, T. Katome et al., "Photoreceptor impairment and restoration on optical coherence tomographic image," *Journal of Ophthalmology*, vol. 2013, Article ID 518170, 7 pages, 2013.

[51] I. Y. Wong, L. P. Iu, H. Koizumi, and W. W. Lai, "The inner segment/outer segment junction: what have we learnt so far?," *Current Opinion in Ophthalmology*, vol. 23, no. 3, pp. 210–218, 2012.

[52] C. Y. Tsai, Y. T. Hsieh, and C. M. Yang, "Epiretinal membrane–induced full-thickness macular holes: the clinical features and surgical outcomes," *Retina*, vol. 36, no. 9, pp. 1679–1687, 2016.

[53] C. E. Pang, R. F. Spaide, and K. B. Freund, "Epiretinal proliferation seen in association with lamellar macular holes: a distinct clinical entity," *Retina*, vol. 34, no. 8, pp. 1513–1523, 2014.

[54] V. Mester and F. Kuhn, "Internal limiting membrane removal in the management of full-thickness macular holes," *American Journal of Ophthalmology*, vol. 129, no. 6, pp. 769–777, 2000.

[55] D. Tognetto, R. Grandin, G. Sanguinetti et al., "Internal limiting membrane removal during macular hole surgery: results of a multicenter retrospective study," *Ophthalmology*, vol. 113, no. 8, pp. 1401–1410, 2006.

[56] K. Spiteri Cornish, N. Lois, N. Scott et al., "Vitrectomy with internal limiting membrane (ILM) peeling versus vitrectomy with no peeling for idiopathic full-thickness macular hole (FTMH)," *Cochrane Database of Systematic Reviews*, vol. 5, no. 6, 2013.

[57] A. Almony, E. Nudleman, G. K. Shah et al., "Techniques, rationale, and outcomes of internal limiting membrane peeling," *Retina*, vol. 32, no. 5, pp. 877–891, 2012.

[58] F. Morescalchi, C. Costagliola, E. Gambicorti, S. Duse, M. R. Romano, and F. Semeraro, "Controversies over the role of internal limiting membrane peeling during vitrectomy in macular hole surgery," *Survey of Ophthalmology*, vol. 62, no. 1, pp. 58–69, 2016.

[59] F. Pichi, A. Lembo, M. Morara et al., "Early and late inner retinal changes after inner limiting membrane peeling," *International Ophthalmology*, vol. 34, no. 2, pp. 437–446, 2014.

[60] A. Modi, A. Giridhar, and M. Gopalakrishnan, "Comparative analysis of outcomes with variable diameter internal limiting membrane peeling in surgery for idiopathic macular hole repair," *Retina*, vol. 37, no. 2, pp. 265–273, 2016.

[61] A. Clark, N. Balducci, F. Pichi et al., "Swelling of the arcuate nerve fiber layer after internal limiting membrane peeling," *Retina*, vol. 32, no. 8, pp. 1608–1613, 2012.

[62] R. F. Spaide, ""Dissociated optic nerve fiber layer appearance" after internal limiting membrane removal is inner retinal dimpling," *Retina*, vol. 32, no. 9, pp. 1719–1726, 2012.

[63] T. C. Ho, C. M. Yang, J. S. Huang, C. H. Yang, and M. S. Chen, "Foveola nonpeeling internal limiting membrane surgery to prevent inner retinal damages in early stage 2 idiopathic macula hole," *Graefe's Archive for Clinical and Experimental Ophthalmology*, vol. 252, no. 10, pp. 1553–1560, 2014.

[64] Y. Morizane, F. Shiraga, S. Kimura et al., "Autologous transplantation of the internal limiting membrane for refractory macular holes," *American Journal of Ophthalmology*, vol. 157, no. 4, pp. 861–869.e1, 2014.

[65] Z. Michalewska and J. Nawrocki, "Macular hole surgery in a patient who cannot maintain facedown positioning," *Case Reports in Ophthalmology*, vol. 4, no. 1, pp. 1–6, 2013.

[66] H. Hayashi and S. Kuriyama, "Foveal microstructure in macular holes surgically closed by inverted internal limiting membrane flap technique," *Retina*, vol. 34, no. 12, pp. 2444–2450, 2014.

[67] M. Hirano, Y. Morizane, T. Kawata et al., "Case report: successful closure of a large macular hole secondary to uveitis using the inverted internal limiting membrane flap technique," *BMC Ophthalmology*, vol. 15, no. 83, 2015.

[68] Z. Michalewska, J. Michalewski, K. Dulczewska-Cichecka, and J. Nawrocki, "Inverted internal limiting membrane flap technique for surgical repair of myopic macular holes," *Retina*, vol. 34, no. 4, pp. 664–669, 2014.

[69] Z. Chen, C. Zhao, J. J. Ye, X. Q. Wang, and R. F. Sui, "Inverted internal limiting membrane flap technique for repair of large macular holes: a short-term follow-up of anatomical and functional outcomes," *Chinese Medical Journal*, vol. 129, no. 5, pp. 511–517, 2016.

[70] S. Kase, W. Saito, S. Mori et al., "Clinical and histological evaluation of large macular hole surgery using the inverted internal limiting membrane flap technique," *Clinical Ophthalmology*, vol. 11, pp. 9–14, 2017.

[71] A. Oleñik, J. Rios, and C. Mateo, "Inverted internal limiting membrane flap technique for macular holes in high myopia with axial length ≥30 mm," *Retina*, vol. 36, no. 9, pp. 1688–1693, 2016.

[72] Y. Shiode, Y. Morizane, R. Matoba et al., "The role of inverted internal limiting membrane flap in macular hole closure," *Investigate Ophthalmology & Visual Science*, vol. 58, no. 11, pp. 4847–4855, 2017.

[73] Z. Song, M. Li, J. Liu, X. Hu, Z. Hu, and D. Chen, "Viscoat assisted inverted internal limiting membrane flap technique for large macular holes associated with high myopia," *Journal of Ophthalmology*, vol. 2016, Article ID 8283062, 7 pages, 2016.

[74] S. N. Chen, "Large semicircular inverted internal limiting membrane flap in the treatment of macular hole in high myopia," *Graefes Archive for Clinical and Experimental Ophthalmology*, vol. 255, no. 12, pp. 2337–2345, 2017.

[75] K. Y. Pak, J. Y. Park, S. W. Park, I. S. Byon, and J. E. Lee, "Efficacy of the perfluoro-N-octane-assisted single-layered inverted internal limiting membrane flap technique for large macular holes," *Ophthalmologica*, vol. 238, no. 3, pp. 133–138, 2017.

[76] Z. Michalewska, J. Michalewski, K. Dulczewska-Cichecka, R. A. Adelman, and J. Nawrocki, "Temporal inverted internal limiting membrane flap technique versus classic inverted internal limiting membrane flap technique: a comparative study," *Retina*, vol. 35, no. 9, pp. 1844–1850, 2015.

[77] S. N. Chen and C. M. Yang, "Lens capsular flap transplantation in the management of refractory macular hole from multiple etiologies," *Retina*, vol. 36, no. 1, pp. 163–170, 2016.

[78] D. S. Grewal and T. H. Mahmoud, "Autologous neurosensory retinal free flap for closure of refractory myopic macular holes," *JAMA Ophthalmology*, vol. 134, no. 2, pp. 229–230, 2016.

[79] V. B. Mahajan, E. K. Chin, R. M. Tarantola et al., "Macular hole closure with internal limiting membrane abrasion technique," *JAMA Ophthalmology*, vol. 133, no. 6, pp. 635–641, 2015.

[80] D. R. Almeida, E. K. Chin, R. M. Tarantola et al., "Effect of internal limiting membrane abrasion on retinal tissues in macular holes," *Investigative Ophthalmology & Visual Science*, vol. 56, no. 5, pp. 2783–2789, 2015.

[81] E. Abdelkader and N. Lois, "Internal limiting membrane peeling in vitreo-retinal surgery," *Survey of Ophthalmology*, vol. 53, no. 4, pp. 368–396, 2008.

[82] A. Gandorfer, C. Haritoglou, and A. Kampik, "Toxicity of indocyanine green in vitreoretinal surgery," *Developments in Ophthalmology*, vol. 42, pp. 69–81, 2008.

[83] J. Bainbridge, E. Herbert, and Z. Gregor, "Macular holes: vitreoretinal relationships and surgical approaches," *Eye*, vol. 22, no. 10, pp. 1301–1309, 2008.

[84] Y. Wu, W. Zhu, D. Xu et al., "Indocyanine green-assisted internal limiting membrane peeling in macular hole surgery: a meta-analysis," *PLoS One*, vol. 7, no. 11, article e48405, 2012.

[85] E. B. Rodrigues and C. H. Meyer, "Meta-analysis of chromovitrectomy with indocyanine green in macular hole surgery," *Ophthalmologica*, vol. 222, no. 2, pp. 123–129, 2008.

[86] M. Nakazawa, H. Terasaki, T. Yamashita, A. Uemura, and T. Sakamoto, "Changes in visual field defects during 10-year follow-up for indocyanine green-assisted macular hole surgery," *Japanese Journal of Ophthalmology*, vol. 60, no. 387, pp. 383–5, 2016.

[87] D. Shukla, J. Kalliath, N. Neelakantan, K. B. Naresh, and K. Ramasamy, "A comparison of brilliant blue G, trypan blue, and indocyanine green dyes to assist internal limiting membrane peeling during macular hole surgery," *Retina*, vol. 31, no. 10, pp. 2021–2025, 2011.

[88] C. Bellerive, B. Cinq-Mars, M. Louis et al., "Retinal function assessment of trypan blue versus indocyanine green assisted internal limiting membrane peeling during macular hole surgery," *Canadian Journal of Ophthalmology*, vol. 48, no. 2, pp. 104–109, 2013.

[89] E. A. Abdelkader, M. B. VA, M. Anand, N. W. Scott, M. A. Rehman Siddiqui, and N. Lois, "In vivo safety of trypan blue use in vitreoretinal surgery," *Retina*, vol. 31, no. 6, pp. 1122–1127, 2011.

[90] Y. Jin, S. Uchida, Y. Yanagi, M. Aihara, and M. Araie, "Neurotoxic effects of trypan blue on rat retinal ganglion cells," *Experimental Eye Research*, vol. 81, no. 4, pp. 395–400, 2005.

[91] L. Kodjikian, T. Richter, M. Halberstadt et al., "Toxic effects of indocyanine green, infracyanine green, and trypan blue on the human retinal pigmented epithelium," *Graefe's Archive for Clinical and Experimental Ophthalmology*, vol. 243, no. 9, pp. 917–925, 2005.

[92] S. Jain, K. Kishore, and Y. R. Sharma, "Progressive atrophy of retinal pigment epithelium after trypan-blue-assisted ILM peeling for macular hole surgery," *Indian Journal of Ophthalmology*, vol. 61, no. 5, pp. 235–237, 2013.

[93] M. U. Saeed and H. Heimann, "Atrophy of the retinal pigment epithelium following vitrectomy with trypan blue," *International Ophthalmology*, vol. 29, no. 4, pp. 239–241, 2009.

[94] M. S. Tsipursky, M. A. Heller, S. A. de Souza et al., "Comparative evaluation of no dye assistance, indocyanine green and triamcinolone acetonide for internal limiting membrane peeling during macular hole surgery," *Retina*, vol. 33, no. 6, pp. 1123–1131, 2013.

[95] R. Ejstrup, M. la Cour, S. Heegaard, and J. F. Kiilgaard, "Toxicity profiles of subretinal indocyanine green, brilliant blue G, and triamcinolone acetonide: a comparative study," *Graefes Archive for Clinical & Experimental Ophthalmology*, vol. 250, no. 5, pp. 669–677, 2012.

[96] S. Taiji and T. Ishibashi, "Visualizing vitreous in vitrectomy by triamcinolone," *Graefes Archive for Clinical & Experimental Ophthalmology*, vol. 247, no. 9, pp. 1153–1163, 2009.

[97] S. Machida, Y. Toba, T. Nishimura, T. Ohzeki, K. Murai, and D. Kurosaka, "Comparisons of cone electroretinograms after indocyanine green-, brilliant blue G-, or triamcinolone acetonide-assisted macular hole surgery," *Graefe's Archive for Clinical and Experimental Ophthalmology*, vol. 252, no. 9, pp. 1423–1433, 2014.

[98] R. Narayanan, J. K. Mungcal, M. C. Kenney, G. M. Seigel, and B. D. Kuppermann, "Toxicity of triamcinolone acetonide on retinal neurosensory and pigment epithelial cells," *Investigative Ophthalmology & Visual Science*, vol. 47, no. 2, pp. 722–728, 2006.

[99] B. Ghosh, S. Arora, N. Goel et al., "Comparative evaluation of sequential intraoperative use of whole blood followed by brilliant blue versus conventional brilliant blue staining of internal limiting membrane in macular hole surgery," *Retina*, vol. 36, no. 8, pp. 1463–1468, 2016.

[100] H. Enaida and T. Ishibashi, "Brilliant blue in vitreoretinal surgery," *Developments in Ophthalmology*, vol. 42, pp. 115–125, 2008.

[101] A. Ueno, T. Hisatomi, H. Enaida et al., "Biocompatibility of brilliant blue G in a rat model of subretinal injection," *Retina*, vol. 27, no. 4, pp. 499–504, 2007.

[102] C. Creuzotgarcher, N. Acar, M. Passemard, S. Bidot, A. Bron, and L. Bretillon, "Functional and structural effect of intravitreal indocyanine green, triamcinolone acetonide, trypan blue, and brilliant blue G on rat retina," *Retina*, vol. 30, no. 8, pp. 1294–1301, 2010.

[103] S. Machida, T. Nishimura, T. Ohzeki, K. I. Murai, and D. Kurosaka, "Comparisons of focal macular electroretinograms after indocyanine green-, brilliant blue G-, or triamcinolone acetonide-assisted macular hole surgery," *Graefes Archive for Clinical & Experimental Ophthalmology*, vol. 255, no. 3, pp. 485–492, 2017.

[104] K. Azuma, Y. Noda, K. Hirasawa, and T. Ueta, "Brilliant blue G-assisted internal limiting membrane peeling for macular hole: a systematic review of literature and meta-analysis," *Retina*, vol. 36, no. 5, pp. 851–858, 2016.

[105] A. Chandra, D. G. Charteris, and D. Yorston, "Posturing after macular hole surgery: a review," *Ophthalmologica*, vol. 226, Supplement 1, pp. 3–9, 2011.

[106] M. Alberti and C. M. La, "Nonsupine positioning in macular hole surgery: a noninferiority randomized clinical trial," *Retina*, vol. 36, no. 11, pp. 2072–2079, 2016.

[107] Z. Hu, P. Xie, Y. Ding, X. Zheng, D. Yuan, and Q. Liu, "Facedown or no face-down posturing following macular hole surgery: a meta-analysis," *Acta Ophthalmologica*, vol. 94, no. 4, pp. 326–333, 2016.

[108] R. W. Essex, Z. S. Kingston, M. Moreno-Betancur et al., "The effect of postoperative face-down positioning and of long- versus short-acting gas in macular hole surgery," *Ophthalmology*, vol. 123, no. 5, pp. 1129–1136, 2016.

[109] T. Xirou, P. G. Theodossiadis, M. Apostolopoulos et al., "Macular hole surgery with short-acting gas and short-duration face-down positioning," *Clinical Ophthalmology*, vol. 6, pp. 1107–1112, 2012.

[110] Y. Hasegawa, Y. Hata, Y. Mochizuki et al., "Equivalent tamponade by room air as compared with SF_6 after macular hole surgery," *Graefe's Archive for Clinical and Experimental Ophthalmology*, vol. 247, no. 11, pp. 1455–1459, 2009.

[111] H. Usui, T. Yasukawa, Y. Hirano, H. Morita, M. Yoshida, and Y. Ogura, "Comparative study of the effects of room air and sulfur hexafluoride gas tamponade on functional and morphological recovery after macular hole surgery: a retrospective study," *Ophthalmic Research*, vol. 50, no. 4, pp. 227–230, 2013.

[112] S. S. Kim, W. E. Smiddy, W. J. Feuer, and W. Shi, "Outcomes of sulfur hexafluoride (SF6) versus perfluoropropane (C3F8) gas tamponade for macular hole surgery," *Retina*, vol. 28, no. 10, pp. 1408–1415, 2008.

[113] S. Briand, E. Chalifoux, E. Tourville et al., "Prospective randomized trial: outcomes of SF_6 versus C_3F_8 in macular hole surgery," *Canadian Journal of Ophthalmology*, vol. 50, no. 2, pp. 95–100, 2015.

[114] A. Modi, A. Giridhar, and M. Gopalakrishnan, "Sulfurhexafluoride (sf6) versus perfluoropropane (c3f8) gas as tamponade in macular hole surgery," *Retina*, vol. 37, no. 2, pp. 283–290, 2017.

[115] N. B. Kannan, O. O. Adenuga, K. Kumar, and K. Ramasamy, "Outcome of 2 cc pure sulfur hexafluoride gas tamponade for macular hole surgery," *BMC Ophthalmology*, vol. 16, no. 1, p. 73, 2016.

[116] L. Wagenfeld, O. Zeitz, C. Skevas, and G. Richard, "Long-lasting endotamponades in vitreoretinal surgery," *Ophthalmologica*, vol. 224, no. 5, pp. 291–300, 2010.

[117] X. Valldeperas and J. Lorenzo-Carrero, "Vitreous tamponades in highly myopic eyes," *BioMed Research International*, vol. 2014, Article ID 420380, 7 pages, 2014.

[118] V. Romano, F. Semeraro, M. R. Romano, M. Cruciani, and C. Costagliola, "Development of ocular hypertension secondary to tamponade with light versus heavy silicone oil: a systematic review," *Indian Journal of Ophthalmology*, vol. 63, no. 3, pp. 227–232, 2015.

[119] T. Avitabile, V. Bonfiglio, D. Buccoliero et al., "Heavy versus standard silicone oil in the management of retinal detachment with macular hole in myopic eyes," *Retina*, vol. 31, no. 3, pp. 540–546, 2011.

[120] H. Heimann, T. Stappler, and D. Wong, "Heavy tamponade 1: a review of indications, use, and complications," *Eye*, vol. 22, no. 10, pp. 1342–1359, 2008.

[121] B. Ivanovska-adjievska, S. Boskurt, F. Semiz, H. Yuzer, and V. Dimovska-Jordanova, "Treatment of idiopathic macular hole with silicone oil tamponade," *Clinical Ophthalmology*, vol. 6, pp. 1449–1454, 2012.

[122] H. Heimann, "Alternative indications for the use of heavy silicone oil tamponades," *Klinische Monatsbltter Für Augenheilkunde*, vol. 226, no. 9, pp. 713–717, 2009.

[123] J. C. Lai, S. S. Stinnett, and B. W. Mccuen, "Comparison of silicone oil versus gas tamponade in the treatment of idiopathic full-thickness macular hole," *Ophthalmology*, vol. 110, no. 6, pp. 1170–1174, 2003.

[124] H. H. Ghoraba, A. F. Ellakwa, and A. A. Ghali, "Long term result of silicone oil versus gas tamponade in the treatment of traumatic macular holes," *Clinical Ophthalmology*, vol. 6, pp. 49–53, 2012.

[125] M. E. Tafoya, H. M. Lambert, L. Vu, and M. Ding, "Visual outcomes of silicone oil versus gas tamponade for macular hole surgery," *Seminars in Ophthalmology*, vol. 18, no. 3, pp. 127–131, 2003.

[126] S. S. Couvillion, W. E. Smiddy, H. W. Flynn Jr, C. W. Eifrig, and G. Gregori, "Outcomes of surgery for idiopathic macular hole: a case-control study comparing silicone oil with gas tamponade," *Ophthalmic Surgery, Lasers & Imaging Retina*, vol. 36, no. 5, pp. 365–371, 2006.

[127] M. Chakrabarti, P. Benjamin, K. Chakrabarti, and A. Chakrabarti, "Closing macular holes with "macular plug" without gas tamponade and postoperative posturing," *Retina*, vol. 37, no. 3, pp. 451–459, 2016.

[128] K. Masuyama, K. Yamakiri, N. Arimura, Y. Sonoda, N. Doi, and T. Sakamoto, "Posturing time after macular hole surgery modified by optical coherence tomography images: a pilot study," *American Journal of Ophthalmology*, vol. 147, no. 3, pp. 481–488.e2, 2009.

[129] D. Gupta, "Face-down posturing after macular hole surgery: a review," *Retina*, vol. 29, no. 4, pp. 430–443, 2009.

[130] C. Eckardt, T. Eckert, U. Eckardt, U. Porkert, and C. Gesser, "Macular hole surgery with air tamponade and optical coherence tomography-based duration of face-down positioning," *Retina*, vol. 28, no. 8, pp. 1087–1096, 2008.

[131] R. A. Mittra, J. E. Kim, D. P. Han, and J. S. Pollack, "Sustained postoperative face-down positioning is unnecessary for successful macular hole surgery," *The British Journal of Ophthalmology*, vol. 93, no. 5, pp. 664–666, 2009.

[132] A. Tatham and S. Banerjee, "Face-down posturing after macular hole surgery: a meta-analysis," *British Journal of Ophthalmology*, vol. 94, no. 5, pp. 626–631, 2010.

[133] R. Iezzi and K. G. Kapoor, "No face-down positioning and broad internal limiting membrane peeling in the surgical repair of idiopathic macular holes," *Ophthalmology*, vol. 120, no. 10, pp. 1998–2003, 2013.

20

Comparison of 25- and 27-Gauge Pars Plana Vitrectomy in Repairing Primary Rhegmatogenous Retinal Detachment

Keiko Otsuka,[1] Hisanori Imai ⓘ,[1] Ayaka Fujii,[1] Akiko Miki,[1] Mizuki Tagami,[2] Atsushi Azumi,[2] and Makoto Nakamura ⓘ[1]

[1]Division of Ophthalmology, Department of Organ Therapeutics, Kobe University Graduate School of Medicine, 7-5-2 Kusunoki-cho, Chuo-ku, Kobe 650-0017, Japan
[2]Department of Ophthalmology, Kobe Kaisei Hospital, 3-11-15 Shinoharakitamati, Nada-ku, Kobe 657-0068, Japan

Correspondence should be addressed to Hisanori Imai; hisimai@med.kobe-u.ac.jp

Academic Editor: Ala Moshiri

Aim. To compare the anatomic and visual outcomes of 25-gauge (25G), and 27-gauge (27G) transconjunctival sutureless pars plana vitrectomy (TSV) for the management of primary rhegmatogeneous retinal detachment (RRD). *Design.* A retrospective nonrandomized clinical trial. *Methods.* A retrospective comparative analysis of 62 consecutive eyes from 62 patients with 6 months of follow-up was performed. *Results.* Thirty two patients underwent 25G TSV, and 30 patients underwent 27G TSV for the treatment of primary RRD. There was no significant difference in baseline demographic and preoperative ocular characteristics between the two groups. The initial and final anatomical success rates were 93.8% and 100% in 25G TSV and 96.7% and 100% in 27G TSV, respectively ($p = 1$ and $p = 1$, resp.). Preoperative best-corrected visual acuity (BCVA) (logMAR) was 0.44 ± 0.69 and 0.38 ± 0.61 for 25G and 27G TSV, respectively ($p = 0.73$). The final follow-up BCVA was 0.07 ± 0.25 and $-0.02\ 0.17$ for 25G and 27G TSV, respectively ($p = 0.16$). The final BCVA was significantly better than the preoperative BCVA in both groups ($p = 0.02$ and $p = 0.002$, resp.). Preoperative intraocular pressure (IOP) (mmHg) was 13.0 ± 3.5 in 25G TSV and 14.3 ± 2.8 in 27G TSV ($p = 0.11$). IOP did not statistically significantly change in both groups during the follow-up period ($p = 0.63$ and $p = 0.21$, resp.). *Conclusion.* The 27G TSV system is safe and useful for RRD treatment as 25G TSV.

1. Introduction

Since the transconjunctival sutureless pars plana vitrectomy (TSV) with 25-gauge (25G) and 23-gauge instrumentation was introduced, there is an accumulating trend toward TSV as the first choice for the treatment of a variety of vitreoretinal surgical indications [1–3]. The advantages of TSV including the small incision, self-sealing, decreased surgical trauma, and less postoperative inflammation provide patients better postoperative comfort, less postoperative astigmatism, and earlier visual recovery compared to the traditional 20-gauge vitrectomy system [4–8]. In 2010, Oshima et al. first reported a preliminary study regarding the safety and practicality of the 27-gauge (27G) instrument system for the vitreoretinal surgery [9]. Although the low rigidity of 27G instruments have been reported, several reports have suggested the clinical outcomes and short-term safety profile of 27G TSV for a variety of surgical indications, including rhegmatogeneous retinal detachment (RRD) [10–14]. However, there remained big concerns whether all surgeons can manage the 27G instrument especially on peripheral vitreoretinal disorders because the low instrument rigidity of 27G sometimes cause the difficulty of the operation and may impact the results especially for inexperienced surgeons.

In this study, we performed a retrospective comparative study to examine the anatomical success rates and complications of 25G and 27G TSV in the repair of primary RRD.

2. Patients and Methods

We performed retrospective analyses of the medical records of 62 consecutive eyes of 62 patients with primary uncomplicated RRD treated with 25G (group A) or 27G (group B) TSV. This study is a nonrandomized, retrospective comparative clinical trial. Our study was performed after obtaining the approval of the institutional review board in Kobe University School of Medicine and Kobe Kaisei Hospital. The procedure used conformed to the Tenets of the Declaration of Helsinki. Patients were enrolled from January 2014 through June 2015. Surgeries were performed by six surgeons. Ophthalmic residents in each hospital assisted all surgeries. Three surgeons who had experienced over 1000 vitreoretinal surgeries are thought to be experienced doctors, and the other three surgeons who had experienced less than 100 vitreoretinal surgeries are thought to be inexperienced doctors. Eyes with giant retinal tears, proliferative vitreoretinopathy, atopic dermatitis, and a history of prior surgery for RRD were excluded. The patients were followed up at least for 6 months after the surgery. The following variables were analyzed: sex, age, primary surgeon, preoperative best-corrected visual acuity (BCVA), postoperative BCVA, preoperative intraocular pressure (IOP), postoperative IOP, the primary anatomical success rate, the final anatomical success rate, the number of retinal breaks, locations of retinal breaks, the number of quadrants involved, the presence or absence of the macular detachment, the number of eyes who needed the suture for sclerotomy sites, the operative time, and the lens status.

2.1. Statistical Methods. The chi-square test and Fisher's exact probability test for dichotomous variables and unpaired t-test for continuous variables were used to compare parameters listed above between the two groups. Paired t-test was used for comparison between pre- and postoperative VA within the same group. We used the Kruskal–Wallis H-test to examine the transition of IOP in each group.

For logistic multiple regression analysis, univariate analysis was performed to establish the relationships between explanatory variables and the primary anatomic success rate, using the chi-square test, Fisher's exact probability test, and unpaired t-test. The level of statistical significance was set at $p < 0.20$. The variables found to be significant in univariate analysis were analyzed with backward logistic multiple regression analysis, using the MedCalc (MedCalc version 12.7.5.0; MedCalc Software, Mariakerke, Belgium). Statistical significance was inferred for $p < 0.05$. The Landolt decimal VA was converted to logarithmic minimum angle of resolution (logMAR) for statistical analysis.

2.2. Surgical Procedures. All surgeries were performed under sub-Tenon anesthesia consisting of approximately 4 mL of 2% lidocaine. The Constellation Vision system (Alcon Laboratories, Inc., Forth Worth, TX, USA) was used for both 25G and 27G TSV with a wide-angle noncontact viewing system (Resight®; Carl Zeiss Meditec AG, Jena, Germany). Three cannulas were created with conjunctival displacement and oblique-angled sclerotomies in the inferotemporal, superotemporal, and superonasal quadrants 3.0–4.0 mm posterior to the limbus. 27G twin chandelier illumination

fibers (Eckardt TwinLight Chandelier, Dorc International, Zuidland, Netherlands) or 29G twin chandelier illumination fibers (Oshima dual, Synergetics USA, Inc.) were placed at 4.0 mm behind the limbus for wide-angle intraocular illumination. Before vitrectomy, for better visualization and shaving of peripheral vitreous, cataract extraction with phacoemulsification using the same machine and intraocular lens implantation were performed for all phakic eyes. Following the core vitrectomy, triamcinolone acetonide (MaQaid, Wakamoto Pharmaceutical, Tokyo, Japan) was injected to visualize vitreous gel during midperipheral vitrectomy. Then, the peripheral vitreous gel was shaved for 360° with scleral indentation under a wide-angle noncontact viewing system. No internal drainage retinotomies was made in the majority of cases to avoid the awareness of a scotoma but made in the most dependent or anterior part of the detached retina if necessary. Subretinal fluid was evacuated from original tears or drainage retinotomy sites and followed by a complete fluid-air exchange. All retinal detachments were reattached intraoperatively. Endolaser photocoagulation was applied to completely surround all retinal breaks and drainage retinotomy sites. At the end of surgery, all eyes were flushed with 50 mL of mix of 20% SF6 gas to assure a complete exchange. Additional gas mixture was injected through the pars plana to adjust IOP if necessary. Any sclerotomy sites that were found to be leaking at the end of the surgery were sutured with 8-0 vicryl suture. Normal IOP was checked by tactile examination. Subconjunctival corticosteroids were injected, and antibiotic ointment was administered at the end of the surgical procedure. All patients were kept in a prone position for 1 to 2 weeks after surgery, at least until less than 50% gas fill.

3. Results

Table 1 summarizes patients' perioperative demographic data. Thirty-two eyes underwent 25G TSV (group A) and 30 eyes with 27G TSV (group B). There were 24 men in group A, and 18 men in group B ($p = 0.32$). The mean ± SD age was 59 ± 13 years in group A and 55 ± 9 years in group B ($p = 0.15$). Their preoperative BCVA (log MAR) was 0.44 ± 0.69 units in group A and 0.38 ± 0.61 in group B ($p = 0.73$). Their postoperative BCVA at the last visit was 0.07 ± 0.25 in group A and -0.02 ± 0.17 in group B ($p = 0.16$). The final BCVA was significantly better than the preoperative BCVA in both groups ($p = 0.02$, $p = 0.002$, resp.). The initial and final anatomical success rates were 93.8% and 100% in group A and 96.7% and 100% in group B, respectively ($p = 1$ and $p = 1$, resp.). The mean ± SD number of retinal beaks was 1.6 ± 1.2 in group A and 1.9 ± 1.2 in group B ($p = 0.30$). Twenty-three eyes had original breaks at the superior quadrant, 8 eyes at the inferior quadrant, and 1 eye at both the quadrants in group A. On the contrary, nineteen eyes had original breaks at the superior quadrant, 9 eyes at the inferior quadrant, and 2 eyes at both the quadrants in group B. There were no statistical differences in the location and the number of the breaks between both groups ($p = 0.96$). Twenty-seven eyes had RRD involving one or two quadrants, and five eyes had more extensive RRD involving three or

TABLE 1: Perioperative demographic data of the patients.

Characteristics	25 gauge	27 gauge	p value
Number of eyes	32	30	—
Sex, male/female	24/8	18/12	0.32
Age (years), mean ± SD	59 ± 13	55 ± 9	0.15
Preoperative visual acuity (logMAR), mean ± SD	0.44 ± 0.69	0.38 ± 0.61	0.73
Visual acuity at the last visit (logMAR), mean ± SD	0.07 ± 0.25	−0.02 ± 0.17	0.16
Preoperative intraocular pressure (mmHg), mean ± SD	13.0 ± 3.5	14.3 ± 2.8	0.11
Initial anatomical success	30 (93.8%)	29 (96.7%)	1
Final anatomical success	32 (100%)	30 (100%)	1
Number of breaks, mean ± SD	1.6 ± 1.2	1.9 ± 1.2	0.30
Location of breaks, superior/inferior/both/undetectable	23/8/1/0	19/9/2/0	0.96
Quadrant of retinal detachment, 1/2/3/4	10/17/4/1	10/17/3/0	0.99
Macular detachment, macular on/macular off	23/9	15/15	0.13
The number of sclerotomies that required sutures	9	4	0.30
Operative time (min), mean ± SD	103.3 ± 39.9	98.4 ± 28.3	0.77
Lens status, phakic/pseudophakic/aphakic	24/7/1	27/3/0	0.61

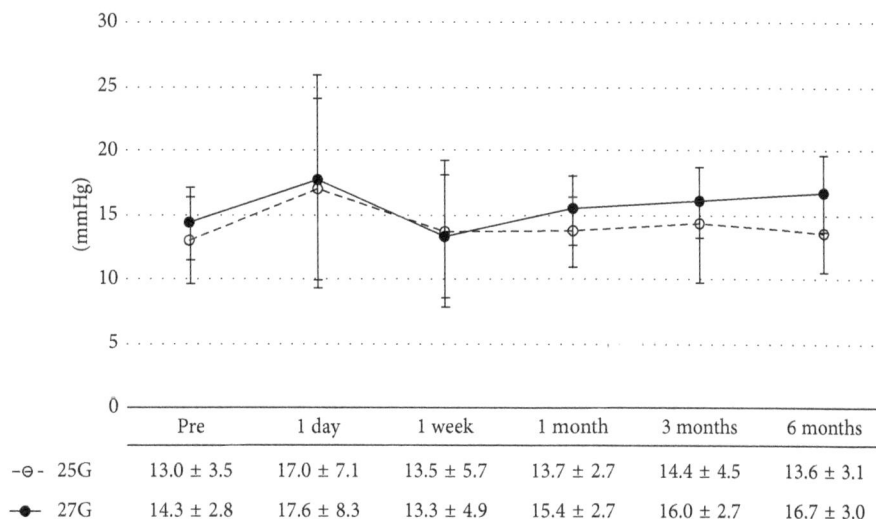

	Pre	1 day	1 week	1 month	3 months	6 months
-⊖- 25G	13.0 ± 3.5	17.0 ± 7.1	13.5 ± 5.7	13.7 ± 2.7	14.4 ± 4.5	13.6 ± 3.1
-●- 27G	14.3 ± 2.8	17.6 ± 8.3	13.3 ± 4.9	15.4 ± 2.7	16.0 ± 2.7	16.7 ± 3.0

FIGURE 1: Time course changes in intraocular pressure (IOP). The mean IOP at baseline was 13.0 ± 3.5 mmHg in group A and 14.3 ± 2.8 mmHg in group B. At 1 day, 1 week, 1 month, 3 months, and 6 months postoperatively, the IOP was 17.0 ± 7.1, 13.5 ± 5.7, 13.7 ± 2.7, 14.4 ± 4.5, and 13.6 ± 3.1 mmHg, respectively, in group A, and 17.6 ± 8.3, 13.3 ± 4.9, 15.4 ± 2.7, 16.0 ± 2.7, and 16.7 ± 3.0 mmHg, respectively, in group B. IOP did not statistically significantly change in both groups during the follow-up period ($p = 0.63$ and $p = 0.21$, resp.).

four quadrants in group A. Twenty-seven eyes had RRD involving one or two quadrants, and three eyes had more extensive RRD involving three or four quadrants in group B. There was no statistical difference in the location and extent of RRD between both groups ($p = 0.99$). The macula was attached preoperatively in 23 (71.9%) eyes in group A and 15 (50%) in group B ($p = 0.13$). The number of wounds that required sutures was 9/96 in group A and 4/90 in group B ($p = 0.30$). The operative time (minutes) was 103.3 ± 39.9 in group A and 98.4 ± 28.3 in group B ($p = 0.77$).

We evaluated time course changes in IOP during the follow-up period. Preoperative IOP (mmHg) was 13.0 ± 3.5 in group A and 14.3 ± 2.8 in group B ($p = 0.11$). IOP did not statistically significantly change in both groups during the

follow-up period ($p = 0.63$ and $p = 0.21$, resp.) (Figure 1). No eye developed postoperative hypotony in both groups.

We experienced retinal redetachment in both groups (Table 2). The rate of these complications was similar between the two groups. We performed additional 27G TSV with 20% sulfur hexafluoride gas tamponade for the treatment of retinal redetachment by experienced doctors, and all eyes obtained the final retinal attachment.

As a result of univariate analysis, the following variables were selected to perform backward logistic multiple regression analysis: age, number of quadrants involved, and lens status. The logistic multiple regression analysis revealed that all variables were not associated with the primary anatomic success (Table 3).

TABLE 2: Details of patients with postoperative complications.

Complication	25 gauge	27 gauge	Second treatment
Retinal redetachment	2	1	27GPPV + SF6 tamponade

27GPPV = 27-gauge pars plana vitrectomy; SF6 = sulfur hexafluoride.

TABLE 3: Analysis for the establishment of the relationships between explanatory variables and the primary anatomic success.

Explanatory variables	Univariate analysis	Logistic regression analysis	
	p value	p value	OR (95% CI)
Sex	0.26	NE	
Age	0.04	0.054	0.88 (0.78–1.00)
Preoperative visual acuity	0.31	NE	
Visual acuity at the last visit	0.42	NE	
Primary surgeon	0.24	NE	
Number of breaks	0.91	NE	
Location of breaks	0.44	NE	
Quadrant of retinal detachment	0.19	Not included in the model	
Macular detachment	0.28	NE	
Operative time	0.54	NE	
Lens status	0.08	Not included in the model	
Gauge of vitreous cutter	1	NE	

OR = odds ratio; CI = confidence interval; NE = not entered into multiple regression analysis.

4. Discussion

As previously reported [9, 15], in 27G TSV, the vitreous cutter used is short in length and low in stiffness, which bears clinicians, especially for surgically inexperienced doctors, concern regarding the possibility of compromised safety and operability in applying the 27G TSV system on the peripheral vitreoretinal diseases compared with the established larger-gauge TSV systems. In this study, we reported that the 27G TSV system provided anatomical results comparable to those obtained in 25G TSV. This result is compatible with the previous reports [13, 14]. In addition, the result of logistic regression analysis did not indicate any association between the primary anatomic success rate and explanatory variables, including the primary surgeon and gauge of vitreous cutter. These results indicate that 27G TSV have a potential for the practical use in the treatment of RRD for all surgeons, including inexperienced doctors.

Other concerns related to 27G TSV has been the low aspiration efficiency [15], which may extend the operation time. Mitsui et al. reported that, in 27G TSV, the operation time was significantly longer than that in 25G TSV for the epiretinal membrane [12]. On the contrary, previous reports suggested that the duration of vitreous removal is not different between 25G and 27G TSV for RRD [13, 14]. Our results also did not show a significant difference in operation time between 25G and 27G TSV for RRD. In terms of the core vitreoctomy process, the surgeon indeed felt that the aspiration efficiency of 27G TSV was obviously inferior to that of 25G TSV, as

theoretically anticipated [15]. However, during the vitreous gel shaving in the vicinity of a detached retina, the critical procedure of the peripheral vitrectomy for RRD, 27G TSV was rather safe because of less frequent flapping of the retina due to lower aspiration efficiency compared with the 25G TSV. As a result, the total operation time did not differ between the two systems. Moreover, in the epiretinal membrane surgery reported by Mitsui et al. [12], peripheral vitrectomy was not as strenuous as that in RRD surgery. This difference in the required procedures could also account for the discrepant results obtained between the studies. Collectively, we believe that our results indicate the equivalency between 25G and 27G TSV for the RRD treatment. Accumulating cases are needed to confirm our preliminary observations.

Generally, 27G TSV requires a smaller incision, which suggests the possibility of excellent self-closing of the wound, compared to other vitrectomies with larger gauges [9, 15]. We monitored IOP for 6 months after surgery and found no significant difference during the follow-up period. We also found no significant difference in the number of wounds that required sutures between the two systems. In the 27G TSV performed by Mitsui et al. [12], as the stiffness of the cutter was low, the cutter had to be manipulated more dynamically; thus, wound closing might not have been as good as expected. For RRD, the cutter had to be manipulated more dynamically for the peripheral vitrectomy. This may be the reason why no difference was found between the two gauges with regard to the number of wounds that required sutures. In addition, as this research focused on the RRD, the surgery was completed by filling the vitreous cavity with SF6 gas in all the cases. Previous reports have indicated that when a gas tamponade was performed, the postoperative IOP was more stable than when it was not used [9, 16]. Therefore, the use of a gas tamponade may be a reason why the two gauges did not differ in IOP.

This study has potential limitations. First, it is a retrospective study, and there may have been a bias of patient selection. Another problem is that the sample size was relatively small. The results of large-scale, prospective research studies in the future are needed.

In conclusions, we performed a comparative study of outcomes between 25G and 27G TSV for RRD. The surgical results of the two gauges were equivalent with the similar effectiveness. We believe that 27G TSV is as useful as 25G for RRD, which is a disease of the peripheral retina.

Conflicts of Interest

The authors declare that there are no conflicts of interest regarding the publication of this paper.

References

[1] C. I. Falkner-Radler, J. S. Myung, S Moussa et al., "Trends in primary retinal detachment surgery: results of a bicenter study," *Retina*, vol. 31, no. 5, pp. 928–936, 2011.

[2] J. D. Ho, S. W. Liou, C. Y. Tsai, R. J. Tsai, and H. C. Lin, "Trends and outcomes of treatment for primary rhegmatogenous retinal detachment: a 9-year nationwide population-based study," *Eye*, vol. 23, no. 3, pp. 669–675, 2009.

[3] C. W. Wong, W. L. Wong, I. Y. Yeo et al., "Trends and factors related to outcomes for primary rhegmatogenous retinal detachment surgery in a large Asian tertiary eye center," *Retina*, vol. 34, no. 4, pp. 684–692, 2014.

[4] Y. H. Yoon, D. S. Kim, J. G. Kim, and J. U. Hwang, "Sutureless vitreoretinal surgery using a new 25-gauge transconjunctival system," *Ophthalmic Surgery, Lasers & Imaging*, vol. 37, no. 1, pp. 12–19, 2006.

[5] S. Rizzo, F. Genovesi-Ebert, S. Murri et al., "25-gauge, sutureless vitrectomy and standard 20-gauge pars plana vitrectomy in idiopathic epiretinal membrane surgery: a comparative pilot study," *Graefe's Archive for Clinical and Experimental Ophthalmology*, vol. 244, no. 4, pp. 472–479, 2006.

[6] K. Kadonosono, T. Yamakawa, E. Uchio, Y. Yanagi, Y. Tamaki, and M. Araie, "Comparison of visual function after epiretinal membrane removal by 20-gauge and 25-gauge vitrectomy," *American Journal of Ophthalmology*, vol. 142, no. 3, pp. 513–515, 2006.

[7] D. H. Park, J. P. Shin, and S. Y. Kim, "Surgically induced astigmatism in combined phacoemulsification and vitrectomy: 23-gauge transconjunctival sutureless vitrectomy versus 20-gauge standard vitrectomy," *Graefe's Archive for Clinical and Experimental Ophthalmology*, vol. 247, no. 10, pp. 1331–1337, 2009.

[8] G. Galway, B. Drury, B. G. Cronin, and R. D. Bourke, "A comparison of induced astigmatism in 20- vs 25-gauge vitrectomy procedures," *Eye*, vol. 24, no. 2, pp. 315–317, 2010.

[9] Y. Oshima, T. Wakabayashi, T. Sato, M. Ohji, and Y. A. Tano, "27-gauge instrument system for transconjunctival sutureless microincision vitrectomy surgery," *Ophthalmology*, vol. 117, no. 1, pp. 93.e2–102.e2, 2010.

[10] M. A. Khan, A. Shahlaee, B. Toussaint et al., "Outcomes of 27 gauge microincision vitrectomy surgery for posterior segment disease," *American Journal of Ophthalmology*, vol. 161, pp. 36.e2–43.e2, 2016.

[11] S. Rizzo, F. Barca, T. Caporossi, and C. Mariotti, "Twenty-seven–gauge vitrectomy for various vitreoretinal diseases," *Retina*, vol. 35, no. 6, pp. 1273–1278, 2015.

[12] K. Mitsui, J. Kogo, H. Takeda et al., "Comparative study of 27-gauge vs 25-gauge vitrectomy for epiretinal membrane," *Eye*, vol. 30, no. 4, pp. 538–544, 2016.

[13] S. Rizzo, S. Polizzi, F. Barca, T. Caporossi, and G. Virgili, "Comparative study of 27-gauge versus 25-gauge vitrectomy for the treatment of primary rhegmatogenous retinal detachment," *Journal of Ophthalmology*, vol. 2017, Article ID 6384985, 5 pages, 2017.

[14] M. R. Romano, G. Cennamo, M. Ferrara, M. Cennamo, and G. Cennamo, "Twenty-seven-gauge versus 25-gauge vitrectomy for primary rhegmatogenous retinal detachment," *Retina*, vol. 37, no. 4, pp. 637–642, 2017.

[15] S. Osawa and Y. Oshima, "27-Gauge vitrectomy," in *Developments in Ophthalmology*, pp. 54–62, Karger Publishers, Basel, Switzerland, 2014.

[16] S. Yamane, K. Kadonosono, M. Inoue, S. Kobayashi, Y. Watanabe, and A. Arakawa, "Effect of intravitreal gas tamponade for sutureless vitrectomy wounds: three-dimensional corneal and anterior segment optical coherence tomography study," *Retina*, vol. 31, no. 4, pp. 702–706, 2011.

21

Reduction in Ocular Hypotensive Eyedrops by Ab Interno Trabeculotomy Improves not only Ocular Surface Condition but also Quality of Vision

Kenji Kashiwagi ⓘ and Mio Matsubara

Department of Ophthalmology, University of Yamanashi Faculty of Medicine, Chuo, Yamanashi, Japan

Correspondence should be addressed to Kenji Kashiwagi; kenjik@yamanashi.ac.jp

Academic Editor: Van C. Lansingh

Purpose. To investigate the effect of ab interno trabeculotomy using the Trabectome surgical system on tear film stability and functional visual acuity (FVA). *Patients and Methods.* Adult glaucoma patients who underwent Trabectome surgery alone or Trabectome surgery combined with phacoemulsification with intraocular lens insertion were included in this study. Corneal epithelial defects, tear film breakup time (TBUT), tear meniscus height, tear film spreading grade, tear interferometry grade, and FVA were assessed before and after surgery in addition to routine ophthalmic examinations. Changes in ocular surface conditions and visual acuity as a result of the Trabectome surgery were investigated. *Results.* Thirty eyes of 22 patients with a mean age of 72.2 ± 7.9 years, including 8 males and 14 females, were enrolled. The Trabectome surgery significantly reduced the intraocular pressure (IOP) from 20.3 ± 5.2 to 15.0 ± 3.3 mmHg ($P < 0.001$) and the number of different types of ocular hypotensive eyedrops used from 3.2 ± 0.7 to 1.1 ± 0.7 types ($P < 0.001$). The surgery significantly improved corneal epithelial defects, the tear spreading grade, the tear interferometry grade, and FVA. The surgery also improved the visual maintenance ratio among all enrolled patients, including those who underwent Trabectome surgery only. *Conclusion.* Trabectome surgery may be beneficial not only for IOP reduction but also for improving ocular surface conditions and FVA.

1. Introduction

Glaucoma is a disease that affects individuals across the lifespan, and many patients are required to use ocular hypotensive ophthalmic solutions. In previous reports, glaucoma patients used approximately two ophthalmic solutions [1], and ocular surface damage was common. Rossi et al. reported that patients with topically treated glaucoma presented with dry eye syndrome more often than the control group [2], Leung et al. reported that approximately 60% of glaucoma patients had symptoms of dry eye and that the number of benzalkonium chloride- (BAC-) containing eyedrops was associated with the severity of ocular surface disease [3].

Because tear film function requires a regular and smooth ocular surface with a stable tear film to form clear visual images, ocular surface damage causes several symptoms including red eye, photophobia, eye itching, blurring, and other discomforts that sometimes deteriorate a patient's quality of life [2, 4].-

A smaller amount of ocular hypotensive ophthalmic solution may result in better ocular surface condition. Trabeculectomy with mitomycin C is major glaucoma surgery and successfully reduces the number of ocular hypotensive eyedrops, but previous papers reported that trabeculectomy with mitomycin C deteriorated ocular surface conditions due to adverse effects of mitomycin D or deterioration of tear film replacement [5]. The Trabectome system (Neomedix, Tustin, CA) is used for performing trabeculotomy via an internal approach. This procedure successfully reduces the number of topical medications in addition to the intraocular pressure (IOP) [6], which may contribute to ocular surface stability. The Trabectome system does not use antimetabolites, and there is less irregularity of tear film formation. We therefore hypothesized that the Trabectome system may be beneficial to the ocular surface.

A functional visual acuity (FVA) test can evaluate continuous visual acuity changes over time, which may be better for evaluating the quality of vision than a conventional visual acuity test. The methodology of FVA testing has evolved since it first emerged as a promising technology to evaluate changes in visual acuity over time [7, 8]. Some ocular conditions have been reported to influence FVA. Goto et al. reported that dry eye decreased FVA among patients who had normal conventional visual acuity [8, 9]. FVA is significantly reflected in the tear functions and ocular surface status of the eye. The FVA test could help detect the masked impairment of visual function among patients in patients who complain of decreased visual acuity despite having normal visual acuity measurements using conventional testing.

In this study, we investigated the effects of ab interno trabeculotomy using the Trabectome system on tear film stability in terms of superficial punctate keratitis, tear film breakup time (TBUT), height of the tear meniscus, and tear film lipid layer interference patterns as well as visual acuity, which was assessed using a conventional visual acuity test and FVA test.

2. Patients and Methods

This study was performed as a prospective cohort study, approved by the Ethics Committee of the University of Yamanashi and conducted in accordance with the Helsinki Declaration and the Ethical Guidelines for Medical and Health Research Involving Human Subjects of the Japanese Ministry of Health, Labor and Welfare. All participants provided written informed consent.

2.1. Inclusion and Exclusion Criteria. Among all glaucoma patients who underwent Trabectome surgery alone or combined surgery with phacoemulsification and intraocular lens insertion from December 2016 to April 2017, subjects who satisfied the following criteria were enrolled: adult age, a history of use of ocular hypotensive eyedrops for one year or longer, provided written informed consent, no complications during the surgery, best-corrected visual acuity of 20/100 or better before and after the surgery, and completion of the study protocol. The exclusion criteria were as follows: a threat of central visual field loss, specifically, two or more of the four central measured points on the Humphrey field analyzer (HFA) (Carl Zeiss Meditec, Dublin, CA) 10-2 program showing less than 10 dB of sensitivity; any diseases that affect tear film stability, including Sjogren's syndrome; any diseases that affect visual acuity, except for cataracts; astigmatism with ≥1.5 diopters of corneal curvature; a history of intraocular surgery, except cataract surgery performed same or more than one year prior to the study; and administration of routine ophthalmic solutions, except ocular hypotensive solutions and hyaluronic acid solutions.

2.2. General Ophthalmic Examinations. The following examinations were performed before and after surgery: best-corrected visual acuity, refractive error measurement, slit-lamp examination, fundus examination, and IOP measurement using a Goldmann applanation tonometer. Visual field test using the HFA10-2 and 24-2 programs, and optic nerve evaluation using an optical coherence tomography CIRRUS HD-OCT (Carl Zeiss Meditec, Inc., Dublin, CA) were performed within three months before surgery.

2.3. Ocular Surface Evaluation. To evaluate the ocular surface, we employed the following tests:

2.4. Tear Film Breakup Time Examination. Trained medical staff evaluated the TBUT using a DR-1α (Kowa, Nagoya, Japan) to assess tear film stability in a blinded protocol. The DR-1α examination was repeated two times, and recorded video images were subject to analysis. A staff member evaluated the TBUT, which was calculated as the mean measurement of two trials.

2.5. Tear Meniscus Evaluation. An expert ophthalmologist (K.K.) evaluated the tear meniscus height using a tear turnover assessment test. The tear meniscus height was evaluated by adjusting the vertical length of a slit beam on the tear meniscus at the center of the lower lid, and the values were read from the slit-lamp scale [10].

2.6. Corneal Erosion Evaluation. Corneal erosion was evaluated by introducing a wetted 0.7 mg fluorescein sodium ophthalmic strip (FLUORES Ocular Examination Test Paper, Ayumi Pharmaceutical Ltd., Tokyo, Japan) into the inferior fornix. The graded corneal erosion system [11] was adopted as the ocular surface damage assessment. Briefly, two parameters of corneal erosion, area and density, were graded on a scale ranging from A0 to A3 and from D0 to D3, respectively.

2.7. Tear Interferometry Test. The tear interferometry test was conducted using DR-1α. Detailed information has been described elsewhere [13]. In brief, this instrument observes the specular reflected light from the tear surface of a circular area 2 mm in diameter of the central cornea. Lipid layer interference images were recorded soon after a complete blink. The interference patterns of the tear film lipid layer were analyzed and graded from I to V according to the Yokoi standards of grading [12, 13].

Grade I or grade II was considered normal, whereas grade III or above was considered abnormal. In addition, the spreading of a tear film lipid layer was evaluated using 4 grades as follows: grade 1: the tear film smoothly spread across all of the corneal area; grade 2: the tear film slowly spread across more than half of the corneal area; grade 3: the tear film slowly spread across less than half of the corneal area; and grade 4: the tear film never spread on the cornea. Representative images of the lipid layer interference pattern and the tear film spreading patterns are shown in Supplementary Figures 1 and 2.

2.8. Functional Visual Acuity Test. We performed FVA testing with natural blinking without topical anesthesia during a 60 s time interval using an AS-28 FVA

TABLE 1: Demographics: comparison of general ophthalmic status before and after the operation (Table 2).

Number of subjects	30 eyes/22 subjects
Male : female	8 : 14
Age	72.2 ± 7.9 yrs
Type of glaucoma	
POAG	18 eyes
PEX	5 eyes
Others	7 eyes
Alone versus combined	8 versus 22
Preoperative VA (logMAR)	0.104 ± 0.179
HFA MD (program 24-2)	−12.7 ± 7.6 dB
mpNFLT	60.3 ± 10.4 μM
Pre-IOP	20.3 ± 5.2 mmHg
Refractive error	−3.2 ± 4.7 diopter
Phakia versus pseudophakia	28 versus 2
Systemic disease	
CKD	2
Basedow	1
HT	1
Total number of eyedrops	3.4 ± 0.8
Number of ocular hypotensive eyedrops	3.2 ± 0.7

POAG: primary open-angle glaucoma; PEX: pseudoexfoliation glaucoma; MAR: minimum angle resolution; HFA: Humphrey field analyzer; MD: mean deviation; mpNFLT: mean peripapillary nerve fiber layer thickness; IOP: intraocular pressure; CKD: chronic kidney disease; HT: hypertension.

measurement system (Kowa, Nagoya, Japan) as described elsewhere [14], in which subjects were allowed to blink naturally without the administration of topical anesthetics. The AS-28 FVA measurement system displays Landolt optotypes automatically for 2 seconds, starting with a size appropriate for the patient's best-corrected visual acuity. The patient uses a joystick to indicate the orientation of each Landolt ring, and the size is decreased automatically when the answer is correct. If the response is incorrect or no response occurs within 2 seconds, a larger optotype is presented. The test lasts for 60 seconds, and the system can measure visual acuity from 40/20 to 20/2000. After instruction from trained medical staff, patients performed a practice test. If a patient had difficulty in taking a test, he/she repeated the same test until the test was performed smoothly. Then, another trial was performed for the study. In this study, two parameters were compared before and after surgery. First, FVA was defined as the average of the visual acuities measured during a 60 s interval. To allow comparisons of changes in visual acuity over time, another parameter, the visual maintenance ratio (VMR), was determined as an objective index calculated by the logMAR values of the FVA scores over the time frame for testing divided by the logMAR baseline visual acuity score. The VMR formula is as follows: VMR = (lowest logMAR VA score−FVA at 60 s)/(lowest logMAR VA score−baseline VA). The VMR is considered to be adequate for statistically comparing groups with different baseline visual acuities [14].

2.9. Study Protocol. After enrollment, patients underwent general ophthalmic examinations before and after surgery. A TBUT examination, tear meniscus evaluation, corneal erosion evaluation, tear interferometry test, and FVA test were performed 1–3 days before and 4 weeks after the surgery.

TABLE 2: Comparison between preoperative and postoperative parameters.

	Preoperative	Postoperative
Total number of eyedrops	3.4 ± 0.8	2.5 ± 1.2
Number of ocular hypotensive eyedrops	3.2 ± 0.7	1.1 ± 0.7
Number of BAC-contained eyedrops	3.3 ± 0.9	1.2 ± 0.7
IOP (mmHg)	20.3 ± 5.2	15.0 ± 3.3
LogMAR	0.104 ± 0.179	0.038 ± 0.123
Tear meniscus height (mm)	0.29 ± 0.18	0.30 ± 0.17
TBUT (sec)	6.5 ± 1.0	6.5 ± 1.0

IOP: intraocular pressure; MAR: minimum angle resolution; TBUT: tear breakup time.

2.10. Statistical Analysis. Data were analyzed using the JMP 12.0 software program (SAS Institute, Cary, NC), and the results are presented as the means ± standard deviation (SD). Differences in the results were determined using a paired *t*-test and contingency table analysis. *P* values <0.05 were considered significant.

3. Results

3.1. Patient Demographics. Thirty eyes of 22 patients satisfied the inclusion criteria and were included in the study protocol. The demographic characteristics of these patients are shown in Table 1. Eight males and 14 females were included. The mean age was 72.2 ± 7.9 years. Primary open-angle glaucoma was the most common type of glaucoma (60% of patients), followed by pseudoexfoliation glaucoma and other types of glaucoma. The total number of eyedrop types and the number of ocular hypotensive eyedrop types used preoperatively were 3.4 ± 0.8 and 3.2 ± 0.7, respectively.

Trabectome surgery significantly improved visual acuity from 0.104 ± 0.179 logMAR to 0.038 ± 0.123 logMAR (*P* < 0.001). Trabectome surgery also significantly reduced IOP from 20.3 ± 5.2 to 15.0 ± 3.3 mmHg (*P* < 0.001) and the number of types of ocular hypotensive eyedrops from 3.2 ± 0.7 to 1.1 ± 0.7 types (*P* < 0.001).

3.2. Changes in Ocular Surface Conditions. Table 2 shows changes in ocular surface conditions. The TBUT and tear meniscus height were very similar before and after the surgery. The surgery significantly improved corneal erosion (*P* < 0.001) (Figures 1(a) and 1(b)), the tear spreading grade (*P* = 0.03) (Figure 2(a)), and the tear interferometry grade (*P* = 0.01) (Figure 2(b)). A representative case is shown in Supplementary Videos 1 and 2. He was a 72-year-old male patient with primary open-angle glaucoma (POAG). His tear interferometry grades before Trabectome and after Trabectome were grade 3 and grade 1, respectively.

3.3. Functional Visual Acuity Changes. Figure 3(a) shows changes in conventional and FVA after Trabectome surgery. The mean conventional visual acuity significantly improved from 0.104 ± 0.179 logMAR to 0.038 ± 0.123 (*P* = 0.01) logMAR, and the mean FVA also significantly improved

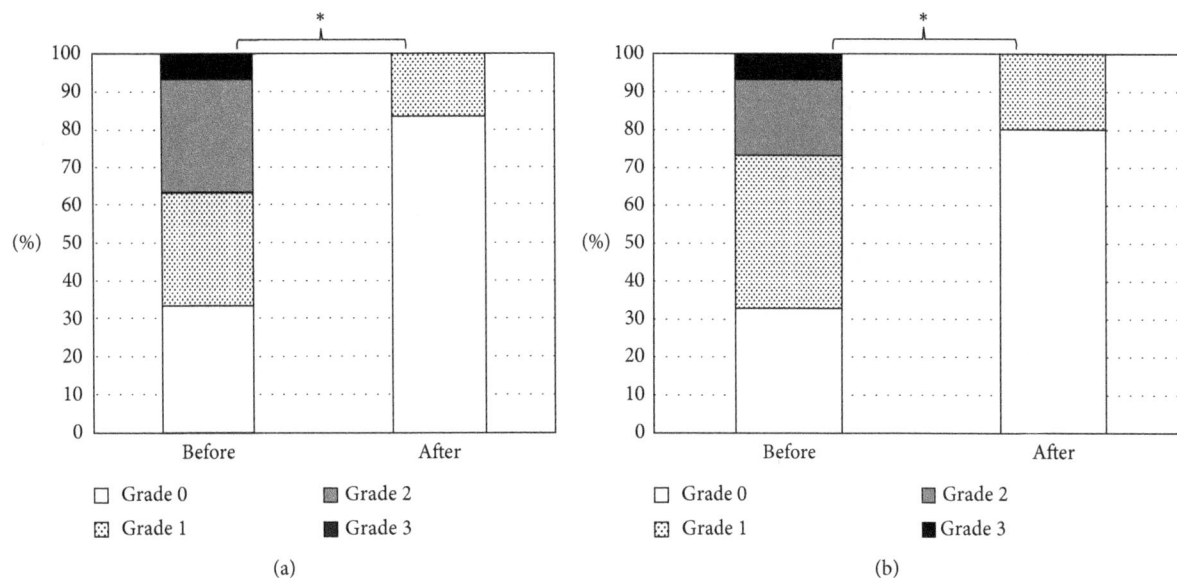

FIGURE 1: Changes in corneal epithelial damage. Changes in distribution of grades of corneal epithelial damage in area (a) and density (b) before and after Trabectome surgery. $^*P < 0.001$, contingency table analysis.

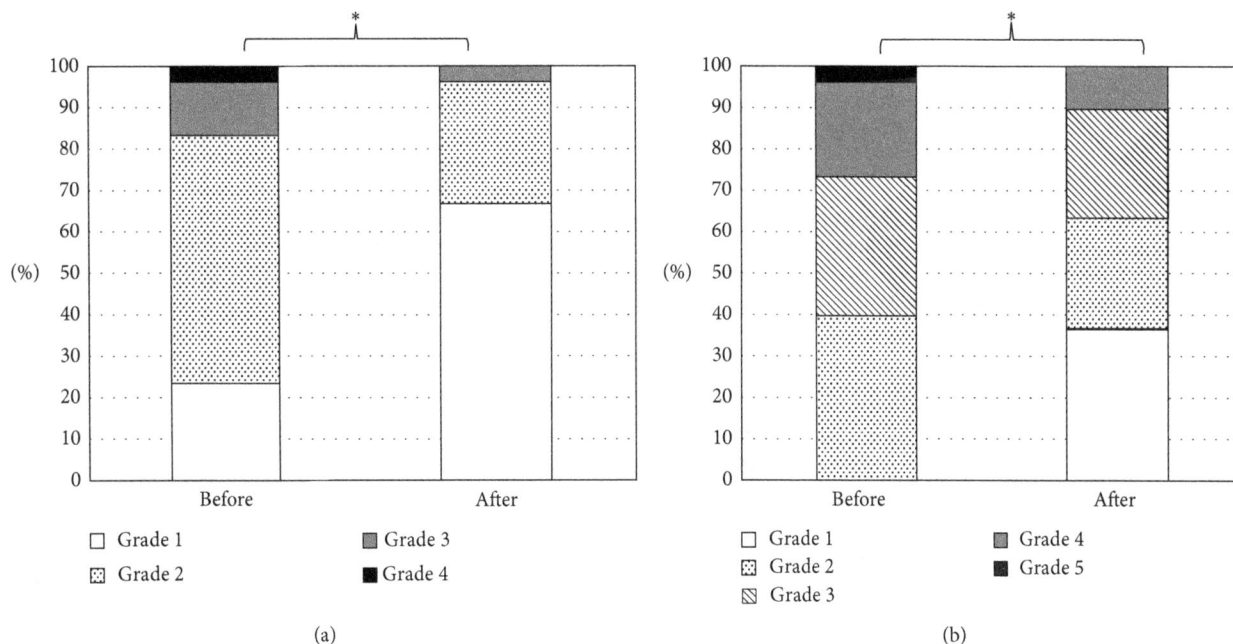

FIGURE 2: Changes in tear film status. Changes in distribution of tear film spreading grade (a) and tear interferometry grade (b) before and after Trabectome surgery. $^*P < 0.05$, contingency table analysis.

from 0.340 ± 0.250 logMAR to 0.241 ± 0.244 logMAR ($P = 0.001$). The mean FVA was significantly worse than the mean conventional visual acuity at the preoperative and postoperative examinations ($P < 0.001$). The difference in conventional visual acuity before surgery was 0.29 ± 0.270 logMAR, while that after surgery was 0.20 ± 0.230 logMAR, which was a significant difference ($P = 0.03$). Trabectome significantly improved the difference in conventional visual acuity and FVA. Trabectome surgery significantly improved the VMR from 0.88 ± 0.06 to 0.92 ± 0.06 among all patients

($P = 0.003$) (Figure 3(b)). To eliminate the effect of cataract surgery on the results, we compared changes in the conventional logMAR and VMR between eyes that underwent the Trabectome surgery only and those that underwent the Trabectome surgery combined with cataract surgery. The combined group showed a significant improvement from the presurgical conventional logMAR value to the postsurgical conventional logMAR value (from 0.145 ± 0.184 to 0.054 ± 0.135) ($P = 0.01$), while the presurgical and postsurgical conventional logMAR values of the Trabectome surgery-alone

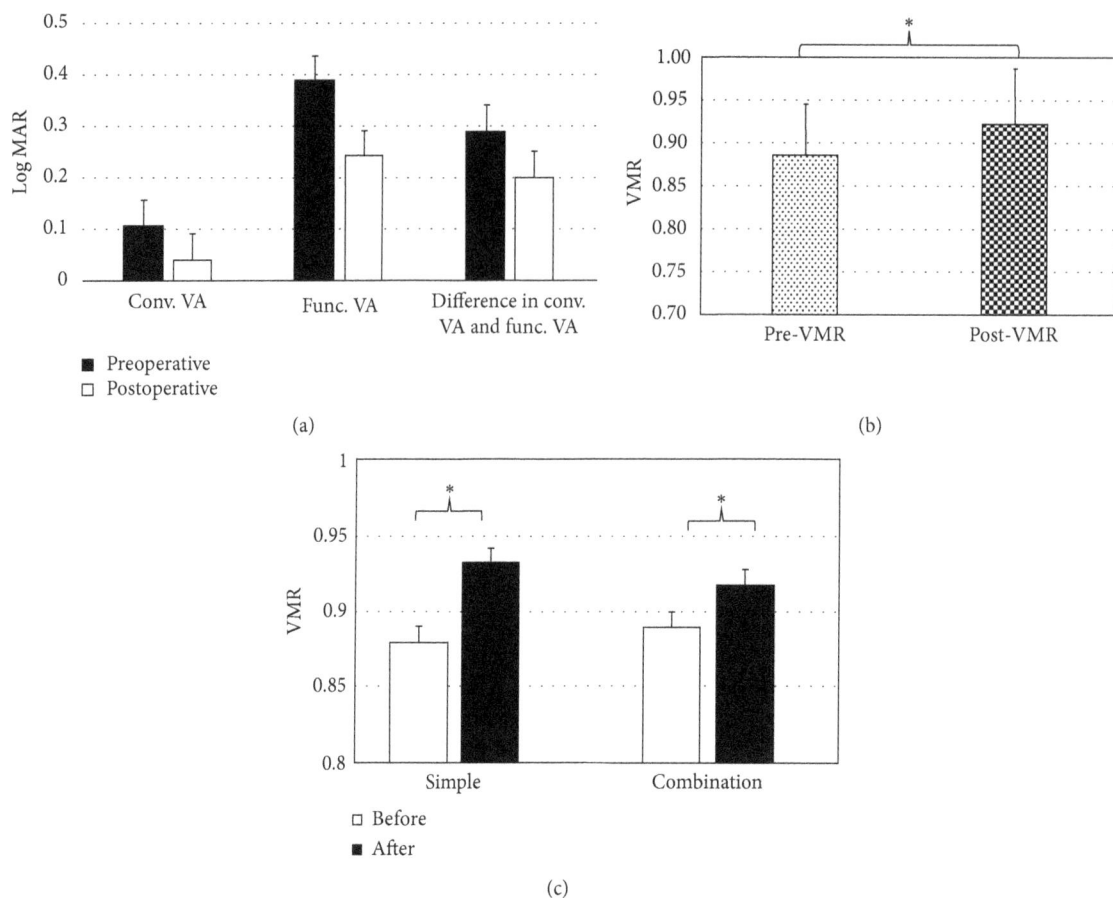

FIGURE 3: Changes in visual acuity. Comparison of conventional visual acuity, functional visual acuity, and the difference in conventional visual acuity and functional visual acuity between preoperative and postoperative conditions (a); change in the VMR after Trabectome surgery (b); and comparison of changes in the VMR between Trabectome surgery only and Trabectome surgery with phacoemulsification with intraocular lens insertion (c). *$P < 0.05$, paired t-test; conv., conventional; func., functional; VA: visual acuity; MAR: minimum angle resolution; VMR: visual maintenance ratio.

group were -0.018 ± 0.050 and -0.008 ± 0.045, respectively, ($P = 0.29$). In contrast, both eyes with Trabectome surgery only and those with Trabectome with cataract surgery showed a significant improvement in VMR from 0.88 ± 0.06 to 0.93 ± 0.06 ($P = 0.04$) and from 0.89 ± 0.06 to 0.92 ± 0.07 ($P = 0.04$), respectively. Both groups showed significant improvements in the VMR of a similar magnitude (Figure 3(c)). A representative case is shown in Supplementary Figure 3. She was a 74-year-old female patient with POAG. Trabectome surgery alleviated the decrease in visual acuity during the test period.

4. Discussion

The current study revealed a new aspect of ab interno trabeculotomy using the Trabectome system in addition to that of IOP reduction. The Trabectome surgery improved not only the ocular surface condition, as evidenced by changes in corneal superficial keratitis, tear spreading, and tear interferometry, but also FVA, which may be highly involved in visual function related to daily life. Together, these positive effects of Trabectome surgery could improve the quality of vision.

Instability of the precorneal tear layer causing corneal epithelial damage is related to factors produced by the lacrimal glands and conjunctival goblet cells. In addition, inflammatory mediators may participate in the development of corneal epithelial damage. Ocular hypotensive eyedrops have been reported to deteriorate ocular surface conditions. Rossi et al. reported that the number of medications used, prolonged use of reserved medications, and total BAC exposure were significantly associated with ocular surface disease [15]. Valente et al. also reported that approximately half of glaucoma patients using preserved ocular hypotensive eyedrops showed symptoms of tear film dysfunction and that ocular surface damage seemed to be greater in patients using more than two medications [16]. Lee et al. reported that compared to normal controls, chronically medicated glaucoma patients were more likely to have an increase in tear film osmolarity, which commonly results in dry eye symptoms [17]. Approximately two-thirds of the enrolled eyes in the current study showed a corneal epithelial defect upon enrollment in the study, which is consistent with the previous reports.

Since the tear meniscus height and TBUT did not show any significant change, the role of superficial punctate keratitis, or SPK, improvement might not be due to an increase in tear volume but to alleviation of drug-induced cytotoxicity and/or tear film formation. Chen et al. reported that commercial latanoprost, travoprost, and bimatoprost damaged the corneal epithelium by breaking down the barrier integrity, cell junction, and cytoskeleton but did not affect aqueous tear production or the TBUT [18], which is consistent with the current results. Lee et al. also reported no significant difference in the TBUT and Schirmer's test between chronically medicated patients and patients who underwent trabeculectomy [17]. However, Villani et al. presented a controversial report that showed that the use of preserved ocular hypotensive eyedrops reduced the TBUT [19]. Taken together, ocular hypotensive eyedrops may damage the ocular surface either through direct action on the corneal epithelial cells or by reducing precorneal tear film stability.

Trabectome surgery significantly reduced the number of different types of ocular hypotensive eyedrops used by patients, which may be related to improvement in the damage of the ocular surface. Zhang et al. reported that pilocarpine and timolol have direct effects on human meibomian gland epithelial cells that may influence their morphology, survival, and proliferative capacity [20]. Arita et al. reported that long-term use of antiglaucoma eyedrops was associated with alterations in meibomian gland morphology and function [21]. The number of eyedrop types containing BAC was also significantly reduced by Trabectome surgery (Table 2). BAC contained in eyedrops has been known to possibly damage the ocular surface [22–24]. BAC-preserved ophthalmic formulations could induce acute cytotoxic effects even during a clinically relevant exposure time [24]. Previous papers have reported that compared to preserved eyedrops, preservative-free eyedrops are significantly less associated with ocular symptoms and signs of irritation [22, 23]. Taken together, ocular surface damage may be induced by the additive effect of ocular hypotensive reagents and BAC, although it is impossible to know the exact cause of ocular surface damage.

All patients used antibacterial eyedrops and/or non-steroidal anti-inflammatory eyedrops at the postoperative examination, which may have influenced the current results. Ayaki et al. reported that ophthalmic antibiotic solutions damaged the corneal epithelium [25], but Price et al. reported that use of ophthalmic solutions containing 0.3% gatifloxacin or 0.5% moxifloxacin did not result in clinically significant epithelial toxicity in healthy human corneas [26]. It is not possible to conclude that ocular hypotensive eyedrops exert a more toxic effect on the ocular surface than other eyedrops because the number of eyedrop types used by patients was not the same between the preoperative and postoperative condition. However, it should be noted that a reduction in the number of ocular hypotensive eyedrop types used may alleviate ocular surface damage.

In the current study, conventional visual acuity and FVA were improved in the eyes that underwent Trabectome surgery combined with cataract surgery; however, the eyes that underwent Trabectome surgery alone did not show any change in conventional visual acuity. In contrast, Trabectome surgery resulted in improvement in the VMR both in eyes treated with Trabectome surgery alone and in those

treated with Trabectome surgery combined with cataract surgery. Interestingly, the magnitude of improvement in the VMR was similar between these two groups. The VMR is proposed as a parameter that can be used to compare FVA among eyes with different conventional visual acuity [7, 8]. Patients who have an unstable tear film showed a decreased VMR [8], which reflects the performance ability of specific daily activities that involve visual tasks.

Currently, medical therapy has been considered the first choice for the care for patients with glaucoma. The number of ocular hypotensive eyedrop types used by patients has been increased. Indeed, the previous studies showed an average of approximately 2 types of ocular hypotensive eyedrops being used by patients [1]. Medical therapy has some drawbacks, such as poor adherence to the drug regimen, adverse effects, and low persistency. Ocular hypotensive eyedrops have been reported to induce an adverse effect when the number of different types of ocular hypotensive eyedrops is increased and the prescribing period is prolonged [15]. Since glaucoma is a lifelong disease, a safe and stable treatment regimen is required. Eliminating ocular hypotensive eyedrops by adopting surgeries including the Trabectome procedure could be an option from the view point of ocular safety and quality of vision, in addition to IOP control.

This study has some limitations. The number of enrolled patients was relatively small, and the observation period was short. We evaluated the ocular surface condition and FVA only once after the surgery. To confirm the current results, additional studies utilizing a larger sample size and multiple tests with a long follow-up period after the surgery should be conducted. It is unclear whether Trabectome surgery itself improved ocular surface condition and FVA. The reduction in hypotensive ophthalmic solutions may have played a role in the current results. It has been reported that mitomycin C-augmented trabeculectomy deteriorated ocular surface condition, which was mainly due to increased irregularity of ocular surface configuration and mitomycin C toxicity. MIGS, including Trabectome, may alleviate ocular surface damage, resulting in improved ocular surface condition and visual function. It is necessary to investigate the effects of other MIGS on the ocular surface and visual function. The learning effect for performing the FVA test could not be completely eliminated, although participating patients repeated the FVA test until becoming sufficiently familiar with it that they could perform the test for the study; the reproducibility of this system has been confirmed previously [14]. Masked examiners independently evaluated the ocular surface conditions; however, the accuracy of the evaluations may not be completely accurate because these evaluation methods included subjective classifications.

In conclusion, applying Trabectome surgery may be beneficial not only for IOP reduction but also for improving ocular surface conditions and visual acuity, which may contribute to improvement in the quality of vision. Although it is unclear whether the ocular hypotonic reagent or BAC play a main role in ocular hypotensive eyedrop-related ocular complications, ophthalmologists should consider reducing the number of different types of ocular hypotonic eyedrops used and/or the BAC concentration as much as possible. Introduction of minimally invasive glaucoma surgeries, including the Trabectome approach, may be a good option for improving the quality of vision, although the current results should be confirmed by further studies with longer observation periods and larger sample sizes.

Conflicts of Interest

The authors have no proprietary or commercial interests in any materials discussed in this article.

Acknowledgments

The authors appreciate the kind cooperation of Ms. Naoko Kaji, Yuko Tazawa, Jun Kaneshige, and Mika Komagata for measuring functional visual acuity and tear interferometry test.

Supplementary Materials

Supplementary 1. Figure 1: representative images of the lipid layer interference pattern (modified from reports of Yokoi et al. [12, 13]).

Supplementary 2. Figure 2: representative images of the tear film spreading patterns (modified from reports of Yokoi et al. [12, 13]).

Supplementary 3. Figure 3: a representative case indicating changes in functional visual acuity after Trabectome surgery.

Supplementary 4. Video 1: a representative case indicating changes in the lipid layer interference pattern before Trabectome.

Supplementary 5. Video 2: a representative case indicating changes in the lipid layer interference pattern after Trabectome.

References

[1] K. Kashiwagi, "Changes in trend of newly prescribed anti-glaucoma medications in recent nine years in a Japanese local community," *Open Ophthalmology Journal*, vol. 4, no. 1, pp. 7–11, 2010.

[2] G. C. Rossi, C. Tinelli, G. M. Pasinetti et al., "Dry eye syndrome-related quality of life in glaucoma patients," *European Journal of Ophthalmology*, vol. 19, no. 4, pp. 572–579, 2009.

[3] E. W. Leung, F. A. Medeiros, and R. N. Weinreb, "Prevalence of ocular surface disease in glaucoma patients," *Journal of Glaucoma*, vol. 17, no. 5, pp. 350–355, 2008.

[4] W. C. Stewart, J. A. Stewart, and L. A. Nelson, "Ocular surface disease in patients with ocular hypertension and glaucoma," *Current Eye Research*, vol. 36, no. 5, pp. 391–398, 2011.

[5] J. Lam, T. T. Wong, and L. Tong, "Ocular surface disease in posttrabeculectomy/mitomycin C patients," *Clinical Ophthalmology*, vol. 9, pp. 187–191, 2015.

[6] J. F. Jordan, T. Wecker, C. van Oterendorp et al., "Trabectome surgery for primary and secondary open angle glaucomas," *Graefe's Archive for Clinical and Experimental Ophthalmology*, vol. 251, no. 12, pp. 2753–2760, 2013.

[7] R. Ishida, T. Kojima, M. Dogru et al., "The application of a new continuous functional visual acuity measurement system in dry eye syndromes," *American Journal of Ophthalmology*, vol. 139, no. 2, pp. 253–258, 2005.

[8] E. Goto, Y. Yagi, Y. Matsumoto et al., "Impaired functional visual acuity of dry eye patients," *American Journal of Ophthalmology*, vol. 133, no. 2, pp. 181–186, 2002.

[9] H. Sagara, T. Sekiryu, H. Noji et al., "Meibomian gland loss due to trabeculectomy," *Japanese Journal of Ophthalmology*, vol. 58, no. 4, pp. 334–341, 2014.

[10] H. Imamura, H. Tabuchi, S. Nakakura, D. Nagasato, H. Baba, and Y. Kiuchi, "Usability and reproducibility of tear meniscus values generated via swept-source optical coherence tomography and the slit lamp with a graticule method," *International Ophthalmology*, vol. 38, no. 2, pp. 679–686, 2017.

[11] K. Miyata, S. Amano, M. Sawa et al., "A novel grading method for superficial punctate keratopathy magnitude and its correlation with corneal epithelial permeability," *Archives of Ophthalmology*, vol. 121, no. 11, pp. 1537–1539, 2003.

[12] N. Yokoi, Y. Takehisa, and S. Kinoshita, "Correlation of tear lipid layer interference patterns with the diagnosis and severity of dry eye," *American Journal of Ophthalmology*, vol. 122, no. 6, pp. 818–824, 1996.

[13] N. Yokoi and A. Komuro, "Non-invasive methods of assessing the tear film," *Experimental Eye Research*, vol. 78, no. 3, pp. 399–407, 2004.

[14] M. Kaido, R. Ishida, M. Dogru et al., "The relation of functional visual acuity measurement methodology to tear functions and ocular surface status," *Japanese Journal of Ophthalmology*, vol. 55, no. 5, pp. 451–459, 2011.

[15] G. C. Rossi, G. M. Pasinetti, L. Scudeller et al., "Risk factors to develop ocular surface disease in treated glaucoma or ocular hypertension patients," *European Journal of Ophthalmology*, vol. 23, no. 3, pp. 296–302, 2013.

[16] C. Valente, M. Iester, E. Corsi et al., "Symptoms and signs of tear film dysfunction in glaucomatous patients," *Journal of Ocular Pharmacology and Therapeutics*, vol. 27, no. 3, pp. 281–285, 2011.

[17] S. Y. Lee, T. T. Wong, J. Chua et al., "Effect of chronic anti-glaucoma medications and trabeculectomy on tear osmolarity," *Eye*, vol. 27, no. 10, pp. 1142–1150, 2013.

[18] W. Chen, N. Dong, C. Huang et al., "Corneal alterations induced by topical application of commercial latanoprost, travoprost and bimatoprost in rabbit," *PLoS One*, vol. 9, no. 3, Article ID e89205, 2014.

[19] E. Villani, M. Sacchi, F. Magnani et al., "The ocular surface in medically controlled glaucoma: an in vivo confocal study," *Investigative Opthalmology & Visual Science*, vol. 57, no. 3, pp. 1003–1010, 2016.

[20] Y. Zhang, W. R. Kam, Y. Liu et al., "Influence of pilocarpine and timolol on human meibomian gland epithelial cells," *Cornea*, vol. 36, no. 6, pp. 719–724, 2017.

[21] R. Arita, K. Itoh, S. Maeda et al., "Comparison of the long-term effects of various topical antiglaucoma medications on meibomian glands," *Cornea*, vol. 31, no. 11, pp. 1229–1234, 2012.

[22] M. Aihara, H. Oshima, and M. Araie, "Effects of SofZia-preserved travoprost and benzalkonium chloride-preserved latanoprost on the ocular surface-a multicentre randomized single-masked study," *Acta Ophthalmologica*, vol. 91, no. 1, pp. e7–e14, 2013.

[23] N. Jaenen, C. Baudouin, P. Pouliquen et al., "Ocular symptoms and signs with preserved and preservative-free glaucoma medications," *European Journal of Ophthalmology*, vol. 17, no. 3, pp. 341–349, 2007.

[24] J. J. Hakkarainen, M. Reinisalo, S. Ragauskas et al., "Acute cytotoxic effects of marketed ophthalmic formulations on human corneal epithelial cells," *International Journal of Pharmaceutics*, vol. 511, no. 1, pp. 73–78, 2016.

[25] M. Ayaki, A. Iwasawa, and Y. Niwano, "In vitro assessment of the cytotoxicity of six topical antibiotics to four cultured ocular surface cell lines," *Biocontrol Science*, vol. 17, no. 2, pp. 93–99, 2012.

[26] M. O. Price, F. W. Price Jr., and D. Maclellan, "Effect of gatifloxacin 0.3% and moxifloxacin 0.5% ophthalmic solutions on human corneal epithelium following 2 dosing regimens," *Journal of Cataract and Refractive Surgery*, vol. 31, no. 11, pp. 2137–2141, 2005.

22

Vector Analysis of the Effects of FS-LASIK and Toric ICL for Moderate to High Astigmatism Correction

Kaijian Chen ⓘ, Zongli Hu, Jihan Zhou, Ting Yu, Jie Xu, Ji Bai ⓘ, and Jian Ye ⓘ

Department of Ophthalmology, Research Institute of Surgery and Daping Hospital, Army Medical University, Chongqing, China

Correspondence should be addressed to Jian Ye; yejian1979@163.com

Academic Editor: Michele Figus

Purpose. To estimate the treatment effectiveness of femtosecond-assisted laser in situ keratomileusis (FS-LASIK) and Toric implantable collamer lens (Toric ICL) for moderate and high astigmatism via vector analysis. *Materials and Methods.* The study involved 44 eyes from 44 patients who had a preoperative refractive cylinder ≥1.0 diopters (D) and underwent bilateral FS-LASIK or Toric ICL surgery. The examinations included corrected distance visual acuity measurement and subjective refraction before and 3 months after surgery. The astigmatic changes were estimated using vector analysis. *Results.* No statistically significant differences were found in cylindrical refraction and percentage of spherical equivalent within 0 D, ±0.50 D, ±1.00 D, and ±1.50 D between the FS-LASIK and Toric ICL groups at 3 months after surgery. The parameters of the vector analysis included intended refractive correction, surgically induced refractive correction, error vector, correction ratio, error ratio, error of magnitude, and error of angle, with no significant differences between the groups. However, error ratio the of the off-axis correction in the FS-LASIK and Toric ICL groups was 4.11 ± 3.02 and 8.11 ± 3.82, respectively, and the difference was significant ($t = -2.46$, $p = 0.02$). *Conclusion.* Both FS-LASIK and Toric ICL were effective for correcting moderate and high astigmatism, although Toric ICL might produce a larger error of angle than FS-LASIK when an off-axis correction occurs.

1. Introduction

Astigmatism is a vital factor leading to visual quality decline besides myopia, and it should be corrected via refractive surgery. Currently, there are two ways of surgery to treat astigmatism combined with myopia, corneal refractive surgery and Toric implantable collamer lens (Toric ICL) surgery [1–3]. Both treatments may be selected for the treatment of moderate and high astigmatism. Generally, corneal refractive surgery requires the ablation of corneal tissue, which could induce a change in corneal biomechanics [4] and lead to high-order aberrations [5]. However, Toric ICL avoids the complications associated with ablation, although the postoperative rotation of the lens could influence visual quality [6, 7]. For corneal refractive surgery, both femtosecond-assisted laser in situ keratomileusis (FS-LASIK) and small incision lenticule extraction (SMILE) have been shown to be safe and effective in the treatment of astigmatism [8]. SMILE has the advantages of fast nerve recovery and biomechanical stability but lacks pupil tracking and iris recognition

technology, which can be used to obtain more accurate alignment and correction [9, 10]. For accurate axial requirements in astigmatism correction, FS-LASIK is favored over SMILE in low to moderate astigmatism correction because the latter requires more alignment of the treatment [11]. Zhang suggested that SMILE should adjust the nomograms for astigmatism correction [12]. In addition, FS-LASIK implementation is more extensive than SMILE. Consequently, the choice for moderate to high astigmatism treatment is generally between FS-LASIK and Toric ICL, with the cornea treated via FS-LASIK and the inside of the eye treated via Toric ICL.

Vector analysis is considered a standard method for analyzing the correction effect of astigmatism by the American National Standards Institute (ANSI) [13]. This method is widely used to evaluate the treatment effect of astigmatism in corneal refractive surgery, cataract phacoemulsification combined with Toric intraocular lens implantation, and Toric ICL implantation, and it can comprehensively assess the effectiveness of astigmatism correction using the treatment magnitude, treatment angle deviation, and so on.

Because the principles of FS-LASIK and Toric ICL are completely different, few studies have compared the effect of astigmatism correction between these surgeries. Therefore, the effect of FS-LASIK and Toric ICL for moderate and high astigmatism correction was compared by vector analysis in our study.

2. Materials and Methods

This comparative, randomized, and retrospective study included 44 eyes from 44 subjects who had preoperative astigmatism ranging from −1.00 diopters (D) to −4.50 D [7]. In total, 22 eyes of 22 patients underwent bilateral FS-LASIK, and 22 eyes of 22 patients received bilateral Toric ICL. This prospective study obtained Institutional Review Board approval from the Ethics Committee of the Research Institute of Field Surgery, Daping Hospital of the Army Medical University, Chongqing, China, and it was performed in accordance with the tenets of the Declaration of Helsinki. All of the study participants provided written informed consent.

The common inclusion criteria were as follows: minimum age of 18 years, stable refraction for at least 1 year, myopia with a minimum astigmatism of −1.0 D, corrected distant visual acuity (CDVA) of 20/30 or better, healthy tear film and ocular surface, absence of corneal ectatic diseases, and corneal scars and retinal pathology. Patients using soft and rigid contact lenses were instructed to discontinue use for at least 2 and 4 weeks, respectively. For the Toric ICL patients, the anterior chamber depth was greater than 2.8 mm, and the endothelial cell density was greater than 2000 cells/mm [2]. In addition, for the FS-LASIK patients, the central corneal thickness was more than 500 μm, and the residual stroma was thicker than 280 μm.

2.1. Surgical Procedure.
For FS-LASIK, the flap was created with a WaveLight FS200 femtosecond laser system (Alcon, USA). The parameters were performed with an intended flap diameter of 8.5 mm, a thickness of 110 μm, a superior hinge, and a side angle cut of 90°. Excimer laser ablation was performed using a WaveLight EX500 Excimer Laser system (Alcon, USA) with an optical zone of 6 mm and pupil tracking technology. The kappa angle of the treatment centration was adjusted based on the Pentacam HR (Oculus Optikgeräte GmbH) before surgery, and the center was fixated intraoperatively.

For Toric ICL implantation, all of the patients underwent 2 preoperative peripheral iridotomies with a neodymium-YAG laser. Patients were marked on the 0°–180° axis using a slit lamp before surgery. After topical anesthesia was administered, a Toric ICL was inserted through a 2.8 mm clear corneal incision with the use of an injector cartridge (STAAR Surgical) after placement of a viscosurgical device (Opegan™; Santen, Osaka, Japan) into the anterior chamber. Then, the Toric ICL was placed in the posterior chamber and rotated to the intended axis using the manipulator.

2.2. Data Collection.
The examinations included slit-lamp biomicroscopy, CDVA measurement, and subjective refraction before and 3 months after surgery. For all patients, sphere and cylinder were assessed by the same optometrists, and spherical equivalent (SE) values were calculated as the sphere power plus 1/2 of the cylinder power. The eye with the greater cylinder was collected for the study [14]. When both the eyes had an equal cylinder, the right eye was collected.

2.3. Vector Analysis

Preparation for Vector Analysis. Astigmatism data from the spectacle to the corneal plane were converted, the cylinder axes of the left eyes were flipped around to the vertical axis, and all axis angles were then doubled. The parameters of the vector analysis were as follows: the intended refractive correction (IRC) vector, which is defined as the vector difference between the preoperative astigmatic correction vector and the target postoperative cylinder vector (preoperative – target); the surgically induced refractive correction (SIRC), which is the vector difference between the preoperative and postoperative astigmatic correction vectors (preoperative – postoperative); the error vector (EV), which is defined as the vector difference between the intended refractive correction and the surgically induced refractive correction (IRC-SIRC); the error ratio (ER), which is the proportion of the intended correction that was not successfully treated (|EV|/|IRC|); the correction ratio (CR), which is the ratio of the achieved correction magnitude to the required correction (|SIRC|/|IRC|); the error of magnitude (EM), which is the arithmetic difference of the magnitudes between SIRC and IRC (|IRC|-|SIRC|); and the error of angle (EA), which measures whether the treatment was applied at the correct axis.

2.4. Statistical Analysis.
The statistical analysis was performed using PASW software V.18.0 (SPSS/IBM, Chicago, Illinois, USA). The Kolmogorov–Smirnov test was used to analyze the normality of the parameters. Independent sample T-test was used to normal distribution variables, and Mann–Whitney U test was used to abnormal distribution variables between groups. Categorical variables were evaluated using the χ^2 test. A value of $p < 0.05$ was considered statistically significant.

3. Results

Overall, 44 eyes (44 patients) were included in the study, with 22 eyes in the FS-LASIK group and 22 eyes in the Toric ICL group. The mean age of the patients was 22.72 ± 4.85 years and 25.27 ± 5.49 years in FS-LASIK and Toric ICL groups, respectively. Significant differences were not observed in the manifest sphere, manifest cylinder, manifest spherical equivalent, and axial and CDVA between two groups preoperatively or postoperatively (Table 1). All surgeries were uneventful, with no intraoperative complications.

3.1. Safety and Effectiveness Analysis.
At 3 months after surgery, 6 (27.27%) eyes in the FS-LASIK group and 6 (27.27%) eyes in the Toric ICL group gained ≥1 line in the CDVA. In both groups, none of the eyes lost ≥2 lines in the CDVA.

TABLE 1: Demographic data of the FS-LASIK and Toric ICL groups.

	FS-LASIK group	Toric ICL group	p value
Patients/eyes (n)	22/22	22/22	—
Eye, right (%)	54.55	40.91	0.36**
Sex, male (%)	50	31.82	0.38**
Age (y)	22.72 ± 4.85 (18 to 33)	25.27 ± 5.49 (18 to 35)	0.11*
Presphere (D)	−6.97 ± 1.20 (−9.25 to −5.00)	−8.32 ± 3.14 (−14.00 to −2.00)	0.07*
Precylinder (D)	−2.40 ± 0.59 (−3.50 to −1.25)	−2.28 ± 0.88 (−4.00 to −1.00)	0.57*
Pre-SE (D)	−8.18 ± 1.10 (−10.25 to −6.75)	−9.47 ± 2.99 (−15.00 to −3.75)	0.07*
Preaxial	17.50/5.00/172.50 (0 to 175)	5.00/0.00/78.75 (0 to 175)	0.06#
Pre-CDVA (logMAR)	0.04 ± 0.06 (0 to 0.2)	0.06 ± 0.09 (0 to 0.3)	0.31*
Postsphere (D)	−0.08 ± 0.40 (−1.00 to 0.75)	0.13 ± 0.49 (−0.5 to 2.00)	0.14*
Postcylinder (D)	−0.19 ± 0.33 (−1.00 to 0.25)	−0.27 ± 0.37 (−1.25 to 0)	0.45*
Post-SE (D)	−0.18 ± 0.45 (−1.25 to 0.75)	−0.01 ± 0.43 (−0.5 to 1.38)	0.23*
Postaxial	0.00/0.00/85.00 (0 to 155)	0.00/0.00/46.25 (0 to 170)	0.36*
Post-CDVA (logMAR)	0.01 ± 0.03 (0 to 0.1)	0.02 ± 0.04 (0 to 0.1)	0.43#

Pre: preoperative values; SE: spherical equivalent; normal distribution variables: mean ± SD (range); abnormal distribution variables: median/Q25/Q75 (range); **chi-squared test; *independent sample T-test; #Mann–Whitney U test.

The percentage of the eyes with postoperative SE within 0 D, ±0.5 D, ±1.0 D, and ±1.5 D was 18.18% and 36.36%, 77.27% and 95.45%, 95.45% and 95.45%, and 100% and 100% in the FS-LASIK group and Toric ICL group, respectively (Figure 1). The percentage of the eyes with postoperative refractive astigmatism within 0 D, ±0.5 D, ±1.0 D, and ±1.5 D was 45.49% and 59.09%, 86.36% and 81.82%, 100% and 95.45%, and 100% and 100% in the FS-LASIK group and Toric ICL group, respectively (Figure 2). Both the postoperative SE and postoperative refractive astigmatism were not significantly different between the two groups ($\chi^2 = 4.27$ and 1.09; $p = 0.12$ and 0.58, respectively).

3.2. Vector Analysis. The vector analysis results showed that significant differences did not occur in the IRC, SIRC, EV, CR, ER, EM, and EA between the FS-LASIK and Toric ICL groups (Table 2). Significant differences in these parameters were not observed between the two groups.

The percentage of the undercorrection and overcorrection was 36.36% and 27.27% and 18.18% and 13.63% between the FS-LASIK and Toric ICL groups, respectively (Figure 3), and significant differences were not observed ($\chi^2 = 0.82$, $p = 0.66$).

The percentage of correct axes between the achieved treatment and the intended treatment (clockwise and counterclockwise) was 27.27% and 27.27% and 9.1% and 13.64% between the FS-LASIK and Toric ICL groups, respectively (Figures 4 and 5), and significant differences were not observed ($\chi^2 = 0.24$, $p = 0.88$). However, the error angles were 4.11 ± 3.02 (1–10) and 8.11 ± 3.82 (2–14) in the off-axis correction of the LASIK and Toric ICL groups. A significant difference was observed between the groups ($t = -2.46$, $p = 0.02$).

4. Discussion

In this study, our findings suggest that FS-LASIK and Toric ICL presented good safety and efficacy in the treatment of moderate and high astigmatism, which is consistent with the results of previous studies. The CDVA of the patients was

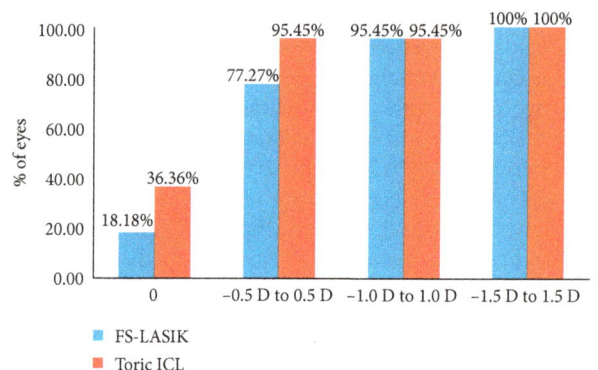

FIGURE 1: Postoperative spherical equivalent in dioptres (D) between FS-LASIK and Toric ICL.

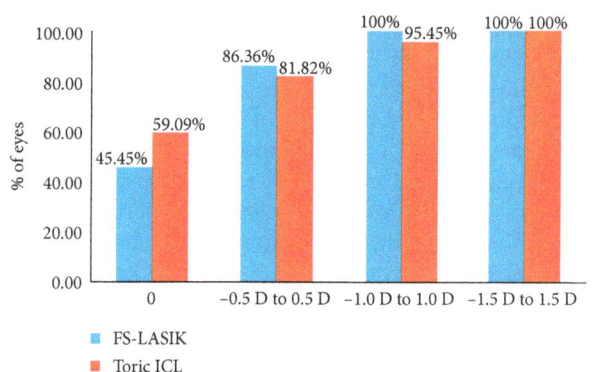

FIGURE 2: Postoperative refractive astigmatism in dioptres (D) between FS-LASIK and Toric ICL.

improved in both groups, and none of the patients lost CDVA. High astigmatism may induce high-order aberrations [15], and high astigmatism corrected using spectacles may generate imaging distortion, which can reduce the patient's CDVA. Topography-guided FS-LASIK and Toric ICL can reduce high-order aberrations [16, 17]. Similarly, correcting myopia and astigmatism also reduces the imaging

TABLE 2: Vector parameters for FS-LASIK and Toric ICL.

	FS-LASIK group ($n = 22$)	Toric ICL group ($n = 22$)	p value
IRC	2.00 ± 0.50 (1.01 to 3.00)	1.86 ± 0.76 (0.77 to 1.86)	0.47*
SIRC	1.95 ± 0.48 (1.01 to 3.00)	1.76 ± 0.81 (0.77 to 3.30)	0.36*
EV	0.25/0.00/0.31 (0 to 0.97)	0.00/0.00/0.49 (0 to 1.29)	0.86#
CR	1.00/0.91/1.00 (0.69 to 1.28)	1.00/1.00/0.92 (0.41 to 1.21)	0.96#
ER	0.12/0.00/0.19 (0 to 0.39)	0.00/0.00/0.30 (0 to 0.61)	0.92#
EM	0.00/0.00/0.17 (-0.47 to 0.77)	0.00/0.00/0.22 (-0.35 to 1.24)	0.98#
EA	0.00/-2.00/0.00 (-10 to 8)	0.00/-4.25/0.00 (-14 to 13)	0.81#

RC: intended refractive correction; SIRC: surgically induced refractive correction; EV: error vector; CR: correction ratio; ER: error ratio; EM: error of the magnitude; normal distribution variables: mean $\pm$ SD (range); abnormal distribution variables: median/Q25/Q75 (range); #Mann–Whitney U test; *independent sample T-test.

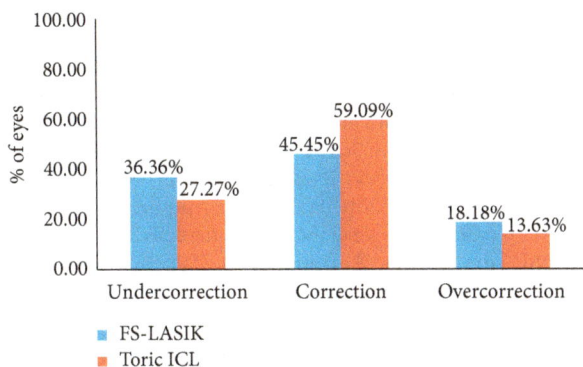

FIGURE 3: Astigmatism correction ratio in FS-LASIK and Toric ICL.

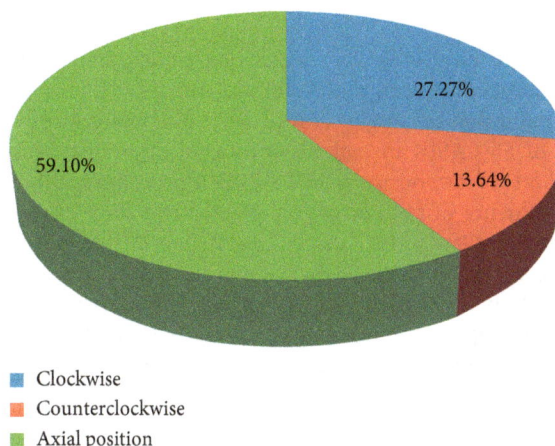

FIGURE 4: Correct axis between the achieved treatment and intended treatment in FS-LASIK.

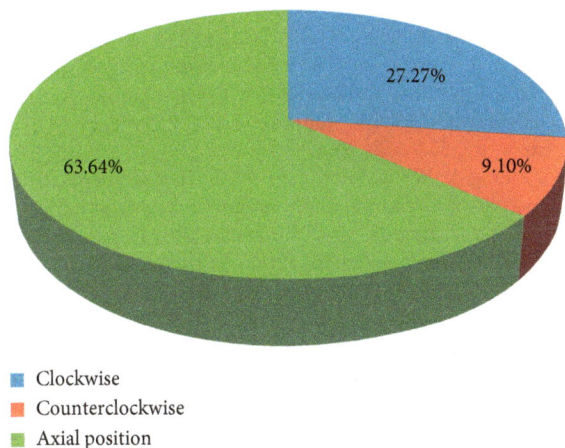

FIGURE 5: Correct axis between the achieved treatment and the intended treatment in Toric ICL.

distortion from spectacles. However, FS-LASIK and Toric ICL have different treatment characteristics. In FS-LASIK, corneal ablation occurs via excimer laser spot superposition at high speeds to achieve therapeutic purposes. In the excimer laser ablation procedure, changes in the circumambient temperature and humidity, attenuation of laser energy, and movement of the laser cutting plane can affect the treatment effect. Toric ICL is a molded lens designed for therapeutic purposes, and it is implanted in the posterior chamber; thus, deviations from the pupil center are rare. The therapeutic gradient of Toric ICL for astigmatism is 0.5D, while FS-LASIK is usually 0.25 D. In addition, undercorrection is more likely

to occur with Toric ICL. For high astigmatism, the treatment may have to be adjusted according to nomograms. Different devices usually have different nomograms, and the success of the adjustment depends on the experience of the surgeon. Although different advantages and limitations were observed between the two surgeries, significant differences were not observed in the correction effect. Ganesh et al. found that the predictability of low to moderate astigmatism correction was not significantly different among FS-LASIK, Toric ICL, and reflex SMILE [17]. Hasegawa et al. found that the predictability in the LASIK group was higher in the moderate refractive cylinder but lower in the high refractive cylinder than that in the Toric phakic intraocular lens group [18]. Therefore, we believe that there are similar treatment effects in moderate to high astigmatism between FS-LASIK and Toric ICL.

Astigmatism correction is based on the magnitude of the astigmatism and on the axis of the astigmatism, which makes the treatment of astigmatism more complicated compared with the treatment of myopia. Alpins found that when the treatment is off the intended axis, then the effect of the astigmatism correction will be reduced [19]. As a result, accurate axial correction is a difficulty associated with astigmatism correction. Zhang et al. found that axial errors may be one of the potential factors for moderate and high astigmatism undercorrection [20]. Our study also found that the patients showing undercorrection or overcorrection had different degrees of axial errors in the treatment according to the vector analysis, and axial errors were not observed in the complete correction cases. Pupil tracking avoided decentration ablation, which resulted from eye movement in FS-LASIK, although the patient's head position and rotation or vertical movement of the eye may still cause off-axis ablation. The treatment must be adjusted according to the nomogram for high astigmatism correction via FS-LASIK, and overcorrection may be related to fewer adjustments for corrections. The effective lens position and posterior corneal astigmatism might represent influencing factors in Toric ICL when the Toric intraocular lens is used to correct for astigmatism in cataract surgery [21].

To our knowledge, few studies have compared the axial offset degree between FS-LASIK and Toric ICL. In our study, we found that the angle error of Toric ICL was greater than that of FS-LASIK in patients with axial migration because axial errors may occur in the FS-LASIK procedure, although the influence of such errors on astigmatism correction may be reduced with the strict supervision of the surgeon. However, the Toric ICL axis was marked before surgery and found to be consistent with the expected intraoperative axis by the surgeons. Nonetheless, Toric ICL rotation is an uncertain postoperative scenario, and repositioning is required when severe rotation occurs. Therefore, we believe that the error angle of Toric ICL may be greater than that of FS-LASIK in patients with off-axis correction.

5. Conclusions

In conclusion, our study found that FS-LASIK and Toric ICL were effective for moderate and high astigmatism correction. However, Toric ICL might create a larger error angle than FS-LASIK when off-axis correction occurs.

Conflicts of Interest

The authors declare that there are no conflicts of interest.

References

[1] A. Barsam and B. D. Allan, "Excimer laser refractive surgery versus phakic intraocular lenses for the correction of moderate to high myopia," *Cochrane Database of Systematic Reviews*, vol. 65, no. 6, article CD007679, 2014.

[2] J. L. Alió, F. Soria, A. Abbouda, and P. Peña-García, "Laser in situ keratomileusis for −6.00 to −18.00 diopters of myopia and up to −5.00 diopters of astigmatism: 15-year follow-up," *Journal of Cataract and Refractive Surgery*, vol. 41, no. 1, pp. 33–40, 2015.

[3] D. R. Sanders, D. Schneider, R. Martin et al., "Toric implantable collamer lens for moderate to high myopic astigmatism," *Ophthalmology*, vol. 114, no. 1, pp. 54–61, 2007.

[4] M. A. Qazi, J. P. Sanderson, A. M. Mahmoud, E. Y. Yoon, C. J. Roberts, and J. S. Pepose, "Postoperative changes in intraocular pressure and corneal biomechanical metrics: laser in situ keratomileusis versus laser-assisted subepithelial

[5] W. Wu and Y. Wang, "Corneal higher-order aberrations of the anterior surface, posterior surface, and total cornea after SMILE, FS-LASIK, and FLEx surgeries," *Eye and Contact Lens: Science and Clinical Practice*, vol. 42, no. 6, pp. 358–365, 2016.

[6] K. Kamiya, K. Shimizu, H. Kobashi, A. Igarashi, and M. Komatsu, "Three-year follow-up of posterior chamber Toric phakic intraocular lens implantation for moderate to high myopic astigmatism," *PLoS One*, vol. 8, no. 2, Article ID e56453, 2013.

[7] E. S. Sari, D. P. Pinero, A. Kubaloglu et al., "Toric implantable collamer lens for moderate to high myopic astigmatism: 3-year follow-up," *Graefe's Archive for Clinical and Experimental Ophthalmology*, vol. 251, no. 5, pp. 1413–1422, 2013.

[8] M. Liu, Y. Chen, D. Wang et al., "Clinical outcomes after SMILE and femtosecond laser-assisted LASIK for myopia and myopic astigmatism: a prospective randomized comparative study," *Cornea*, vol. 35, no. 2, pp. 210–216, 2015.

[9] M. N. Karim, A. K. Riau, N. C. Lwin, S. S. Chaurasia, D. T. Tan, and J. S. Mehta, "Early corneal nerve damage and recovery following small incision lenticule extraction (SMILE) and laser in situ keratomileusis (LASIK)," *Investigative Ophthalmology and Visual Science*, vol. 55, no. 3, pp. 1823–1834, 2014.

[10] D. Wu, Y. Wang, L. Zhang, S. Wei, and X. Tang, "Corneal biomechanical effects: small-incision lenticule extraction versus femtosecond laser-assisted laser in situ keratomileusis," *Journal of Cataract and Refractive Surgery*, vol. 40, no. 6, pp. 954–962, 2014.

[11] T. C. Chan, A. L. Ng, G. P. Cheng et al., "Vector analysis of astigmatic correction after small-incision lenticule extraction and femtosecond-assisted LASIK for low to moderate myopic astigmatism," *British Journal of Ophthalmology*, vol. 100, no. 4, pp. 553–559, 2015.

[12] J. Zhang, Y. Wang, W. Wu, L. Xu, X. Li, and R. Dou, "Vector analysis of low to moderate astigmatism with small incision lenticule extraction (SMILE): results of a 1-year follow-up," *BMC Ophthalmology*, vol. 15, no. 1, pp. 1–10, 2015.

[13] M. B. Eydelman, B. Drum, J. Holladay et al., "Standardized analyses of correction of astigmatism by laser systems that reshape the cornea," *Journal of Refractive Surgery*, vol. 22, no. 1, pp. 81–95, 2006.

[14] G. Wen, K. Tarczyhornoch, R. Mckeancowdin et al., "Prevalence of myopia, hyperopia and astigmatism in non-Hispanic white and Asian children: multi-ethnic pediatric eye disease study," *Ophthalmology*, vol. 120, no. 10, pp. 2109–2116, 2013.

[15] M. Mohammadpour, Z. Heidari, H. Mohammad-Rabei et al., "Correlation of higher order aberrations and components of astigmatism in myopic refractive surgery candidates," *Journal of Current Ophthalmology*, vol. 28, no. 3, pp. 112–116, 2016.

[16] R. Shetty, R. Shroff, K. Deshpande, R. Gowda, S. Lahane, and C. Jayadev, "A prospective study to compare visual outcomes between wavefront-optimized and topography-guided ablation profiles in contralateral eyes with myopia," *Journal of Refractive Surgery*, vol. 33, no. 1, pp. 6–10, 2017.

[17] S. Ganesh, S. Brar, and A. Pawar, "Matched population comparison of visual outcomes and patient satisfaction between 3 modalities for the correction of low to moderate myopic astigmatism," *Clinical Ophthalmology*, vol. 11, pp. 1253–1263, 2017.

[18] A. Hasegawa, T. Kojima, N. Isoga, A. Tamaoki, T. Nakamura, and K. Ichikawa, "Astigmatism correction: laser in situ

keratectomy," *Journal of Cataract and Refractive Surgery*, vol. 35, no. 10, pp. 1774–1788, 2009.

keratomileusis versus posterior chamber collagen copolymer Toric phakic intraocular lens implantation," *Journal of Cataract and Refractive Surgery*, vol. 38, no. 4, pp. 574–581, 2012.

[19] N. A. Alpins, "Vector analysis of astigmatism changes by flattening, steepening, and torque," *Journal of Cataract and Refractive Surgery*, vol. 23, no. 10, pp. 1503–1514, 1997.

[20] J. Zhang, Y. Wang, and X. Chen, "Comparison of moderate-to high-astigmatism corrections using wavefront-guided laser in situ keratomileusis and small-incision lenticule extraction," *Cornea*, vol. 35, no. 4, pp. 523–530, 2016.

[21] Y. Eom, D. Ryu, D. W. Kim et al., "Development of a program for Toric intraocular lens calculation considering posterior corneal astigmatism, incision-induced posterior corneal astigmatism, and effective lens position," *Graefe's Archive for Clinical and Experimental Ophthalmology*, vol. 254, no. 10, pp. 1977–1986, 2016.

23

Trends in Indications and Techniques of Corneal Transplantation from 1999 through 2015 at a Tertiary Referral Center in Athens, Greece

Konstantinos Droutsas [ID],[1,2] Georgios Bagikos,[3] Dimitrios Miltsakakis,[3] Ilias Georgalas [ID],[1] Apostolos Lazaridis [ID],[1,2] Klio Chatzistefanou,[1] Marilita M. Moschos [ID],[1] Chryssanthi Koutsandrea,[1] and Georgios Kymionis[1,4]

[1]First Department of Ophthalmology, National and Kapodistrian University of Athens, Athens, Greece
[2]Department of Ophthalmology, Philipps University, Marburg, Germany
[3]State Ophthalmology Clinic, General Hospital "G. Gennimatas", Athens, Greece
[4]Jules Gonin Eye Hospital, University of Lausanne, Lausanne, Switzerland

Correspondence should be addressed to Konstantinos Droutsas; konstantinos_droutsas@yahoo.gr

Academic Editor: Van C. Lansingh

Introduction. During the past decade, novel techniques of corneal transplantation allowing faster and better restoration of vision have emerged. The present cohort study describes a shift of indications and techniques that has occurred in the field of corneal transplantation over a 17-year period in Greece. *Methods.* All patients undergoing keratoplasty between January 1999 and December 2015 at an academic tertiary referral center in Athens, Greece, were retrospectively reviewed. The annual incidence of keratoplasty indications and techniques was recorded and analyzed. *Results.* A total of 1382 keratoplasty procedures were included. Leading indications were bullous keratopathy (BK) (37.5%), followed by allograft rejection (17.7%), corneal scar (12%), keratoconus (KC) (10.3%), and Fuchs endothelial dystrophy (FED) (8.8%). A decreasing trend was observed for KC ($P = 0.009$) and an increasing trend for BK ($P = 0.003$) and FED ($P = 0.001$). In 2015, the incidence of penetrating keratoplasty (PK) had decreased from 100% (1999 to 2009) to 21.4%; for cases with isolated pathology of the corneal endothelium, DSAEK was the preferred technique (59.8%), while the respective rate of DMEK was 18.8%. *Conclusion.* Herein, we observed an increasing trend of endothelial pathology among keratoplasty indications as well as a major shift in preferred techniques due to a wide adoption of the new EK procedures.

1. Introduction

Keratoplasty is one of the most common and successful allotransplantations in humans and the only treatment of several corneal pathologies. Since the first successful corneal transplantation by Zirm in 1906 [1], penetrating keratoplasty (PK) was the gold standard. Over the past decade, however, advancements in the field of corneal transplantation changed the preferred practice patterns of corneal surgeons. The more or less selective transplantation of corneal endothelium evolved since the introduction of posterior lamellar keratoplasty in 1998 [2] to safer and more targeted techniques, for example, Descemet (automated) stripping endothelial keratoplasty (DS(A)EK) [3] and Descemet membrane endothelial keratoplasty (DMEK) [4, 5]. Moreover, advancements in the field of keratoconus surgery that may delay or even arrest disease progression, that is, corneal crosslinking (CXL), have reduced the need for keratoplasty [6].

Indeed, recent reports describe both an increase of endothelial pathology and a shift from PK to lamellar keratoplasty techniques [7–9]. However, only limited data on the implementation of DMEK among keratoplasty procedures are available [8, 9]. Purpose of the current paper is therefore to report trends in indications and techniques in a cohort where both DMEK and DSAEK were implemented.

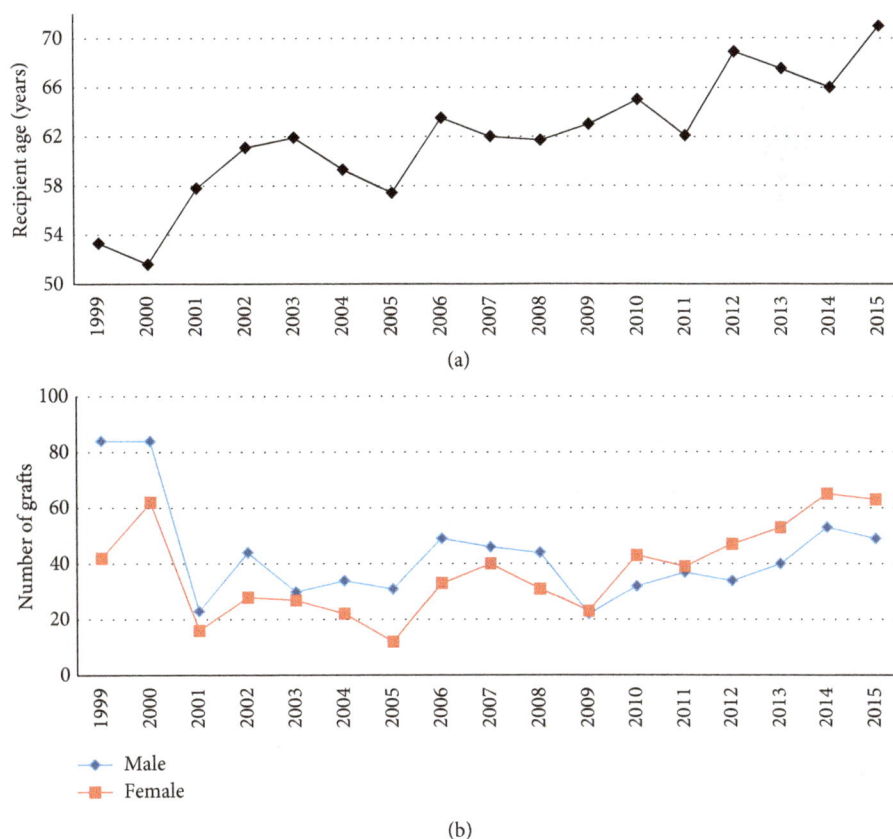

FIGURE 1: Chart depicting distribution of recipient age (a) and gender distribution (b) per calendar year. (a) Recipient age shows a statistically significant increase ($P < 0.001$, $r^2 = 0.79$, univariate linear regression). (b) In addition, a switch from male to female predominance is noted in 2009, the year of EK implementation. This also may be explained by the increase Fuchs endothelial dystrophy that affects mainly women.

2. Materials and Methods

The records of all corneal transplantations conducted between 1999 through 2015 at a referral center in a large hospital in Athens, Greece (First Department of Ophthalmology, National and Kapodistrian University, Athens, and Ophthalmology Department, General Hospital "G. Gennimatas") were reviewed.

All procedures were performed by 3 surgeons in total. The number of surgeons operating during each calendar year varied from 1 to 3.

The present research adhered to the tenets of the Declaration of Helsinki. Due to the observational and retrospective character of the study, IRB approval was not required.

2.1. Data Collection. Indications were grouped according to the following criteria:

(1) "Bullous keratopathy" (BK) included all cases of corneal endothelial decompensation except for cases of Fuchs endothelial dystrophy and failed corneal grafts.

(2) "Regraft" included cases of repeat keratoplasty due to graft failure.

(3) "Corneal scar" included stromal opacities, for example, after herpetic and infectious keratitis, pemphigoid, chemical and mechanical trauma, trachoma, or anesthetic abuse.

(4) "Keratoconus" (KC).

(5) "Fuchs endothelial dystrophy" (FED).

(6) "Sterile melt/perforation" included all cases of non-infectious keratitis leading to corneal perforation.

(7) "Infectious keratitis" included all cases of therapeutic keratoplasty for progressive corneal melt due to bacteria, fungi, or acanthameba. This group also included cases where the pathogen could not be isolated.

(8) "Stromal dystrophies" (SD).

2.2. Statistical Analysis.
All data were collected with Excel software (version 14, Microsoft Corp.). Descriptive and inferential data analysis was performed with SPSS software (version 17.0, SPSS Inc.). Numerical data are presented as mean ± standard deviation. Evolution of recipient age, gender, and surgical indication were assessed using linear regression analysis. The x^2 test was used where appropriate. A P value less than 0.05 was considered statistically significant.

(a)

■ Male
■ Female

(b)

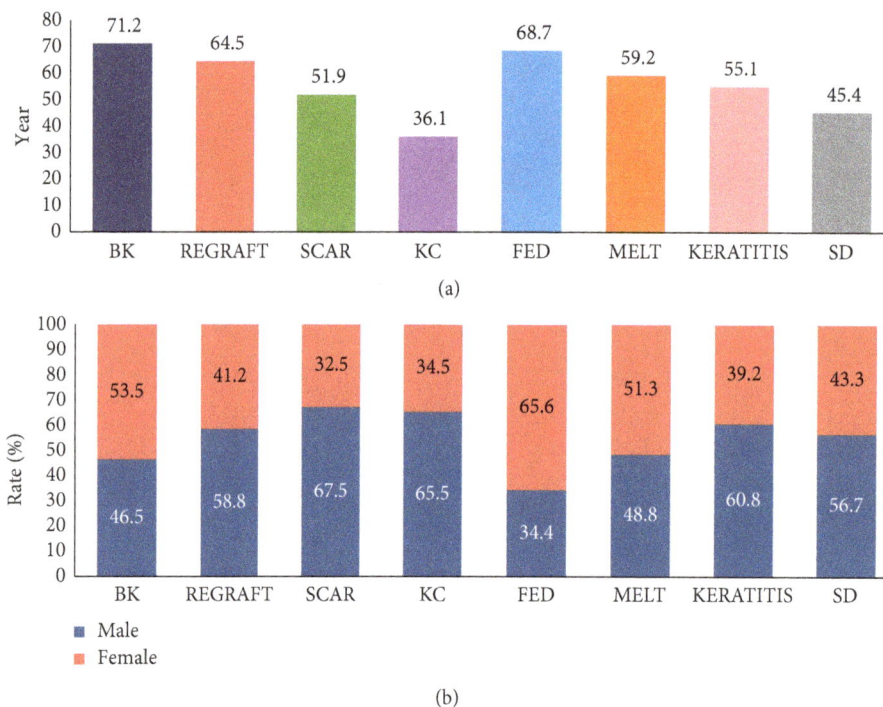

FIGURE 2: Chart depicting recipient age (a) and gender distribution (b) per indication. (a) The lowest age is observed in keratoconus while the highest in Fuchs endothelial dystrophy patients. (b) Significant predominance of men is noted in keratoconus (65.5%) and corneal scar (67.5%) whereas of women in Fuchs endothelial dystrophy patients (65.6%).

3. Results

3.1. Demographics. The present retrospective cohort study includes 1382 eyes undergoing corneal transplantation at a single tertiary referral center with a nationwide patient pool. While the majority of donor tissue (79.4%) was imported from eye banks outside Greece, the rest was retrieved from local multiorgan donors.

Mean recipient age was 61.9 ± 5.1 years with increasing trend, starting at 53.3 ± 20.7 years (1999) and reaching 71.1 ± 12.0 years (2015) ($P < 0.001$, $r^2 = 0.79$, univariate linear regression) (Figure 1(a)).

The present cohort comprises 736 men (53.3%) and 646 women (46.7%) in total. In 2009, a switch of male to female predominance was evident, suggesting an increasing trend for female patients. Indeed, when dividing the observation time into a first (1999 through 2008) and last period (2009 through 2015), an increasing trend for females was found only in the last period ($P = 0.011$, $r^2 = 0.89$, univariate linear regression) (Figure 1(b)).

Patients with keratoconus (KC, mean age 36.1 ± 14.3 years) formed the youngest and patients with BK the oldest group (mean age 71.2 ± 11.5 years) (Figure 2(a)). A significant predominance of men was found in KC ($x^2 = 13.36$, $P < 0.001$), regraft ($x^2 = 7.55$, $P = 0.006$), and scar ($x^2 = 20.27$, $P < 0.001$), while that of women was found in FED ($x^2 = 11.84$, $P = 0.001$) (Figure 2(b)).

3.2. Indications. Leading indication was BK (37.5%), followed by allograft rejection (17.7%), corneal scar (12%), KC

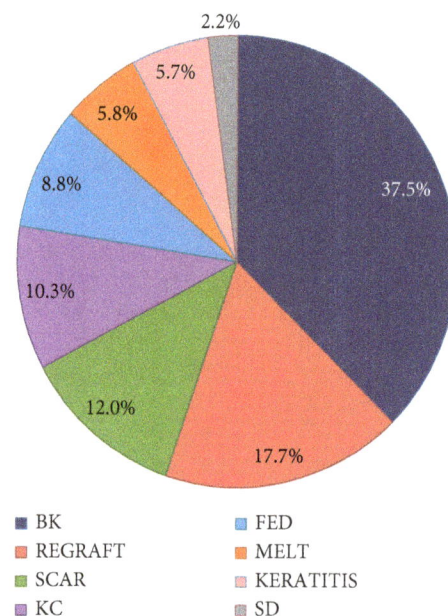

■ BK   ■ FED
■ REGRAFT   ■ MELT
■ SCAR   ■ KERATITIS
■ KC   ■ SD

FIGURE 3: The pie chart illustrates the incidence of all keratoplasty indications from 1999 to 2015. Top 3 indications were bullous keratopathy (37.5%), regraft (17.7%), and corneal scar (12%). Each diagnosis is represented by the same color as in the bar chart in Figure 2.

(10.3%), FED (8.8%), corneal melt (5.8%), infectious keratitis (5.7%), and stromal dystrophy (2.2%) (Figure 3).

Univariate linear regression analysis of the annual incidence for each indication revealed a significant increase of endothelial

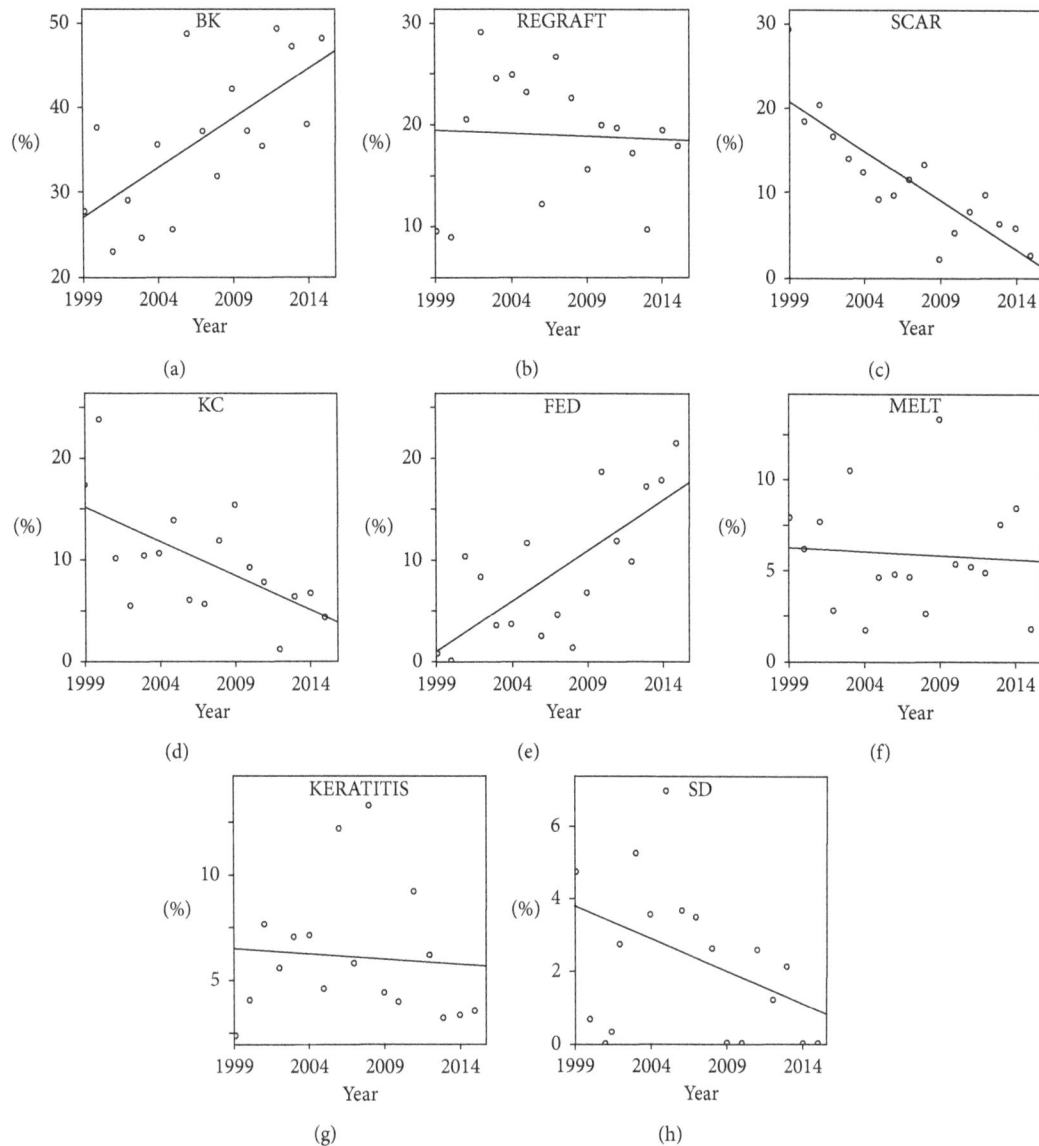

FIGURE 4: Scatter plot depicting the annual incidence of each keratoplasty indication. A significant trend was found for bullous keratopathy (BK; $r^2 = 0.47$, $P = 0.003$), corneal scar ($r^2 = 0.72$, $P < 0.001$), keratoconus (KC; $r^2 = 0.38$, $P = 0.009$), and Fuchs endothelial dystrophy (FED; $r^2 = 0.55$, $P = 0.001$). All others were found not significant (univariate linear regression analysis).

pathologies, that is, BK ($r^2 = 0.47$, $P = 0.003$) and FED ($r^2 = 0.55$, $P = 0.001$) and a significant decrease in corneal scar ($r^2 = 0.72$, $P < 0.001$) and KC ($r^2 = 0.38$, $P = 0.009$). All other indications did not show significant fluctuations (univariate linear regression analysis) (Figure 4).

3.3. Techniques. PK was the only technique applied until 2009, when DSAEK was introduced, starting with 8.9% (2009) and reaching 59.9% (2015) (Figure 5). DMEK was introduced in July 2013 reaching 11.8% in the first (half) year, peaking with 41.5% in the second year, and decreasing to 18.8% in the third year of its implementation (Figure 5).

By the final year of the study, EK was the preferred treatment for BK (89.8% EK versus 11.2% PK) and the only treatment for FED (Figure 6).

4. Discussion

The present study reports trends in keratoplasty indications and techniques from 1999 through 2015 at an academic tertiary referral center in Athens, Greece. As part of this study, the implementation of new endothelial keratoplasty techniques (DMEK and DSAEK) in a large keratoplasty cohort was evaluated.

The leading indication herein was BK (37.7%), being in accordance with a previous Greek multicenter study reporting aphakic/pseudophakic corneal edema (29.1%), keratoconus (26%), and regraft (11.9%) as main indications [10].

The increase of corneal endothelial pathology (BK and FED) among indications may be explained by the early and successful adoption of DSAEK and DMEK in our cohort (Figure 4).

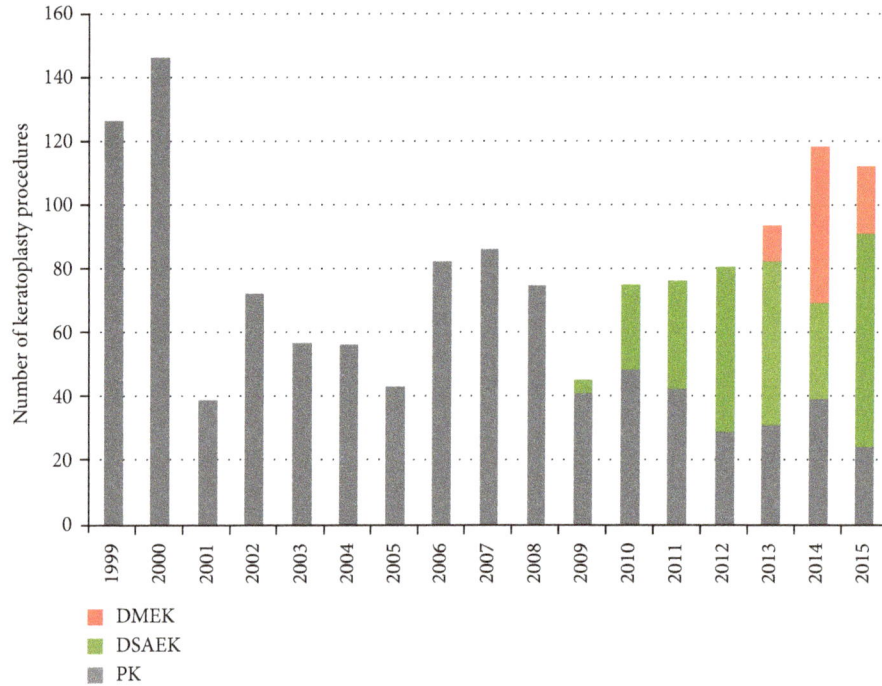

FIGURE 5: Column chart depicting the absolute number of keratoplasty procedures performed in each calendar year from 1999 to 2015. Penetrating keratoplasty (gray columns) was the only technique applied until DSAEK (green columns) and DMEK (red columns) were implemented (2009 and 2013, resp.). In the last year, PK was only performed in 21.4%. Significant fluctuations in the annual number of surgeries were caused by fluctuations in the number of operating surgeons as well as by graft shortage periods.

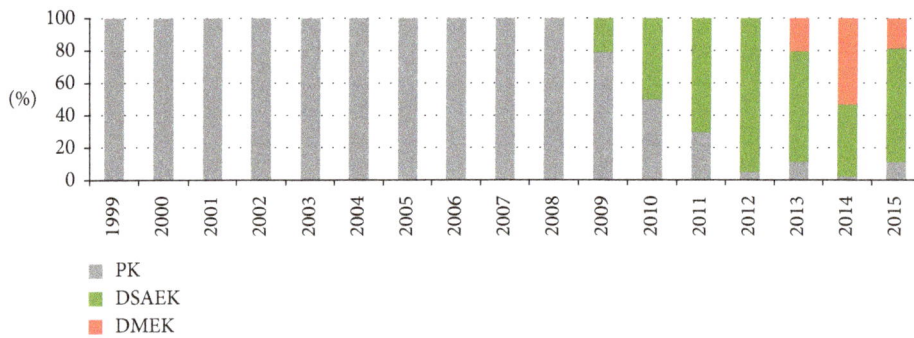

(a)

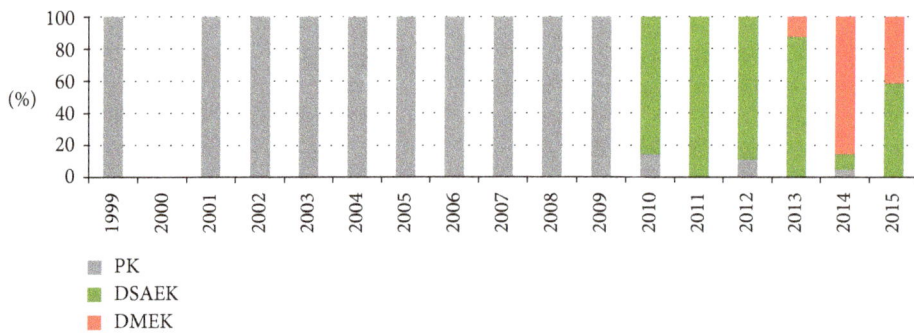

(b)

FIGURE 6: Continued.

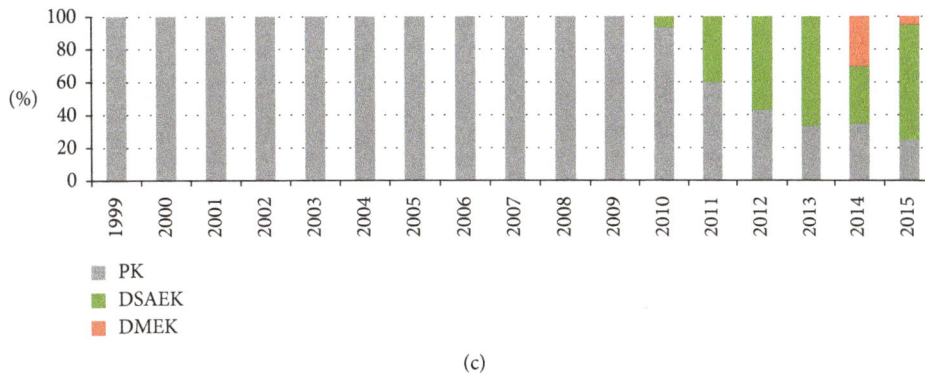

(c)

FIGURE 6: Column chart depicting keratoplasty techniques applied for endothelial pathology, that is, BK (a), FED (b), and regrafts (c). Note that, in the last 3–6 years of the observation period, PK has been replaced to a variable extent by endothelial keratoplasty, that is, DSAEK and DMEK.

On the other hand, KC demonstrated a significant decrease over time that may relate to the introduction of CXL as well as advancements in optical rehabilitation, for example, scleral contact lenses or intracorneal ring segments.

Compared to the global introduction of new lamellar techniques [7], the present cohort keeps up with advancements in endothelial keratoplasty. Thus, although it took three years for EK (DSAEK) to surpass PK, both EK techniques (DSAEK and DMEK) were successfully implemented, with EK accounting for 78.6% of the total keratoplasty procedures performed during the final year of our study (Figure 5). This is in agreement with other studies reporting similar trends in keratoplasty techniques [7–9]. With regard to endothelial pathology, EK procedures have almost completely replaced PK, ranging between 88.9% for BK and 100% for FED cases (Figure 6).

This rapid shift in surgeons' preferences from PK to EK techniques in the treatment of endothelial pathology can easily be explained by several advantages of EK, for example, smaller incisions, fewer or no sutures, and no open sky surgery. The main advantage of EK however is faster and better visual rehabilitation and lower risk for immunologic rejection [8, 11, 12].

Another notable observation is the smooth implementation of DMEK accounting for 36% of EK procedures during the last 3 years of the study, as opposed to a peak rate of 11% for 2014, as recently reported by the Eye Bank Association of America [7].

In conclusion, keratoplasty indications showed remarkable trends over the past 17 years. These changes relate to the introduction of endothelial keratoplasty as well as to new treatment alternatives for KC other than keratoplasty. Respectively, a considerable shift of keratoplasty techniques from PK to DSAEK and DMEK in the treatment of endothelial disorders is evident. Finally, despite being a challenging procedure, DMEK was successfully implemented in our center.

Disclosure

This paper contains results of the thesis of Dr. Georgios Bagikos and has been presented as a poster in the Annual Meeting of the European Society of Cataract and Refractive Surgeons, Copenhagen, 2016.

Conflicts of Interest

The authors declare that there are no conflicts of interest regarding the publication of this paper.

Authors' Contributions

Konstantinos Droutsas and Georgios Bagikos contributed equally to this article.

Acknowledgments

The authors would like to thank Dr. Spyridoula Souki for preoperative control and postoperative follow-up of the patients who underwent corneal transplantation, her assistance with the surgical procedure and postoperative care and management of complications, and her contributions to the department's database organization and digitization.

References

[1] E. K. Zirm, "Eine erfolgreiche totale keratoplastik (A successful total keratoplasty)," *Refractive Corneal Surgery*, vol. 5, no. 4, pp. 258–261, 1989.

[2] G. R. Melles, F. A. Eggink, F. Lander et al., "A surgical technique for posterior lamellar keratoplasty," *Cornea*, vol. 17, no. 6, pp. 618–626, 1998.

[3] F. W. Price and M. O. Price, "Descemet's stripping with endothelial keratoplasty in 200 eyes: early challenges and techniques to enhance donor adherence," *Journal of Cataract and Refractive Surgery*, vol. 32, no. 3, pp. 411–418, 2006.

[4] G. R. Melles, T. S. Ong, B. Ververs, and J. van der Wees, "Descemet membrane endothelial keratoplasty (DMEK)," *Cornea*, vol. 25, no. 8, pp. 987–990, 2006.

[5] I. Dapena, L. Ham, and G. R. Melles, "Endothelial keratoplasty: DSEK/DSAEK or DMEK—the thinner the better?," *Current Opinion in Ophthalmology*, vol. 20, no. 4, pp. 299–307, 2009.

[6] G. D. Kymionis, D. G. Mikropoulos, D. M. Portaliou, I. C. Voudouragkaki, V. P. Ko-zobolis, and A. G. Konstas, "An

overview of corneal collagen cross-linking (CXL)," *Advances in Therapy*, vol. 30, no. 10, pp. 858–869, 2013.

[7] C. Y. Park, J. K. Lee, P. K. Gore, C. Y. Lim, and R. S. Chuck, "Keratoplasty in the United States: a 10-year review from 2005 through 2014," *Ophthalmology*, vol. 122, no. 12, pp. 2432–2442, 2015.

[8] S. J. Lang, M. Bischoff, D. Böhringer, B. Seitz, and T. Reinhard, "Analysis of the changes in keratoplasty indications and preferred techniques," *PLoS One*, vol. 9, no. 11, Article ID e112696, 2014.

[9] U. de Sanctis, C. Alovisi, L. Bauchiero et al., "Changing trends in corneal graft surgery: a ten-year review," *International Journal of Ophthalmology*, vol. 9, no. 1, pp. 48–52, 2016.

[10] C. S. Siganos, N. S. Tsiklis, D. G. Miltsakakis et al., "Changing indications for penetrating keratoplasty in Greece, 1982-2006: a multicenter study," *Cornea*, vol. 29, no. 4, pp. 372–374, 2010.

[11] K. Droutsas, A. Lazaridis, D. Papaconstantinou et al., "Visual outcomes after descemet membrane endothelial keratoplasty versus descemet stripping automated endothelial keratoplasty-comparison of specific matched pairs," *Cornea*, vol. 35, no. 6, pp. 765–771, 2016.

[12] A. Anshu, M. O. Price, and F. W. Price, "Risk of corneal transplant rejection significantly reduced with Descemet's membrane endothelial keratoplasty," *Ophthalmology*, vol. 119, no. 3, pp. 536–540, 2012.

24

The Effect of Strabismus Muscle Surgery on Corneal Biomechanics

Heba A. El Gendy ⓘ,[1] **Noha M. Khalil** ⓘ,[2] **Iman M. Eissa** ⓘ,[2] **and Shireen MA. Shousha**[3]

[1]*Professor of Ophthalmology, Faculty of Medicine, Cairo University, Cairo, Egypt*
[2]*Associate Professor of Ophthalmology, Faculty of Medicine, Cairo University, Cairo, Egypt*
[3]*Lecturer of Ophthalmology, Faculty of Medicine, Cairo University, Cairo, Egypt*

Correspondence should be addressed to Noha M. Khalil; khalilnoha76@gmail.com

Academic Editor: Anna Nowinska

Purpose. Studying the early effect of different extraocular muscle (EOM) surgeries on corneal biomechanics. *Subjects and methods.* This is a prospective, nonrandomized, interventional study, in which 42 eyes of 29 candidates for EOM surgery for strabismus correction at Cairo university hospitals, aged 14–37 years, were recruited. All participants had measuring of the visual acuity, refraction (spherical equivalent (SE)), assessment of the EOM motility and muscle balance, sensory evaluation, fundus examination, and assessing the ocular biomechanics using the Ocular response analyzer (ORA, Reichert, INC., Depew, NY) noting the corneal hysteresis (CH) and corneal resistance factor (CRF) preoperatively. Same patients were reassessed using ORA 4 weeks postoperatively following a different standard EOM surgery (recti weakening/strengthening and inferior oblique weakening either (graded recession) according to the surgical indication, and ΔCH and ΔCRF were calculated, each is the preoperative – the postoperative value. *Results.* ΔCH and ΔCRF = −0.78 ± 1.56 and −0.72 ± 2.15, respectively, and a highly significant difference was found between each of the pre- and postoperative CH and CRF ($p < 0.001$). 18 eyes had single EOM surgery, while 24 had multiple (2 or 3) EOM surgery; ΔCH in the single group = 1.28 1.5, and ΔCH in the multiple group = 0.4 1.49 ($p = 0.07$). 23 eyes had EOM weakening surgery, while 18 had combined weakening and strengthening EOM surgery: ΔCH in the weakening group = 1.24 1.77 and ΔCH in combined group = 0.26 1.07 ($p = 0.04$). A nonsignificant difference was found for ΔCRF ($p = 0.53$). *Conclusion.* A different EOM surgery has an early tendency for increase of the postoperative CH specially for muscle weakening procedures (recti recession/inferior oblique muscle weakening).

1. Introduction

Corneal and ocular biomechanics have been a topic of increasing interest in ophthalmology over the last two decades. The eye has been commonly thought of as an optical rather than a mechanical system; however, biomechanics can still play an important role in a number of different ophthalmic pathologies [1, 2].

Corneal biomechanical properties, namely, corneal hysteresis (CH), corneal resistance factor (CRF), and corneal compensated intraocular pressure (IOPcc), generally reflect corneal deformation and equilibrium under the application of external force. Hence, the structure and properties of corneal tissue are dependent on the nature of the components present in it and their relative amounts. Mechanical properties of a tissue will thus depend on how fibers, cells,

and ground substance are structurally organized into this tissue [3–5]. One commercially available and approved instrument used to measure CH, CRF, and IOPcc is the Ocular Response Analyzer (ORA, Reichert, Inc., Depew, NY) [6, 7].

In the past years, multiple studies have tackled the fact that corneal topography and corneal refractive power can change after strabismus surgery. However, some of the refractive changes were found to be mild and regress with time [8–10].

Recent studies found mild corneal topographic changes after sutureless vitrectomy as well, that most of these changes however, decayed with time [11, 12].

For the current study, the authors wanted to test a new hypothesis triggered by these previous studies as to whether corneal biomechanics can be affected by strabismus muscle surgery. To our knowledge, there is paucity of literature on this point. The authors postulate that if muscle tension forces applied to the global wall were changed, this could have a possible effect on corneal hysteresis, IOPg, IOPcc, and corneal resistance factor.

2. Subjects and Methods

The present study was approved by the Research Ethics Committee of the Faculty of Medicine, Cairo University. Data collection conformed to all local laws, and the study followed the guidelines of the Declaration of Helsinki 1964 [13].

In this prospective, nonrandomized, interventional study, 29 patients, aged 14–37 years, who presented with manifest heterotropias and who met the inclusion criteria for the current study, were scheduled for elective strabismus muscle surgery. All cases were recruited from the outpatient strabismus clinic in Kasr Al Ainy Hospital, Faculty of Medicine, Cairo University, during the period from December 2016 to July 2017.

All patients who met the predetermined inclusion criteria or their guardians were requested to sign a full informed consent regarding their acceptance of participation in the current study, the surgical procedure, the follow-up protocol regimen, and the possible complications.

2.1. Inclusion Criteria. The following are the various inclusion criteria:

   (i) Manifest primary comitant heterotropia

   (ii) No previous history of strabismus surgery or any other ocular surgery

   (iii) No history of ocular conditions that may affect ocular biomechanics, i.e., corneal scars, keratoconus, or glaucoma

   (iv) No history of contact lens wear

   (vi) No history of systemic conditions that may affect the ocular biomechanics, i.e., diabetes mellitus, thyroid dysfunction, or collagen vascular diseases

Full history taking regarding the onset of eye deviation, its duration, history of wearing glasses, amblyopia therapy, and previous ocular surgeries was taken from all patients.

All patients underwent full ophthalmological examination, as well as full motor and sensory assessment of their heterotropias, and cases with paralytic or restrictive strabismus were excluded, as well as cases with previous muscle surgeries.

2.2. Preoperative Measurement of Corneal Biomechanics. Corneal hysteresis (CH), corneal resistance factor (CRF), intraocular pressure Goldmann (IOPg), and cornea compensated intraocular pressure (IOPcc) were measured using Reichert Ocular Response Analyzer (ORA, Reichert Instruments, Depew, New York, USA). Measurements were done for all patients between 10 AM and 12 PM by the same masked operator to avoid bias induced by diurnal variations

in corneal biomechanics [9]. Three consecutive measurements were performed, and the best waveform score (WS) from each patient was included in the statistical analysis.

2.3. The Surgical Intervention. All patients underwent strabismus muscle surgery under general anesthesia in the form of either muscle weakening procedure (recession of recti or inferior oblique graded recession,) or strengthening procedure (muscle resection or plication), with the determined amount of recession and/or resection in millimeters done according to the preoperative angle measurements.

All cases were done using a low magnification power surgical microscope, through fornix-based conjunctival incisions.

Out of 42 eyes that underwent surgery, 17 eyes underwent a combined weakening-strengthening procedure, 24 eyes underwent muscle weakening procedure, and only one eye underwent a single muscle strengthening procedure.

The number of the eyes which underwent single muscle surgery was 18: 17 with muscle weakening procedure and a single eye with a single muscle strengthening procedure, while 24 eyes underwent two or three muscle surgeries: 18 eyes out of 24 underwent combined weakening-strengthening and 6 eyes underwent combined muscle weakening procedures (rectus and oblique muscles).

2.4. Postoperative Follow-Up. All patients were routinely examined 1st day postoperatively, regarding their ocular alignment, ocular motility, and conjunctival wound coaptation.

All patients received routine medications in the form of combined topical steroids and antibiotics preparations 4 times daily for 2 weeks' duration, and all were requested to attend their follow-up visits regularly at 2 weeks and 4 weeks postoperatively.

2.5. Postoperative Measurement of Corneal Biomechanics. All patients underwent a second postoperative measurement of corneal biomechanics at 4 weeks postoperatively, to be compared with those recorded preoperatively, and measurements were done for all patients between 10 AM and 12 PM to avoid bias induced by diurnal variations in corneal biomechanics [9].

The measurements were recorded by the same masked operator who was concerned with the preoperative measurements.

2.6. Data Collection and Statistical Analysis. Statistical analysis was performed using Statistical Package for Social Sciences, version 16 (SPSS 16). All variables were tested for normality using the Kolmogorov–Smirnov test, that was nonsignificant, and normality was accepted for all variables. Accordingly, quantitative data are presented as mean ± standard deviation, while qualitative data are presented as number (percentage). Because all quantitative data were normally distributed, variables were compared between two related samples using 2-sample t-test, and the probability value ($p \leq 0.05$) was considered statistically significant.

Bivariate correlations were performed between different parameters using Pearson's correlation coefficient (r), and Δ for a variable was calculated by subtracting the preoperative value from the postoperative value.

3. Results

In this prospective nonrandomized interventional study, 42 eyes of 29 patients (14 males and 15 females) aged 14–37 years (mean 24.9 ± 6.86 SD), who met the inclusion criteria of the proposed study protocol and scheduled for elective strabismus muscle surgery, were recruited for participation in the study.

Twenty patients presented with exotropia (mean 52.5 ± 1.19 Δ), 6 presented with esotropia (mean 33.75 ± 1.37 Δ), and 3 with hypertropia (mean 21.6 ± 2.9 Δ), whereas the mean preoperative spherical equivalent was -2.56 ± 3.16 D.

All the eyes underwent elective muscle surgeries through either muscle weakening (mean 8.17 ± 1.87 mm) or strengthening procedures (mean 6. 46 ± 0.82 mm and 5.41 ± 0.73 mm) for muscle resection and plication, respectively, according to the preoperative measurements of the angles of deviations.

The preoperative parameters (preoperative intraocular pressure Goldmann (IOPg), preoperative intraocular pressure corneal compensated (IOPcc), corneal hysteresis (pre-op CH), and corneal resistance factor (pre-op CRF)) were compared to the postoperative parameters (post-op IOPg, post-op IOPcc, post-op CH, and post-op CRF) of the same studied eyes, measured at the 4th postoperative week.

A statistically significant difference in CH, CRF, and IOPg was noted, as well as a tendency for a change in IOPcc as well which was close to being significant ($p = 0.06$).

The comparison between preoperative and the postoperative parameters of the same studied eyes is summarized in Table 1.

The change in corneal hysteresis (CH) and in corneal resistance factor (CRF) was calculated as the preoperative-postoperative value (ΔCH and ΔCRF); both were negative values, i.e., -0.78 ± 1.56 and -0.72 ± 2.15, respectively, denoting a postoperative mean increase in CH and CRF.

Bivariate correlations between ΔCH and each of age, sex, refraction, and preoperative CH (Table 2) were all nonsignificant except for a significant fair positive linear correlation to preoperative CH.

Bivariate correlations between ΔCRF and each of age, sex, refraction, and preoperative CRF (Table 3) were all not significant.

Comparison of the differences between pre- and postoperatively studied corneal biomechanics parameters for the eyes with single muscle surgery ($n = 18$), which were mostly muscle recessions—17 out 18 eyes, versus more than 2 or 3 muscle surgeries ($n = 24$) is shown in Table 4 where we recorded higher postoperative mean increase in CH and CRF in the eyes with single muscle surgery compared to multiple muscle surgeries, that was found to be statistically significant regarding CH ($p \leq 0.07$).

Table 1: The comparison between preoperative and postoperative parameters.

Parameter (mmHg)	Preoperative	Postoperative	p value
IOPg	13.32 ± 3.12	13.39 ± 5.76	0.009
IOPcc	14.4 ± 3.01	14.12 ± 5	0.067
CH	9.9 ± 1.78	10.69 ± 1.95	≤ 0.001
CRF	9.33 ± 1.94	10.05 ± 2.6	≤ 0.001

Table 2: Bivariate correlations between ΔCH and each of age, sex, refraction, and preoperative CH.

Variable 1	Variable 2 (mmHg)	$r^{\dagger}$	p
Age (yrs)	ΔCH	0.1	0.52
Sex	ΔCH	0.47	0.77
Refraction (D)	ΔCH	0.2	0.08
Pre-op CH (mmHg)	ΔCH	0.32	0.03

†Pearson's correlation coefficient.

Table 3: Bivariate correlations between ΔCRF and each of age, sex, refraction, and preoperative CRF.

Variable 1	Variable 2 (mmHg)	$r^{\dagger}$	p
Age (yrs)	ΔCRF	0.26	0.09
Sex	ΔCRF	0.17	0.26
Refraction (D)	ΔCRF	-0.04	0.77
Pre-op CRF (mmHg)	ΔCRF	0.19	0.21

†Pearson's correlation coefficient.

Table 4: The mean differences in measured parameters for single muscle surgery versus 2-3 muscle surgeries.

Parameter (mmHg)	Single muscle ($N = 18$)†	2-3 muscles ($N = 24$)	p
ΔCH	-1.28 ± 1.5	-0.4 ± 1.49	0.07
ΔCRF	-0.91 ± 1.81	-0.58 ± 2.4	0.3

†Number of the eyes.

Furthermore, comparison of the differences between pre- and postoperatively studied corneal biomechanics parameters for the eyes with weakening muscle surgery ($n = 23$, recti recession or inferior oblique muscle weakening) versus combined (weakening and strengthening) muscle surgery ($n = 18$) is shown in Table 5, with the results showing a significant postoperative increase in corneal hysteresis for the eyes with muscle weakening surgery compared to those with the combined weakening-strengthening procedure ($p \leq 0.04$), yet no statistically significant difference regarding CRF was shown in the same group of patients.

4. Discussion

Corneal biomechanics are relatively new parameters recently found to have clinical implications when tackling certain ocular conditions including glaucoma and some refractive

TABLE 5: The mean differences in measured parameters for weakening muscle surgery versus combined muscle surgery.

Parameter (mmHg)	Weakening group $(N = 23)^\dagger$	Combined group $(N = 18)$	p
ΔCH	-1.24 ± 1.77	-0.26 ± 1.07	0.04
ΔCRF	-0.93 ± 2.1	-0.5 ± 2.29	0.53

†Number of the eyes.

surgeries. Namely, these corneal biomechanical properties are corneal hysteresis, corneal resistance factor, and corneal compensated IOP [7, 14].

In the current study, CH, CRF, and IOPg were all found to increase significantly early after strabismus surgery, a finding which supports our hypothesis that, if forces applied to the global wall by the extraocular muscles are changed, the corneal biomechanics are likely to change. There was also a tendency for an increase in IOPcc after surgery ($p = 0.06$); however, it was not statistically significant. The significant increase in IOPg could be partially attributed to steroid-induced rise of IOP in three cases which went back to normal with follow-up after cessation of topical steroids.

Despite the fact that to our knowledge no recent studies have tackled the same variables, our hypothesis was inspired based on older studies which stated that, after strabismus surgery, corneal topographic changes were likely to occur [8, 9, 15]. In other studies, transient corneal topographic changes were found to occur after sutureless vitrectomy as well [11, 12]. These changes occurred despite the lack of direct tissue continuity between the cornea and the vitreous body. Similarly, we believe that changing the site of insertion of extraocular muscles and/or changing the area of contact between a muscle and the globe can potentially alter corneal biomechanics.

Moreover, pterygium was noted to affect corneal biomechanical properties [16, 17]. In a recent study by Koç et al., corneal biomechanical changes were also found to occur after pterygium surgery, where all preoperative ORA measured parameters were recorded to be decreased, yet the decrease was statistically nonsignificant [18].

Another study by Mombaerts et al. [19] stated that higher degrees of "with the rule astigmatism" were found in patients under 55 years old who suffered Graves' ophthalmopathy. These patients were examined clinically and by CT and were found to have fibrosis of the orbit as well as restrictive motility disorders. Restrictive motility disorders changes the tension force a muscle exerts on the global wall, to an extent that it may induce with the rule corneal astigmatism in this study.

Furthermore, changes in the corneal biomechanical properties were reported in the eyes with thyroid eye disease (TED), that CH values showed significant lowering in TED patients as compared to controls, that were noted to be correlated to the severity of the disease "as the severity of TED increases, CH decreases" [20]. Similarly, the authors assumed that a weakening or a strengthening muscle procedure could alter the corneal response to external pressure and thus potentially affect corneal biomechanical properties.

In 2017, Jiang et al. [21] conducted a meta-analysis about corneal biomechanical properties after penetrating keratoplasty (PK) or deep anterior lamellar keratoplasty (DALK) using the ORA; they suggested that both CH and CRF had better recovery after corneal transplantation with DALK than PK.

Comparing the effect of small incision cataract surgery and phacoemulsification on corneal biomechanical properties using ORA, significant differences between preoperative and postoperative corneal biomechanical values were found for CH, IOPcc, and IOPg. The 2.2 mm coaxial microincision cataract surgery group seemed to have a faster recovery (1 week) compared to the 3.0 mm standard coaxial phacoemulsification group (took 2 weeks to return to the preoperative values) [22].

The current study found that weakening muscle procedures had a greater effect on overall corneal biomechanics, with a statistically significant postoperative increase ($p = 0.04$) when compared to procedures involving muscle strengthening. Our proposed explanation for that is that the release of forces (the yielding effect of weakening procedures) on the global wall seemed to be transmitted to the corneal tissue as well leading it to become more resilient. Further studies however are needed to validate this preliminary finding.

Our study also found that changes in corneal biomechanical properties tended to be higher with single versus multiple muscle surgeries ($p = 0.07$). However, the difference was only close to being significant. The authors postulate that the unopposed mechanical effect of a single muscle surgery would naturally be more pronounced than if this effect was somehow "neutralized" by multiple muscle surgeries where the weakening of a lateral rectus, for example, is somehow neutralized by strengthening the ipsilateral medial rectus muscle.

There are limitations to the current study; the relatively small number of cases and the short follow-up period are definite limitations. A continuation of this study is planned by the authors where we can include a larger number of patients and repeat follow-up after longer time intervals. The authors intend to do more extensive subgrouping in the upcoming study, where patients undergoing different single muscle procedures can be further compared with each other and with others undergoing multiple muscle procedures and where weakening procedures can be compared to strengthening ones in more detail. A longer follow-up period will shed more light on whether these postoperative changes in corneal biomechanics are temporary and will decay with time or will become permanent postoperative findings.

We believe this study touches upon a potentially interesting finding exploring the relationship between corneal biomechanics and extraocular muscle forces, a point which can have important clinical implications in patients who underwent strabismus muscle surgery and are candidates for refractive surgery or are being evaluated as glaucoma suspects. New parameters derived from understanding the complex relationship between different ocular tissues utilizing corneal biomechanics may act as a tool for guiding better safety and efficacy of different eye healthcare procedures.

Disclosure

The abstract was accepted as an oral presentation and poster presentation for the AAPOS/CAPOS Joint Meeting (Shanghai, China, October 13–15, 2017) and the AAPOS Annual Meeting (Washington, USA, March 18–22, 2018). This study was accepted as a poster in the American Association for Pediatric Ophthalmology and Strabismus (AAPOS) in Washington, DC, USA, March 2018.

Conflicts of Interest

The authors declare that they have no conflicts of interest.

References

[1] M. J. Girard, W. J. Dupps, M. Baskaran et al., "Translating ocular biomechanics into clinical practice: current state and future prospects," *Current Eye Research*, vol. 40, no. 1, pp. 1–18, 2015.

[2] A. Luz, F. Faria-Correia, M. Q. Salomao, B. T. Lopes, and R. Ambrosio Jr., "Corneal biomechanics: where are we?," *Journal of Current Ophthalmology*, vol. 28, no. 3, pp. 97-98, 2016.

[3] F. A. Guarnieri, "Corneal biomechanics," in *Corneal Biomechanics and Refractive Surgery*, F. A. Guarnieri, Ed., pp. 7–31, Springer, Berlin, Germany, 2015.

[4] Z. Jiang, M. Shen, G. Mao et al., "Association between corneal biomechanical properties and myopia in Chinese subjects," *Eye (Lond)*, vol. 25, no. 8, pp. 1083–1089, 2011.

[5] D. Touboul, C. Robert, J. Kerautret et al., "Correlation between corneal hysteresis, intraocular pressure, and corneal pachymetry," *Journal of Cataract and Refractive Surgery*, vol. 34, no. 4, pp. 616–622, 2008.

[6] S. C. Goebels, B. Seitz, and A. Langenbucher, "Precision of ocular response analyzer," *Current Eye Research*, vol. 37, no. 8, pp. 689–693, 2012.

[7] A. Kotecha, R. A. Russell, A. Sinapis, S. Pourjavan, D. Sinapis, and D. F. Garway-Health, "Biomechanical parameters of the cornea measured with the ocular response analyzer in normal eyes," *BMC Ophthalmology*, vol. 14, no. 1, p. 11, 2014.

[8] D. P. Hainsworth, J. R. Bierly, E. T. Schmeisser, and R. S. Baker, "Corneal topographic changes after extraocular muscle surgery," *Journal of American Association for Pediatric Ophthalmology and Strabismus*, vol. 3, no. 2, pp. 80–86, 1999.

[9] M. Nardi, S. Rizzo, G. Pellegrini, and A. Lepri, "Effects of strabismus surgery on corneal topography," *Journal of Pediatric Ophthalmology and Strabismus*, vol. 34, no. 4, pp. 244–246, 1997.

[10] K. C. LaMattina and C. N. DeBenedictis, "Refractive changes after strabismus surgery," *Current Opinion in Ophthalmology*, vol. 27, no. 5, pp. 393–397, 2016.

[11] A. A. Mohamed and M. Abdrabbo, "Corneal topographic changes following trans-conjunctival 20 gauge sutureless vitrectomy (TC20V)," *Clinical Ophthalmology*, vol. 6, pp. 565–569, 2012.

[12] A. Yanyali, E. Celik, F. Horozoglu, and A. Nohutcu, "Corneal topographic changes after transconjunctival (25-gauge) sutureless vitrectomy," *American Journal of Ophthalmology*, vol. 140, no. 5, pp. 939–941, 2005.

[13] World Medical Association, "World medical association declaration of Helsinki: ethical principles for medical research involving human subjects," *Journal of the American Medical Association*, vol. 20, no. 310, pp. 2191–2194, 2013.

[14] N. Terai, F. Raiskup, M. Haustein, L. E. Pillunat, and E. Spoerl, "Identification of biomechanical properties of the cornea: the ocular response analyzer," *Current Eye Research*, vol. 37, no. 7, pp. 553–562, 2012.

[15] I. Kutluturk, Z. Eren, A. Koytak, E. S. Sari, A. Alis, and Y. Ozerturk, "Surgically induced astigmatism following medial rectus recession: short term and long term outcomes," *Journal of Pediatric Ophthalmology and Strabismus*, vol. 51, no. 3, pp. 171–176, 2014.

[16] J. Gros-Otero, C. Perez-Rico, M. A. Montes-Mollon, C. Gutierrez-Ortiz, J. Benitez-Herreros, and M. A. Teus, "Effect of pterygium on the biomechanical properties of the cornea: a pilot study," *Archivos de la Sociedad Española de Oftalmología*, vol. 88, no. 4, pp. 134–138, 2013.

[17] V. Oner, M. Tas, E. Ozkaya, and A. Bulut, "Influence of ptreygium on corneal biomechanical properties," *Current Eye Research*, vol. 41, no. 7, pp. 913–916, 2016.

[18] M. Koç, F. Yavrum, M. M. Uzel, E. Aydemir, K. Ozulken, and P. Yilmazbas, "The effect of pterygium and pterygium surgery on corneal biomechanics," *Seminars in Ophthalmology*, vol. 13, no. 4, pp. 449–453, 2017.

[19] I. Mombaerts, S. Vandelanotte, and L. Koornneef, "Corneal astigmatism in graves' ophthalmopathy," *Eye (Lond)*, vol. 20, no. 4, pp. 440–446, 2006.

[20] G. O. Karabulut, P. Kaynak, C. Altan et al., "Corneal biomechanical properties in thyroid eye disease," *Kaohsiung Journal of Medical Sciences*, vol. 30, no. 6, pp. 299–304, 2014.

[21] M. S. Jiang, J. Y. Zhu, X. Li, N. N. Zhang, and X. D. Zhang, "Corneal biomechanical properties after penetrating keratoplasty or deep anterior lamellar keratoplasty using the ocular response analyzer: a meta-analysis," *Cornea*, vol. 36, no. 3, pp. 310–316, 2017.

[22] Z. Zhang, H. Yu, H. Dong, L. Wang, Y. D. Jia, and S. H. Zhang, "Corneal biomechanical properties changes after coaxial 2.2-mm microincision and standard 3.0-mm phacoemulsification," *International Journal of Ophthalmology*, vol. 9, no. 2, pp. 230–234, 2016.

25

Pediatric Traumatic Retinal Detachment: Clinical Features, Prognostic Factors, and Surgical Outcomes

Dilek Yaşa ⓘ**, Zeynep Gizem Erdem, Ufuk Ürdem, Gökhan Demir, Ali Demircan** ⓘ**, and Zeynep Alkın** ⓘ

Department of Ophthalmology, Beyoğlu Eye Research and Training Hospital, No. 2, Beyoglu, 34421 Istanbul, Turkey

Correspondence should be addressed to Dilek Yaşa; dilekyasa2@gmail.com

Academic Editor: Gonzalo Carracedo

Purpose. We report the clinical characteristics, prognostic factors, and surgical outcomes for 23-gauge pars plana vitrectomy (23-G PPV) in pediatric cases of traumatic retinal detachment (RD). *Methods.* Medical records of pediatric patients who underwent 23-G PPV to treat traumatic retinal detachment were retrospectively reviewed. These patients underwent a follow-up examination at least 1 year following surgery. Associations between various preoperative factors and anatomical and visual outcomes were analyzed. An Ocular Trauma Score (OTS) and a Pediatric Ocular Trauma Score (POTS) were calculated for each patient. Raw scores were converted to their corresponding OTS and POTS categories. Final visual acuities by categories were compared with those in the OTS and POTS studies. *Results.* The mean age of the patients was 9 ± 4 years, and the male-to-female ratio was 4.7 : 1. The mean follow-up time was 23 ± 14 months. Anatomical success was achieved in 72% of the eyes, and functional success (>5/200) was achieved in 37% of the eyes. Functional success was less common among patients with visual acuities less than hand motion, macula-off retinal detachment, proliferative vitreoretinopathy at presentation, and recurrent retinal detachment during follow-up. When we compared the categorical distribution of final visual acuities in all categories, our results were significantly different than those suggested by OTS and POTS. *Conclusions.* Visual outcomes are poorer compared to anatomical outcomes. OTS and POTS do not provide reliable prognostic information if the patient has RD. Presenting visual acuity, the presence of macula-off RD, and PVR are all important predictors of final visual acuity.

1. Introduction

Retinal detachment is relatively uncommon in children, and the major cause of retinal detachment in pediatric populations is ocular trauma [1]. However, clinical features and surgical outcomes for traumatic retinal detachment patients in pediatric populations are not well defined in the literature. They are typically reported retrospectively as a part of all ocular injuries or all retinal detachment case studies, and, thus, are represented by a limited number of patients. Only Sarrazin et al. [2] and Sul et al. [3] evaluated pediatric traumatic retinal detachments as an independent group. As a result, there is a need for additional studies to better describe this subgroup.

Ocular trauma patients are not a homogeneous group, and they present with a great diversity of clinical features. As a result, it is difficult to predict functional outcomes after globe injuries. Kuhn et al. developed the Ocular Trauma Score (OTS) to predict visual outcomes at 6 months after injury [4]. However, the predictive value of the OTS after pediatric trauma is not clear. Acar et al. [5] proposed the Pediatric Ocular Trauma Score (POTS), but to the best of our knowledge, it has only been evaluated in two studies involving a limited number of patients [6, 7]. Studies evaluating the applicability of the OTS and POTS to pediatric cases include a limited number of cases with retinal detachment [5–8]. As a result, there is still a need for studies to evaluate the validity of the OTS and POTS in pediatric patients suffering from traumatic retinal detachment.

In this study, we report clinical features and surgical outcomes following 23-G PPV in a group of consecutive pediatric patients diagnosed with traumatic retinal detachment

TABLE 1: Demographics and trauma type.

	Number	Percentage	p^*
Gender			**<0.001**
Male	47	82.5	
Female	10	17.5	
Age			0.150
0 to <6	13	22.8	
6 to <12	25	43.9	
12 to <18	19	33.3	
Laterality			0.996
Right	29	50.9	
Left	28	49.1	
Trauma type			**0.008**
Open	36	63.2	
Closed	21	36.8	

*Chi-square test.

TABLE 2: Mechanism of injury.

	Number	Percent
Knife	12	30
Stone	10	18
Ball	6	11
Projectile (metallic IOFB)	4	7
Falls	3	5
Blunt assault	3	5
Door handle	2	4
Metal wire	2	4
Explosion	2	4
Gun shot	1	2
Thornbush	1	2
Wood	1	2
Plastic bullet	1	2
Glass	1	2
Tweezers	1	2
Corner of a table	1	2
Fork	1	2
Nail	1	2
Pencil	1	2
Broom handle	1	2
Hair clip	1	2
Motor vehicle accident	1	2

associated with open- or closed-globe trauma. In addition, we evaluate the prognostic value of several preoperative factors and the OTS and POTS in this patient group.

2. Methods

This study was conducted in accordance with the Declaration of Helsinki, and the approval was obtained from the institutional review board. Medical records of patients who underwent 23-G PPV in our clinic from 2013 to 2016 were retrospectively evaluated. Patients younger than 18 years old who underwent follow-up for at least 1 year were included in the study. Patient demographics, etiology, the type and zone of trauma, traumatic pathologies other than retinal detachment, the presence or absence of macular detachment, surgical procedures, preoperative and postoperative visual acuities, and complications were recorded.

Visual acuity tests were performed with an ETDRS chart or LEA symbols, depending on the age or cooperation of the patient. Visual acuities were divided into five groups similar to the OTS study: no light perception (NLP), light perception (LP), hand motion (HM), 1/200 to 19/200, 20/200 to 20/50, and 20/40 or better. Functional success was defined as the distance-corrected visual acuity of 5/200 or more. Anatomical success was defined as complete retinal attachment at the final visit.

The determination of the OTS and POTS is described in detail in the literature. First, raw OTS and POTS were calculated for each patient, and then, numerical values were converted to their corresponding OTS and POTS categories. If preoperative visual acuity was not measured, the OTS was not calculated. Finally, the similarity of final visual acuities by category was compared with those in the OTS and POTS studies.

2.1. Statistical Methods. Statistical analyses were performed using MedCalc for Windows, version 12.7.7 (MedCalc Software, Ostend, Belgium), and categorical variables were described by using frequencies (n) and percentages (%).

The chi-square (χ^2) and chi-square exact (at $r \times c$ contingency tables) tests were used for categorical variables

TABLE 3: Associated ocular pathologies.

	Number	Percent
Endophthalmitis	2	4
Hyphema	12	21
Iridodialysis/cyclodialysis	2	4
Cataract	22	39
Crystalline lens dislocation	4	7
Intravitreal hemorrhage	11	19
Subretinal hemorrhage	1	2
Suprachoroidal hemorrhage	2	4
Macula-off RD	22	37
PVR	21	37

RD: retinal detachment; PVR: proliferative vitreoretinopathy ≥Grade B.

which were expressed as observation counts (and percentages). A two-tailed p value of less than 0.05 was considered statistically significant. Multivariate analysis included anatomical/functional success as the dependent variable. The parameters that were significantly associated with anatomical/functional success in bivariate analysis were included as independent variables in the multiple logistic regression analysis.

3. Results

The mean age of the patients was 9 ± 4 years, and the mean follow-up time was 23 ± 14 months. Demographics and trauma type are presented in Table 1. Most of the patients were male, and there was a male-to-female ratio of 4.7 : 1 ($p < 0.001$). Open-globe trauma was more common ($p = 0.008$).

In patients with open-globe trauma, 17 (47%) had penetrating trauma, 12 (33%) had a globe rupture, and 7 (19%) had an intraocular foreign body ($p = 0.051$, chi-square test, two-tailed). In this patient group, 29 (51%)

TABLE 4: Preoperative and postoperative visual acuities.

	Missing n (%)	NLP n (%)	LP/HM n (%)	1/200–19/200 n (%)	20/200–20/50 n (%)	≥20/40 n (%)
Preoperative	5 (9)	4 (7)	35 (61)	8 (14)	4 (7)	1 (2)
Postoperative	1 (2)	5 (9)	27 (46)	14 (25)	8 (14)	3 (5)

NLP: no light perception; LP: light perception; HM: hand motion; n: number.

TABLE 5: Factors associated with anatomical and functional success.

	n	Anatomical success	p	Functional success	p	OR (95% CI)	p^*
Injury type			0.762		0.572	—	—
Open-globe trauma	36	25/36 (69%)		12/36 (33%)			
Closed-globe trauma	21	16/21 (76%)		9/21 (43%)			
Presenting DCVA			0.472		**0.047**	4.073	**0.031**
>Hand motion	13	11/13 (85%)		8/13 (62%)		(1.091–15.203)	
≤Hand motion	39	27/39 (69%)		11/39 (28%)			
Hyphema			0.287		0.177	—	—
Present	12	7/12 (58%)		2/12 (17%)			
Absent	45	34/45 (76%)		19/45 (42%)			
Crystalline lens dislocation			0.568		1.00	—	—
Present	4	4/4 (%100)		1/4 (25%)			
Absent	53	37/53 (70%)		20/53 (38%)			
Intraocular foreign body			0.660		0.404	—	—
Present	7	6/7 (86%)		4/7 (57%)			
Absent	50	35/50 (70%)		17/50 (34%)			
Intravitreal hemorrhage			1.00		0.511	—	—
Present	11	8/11 (73%)		5/11 (46%)			
Absent	46	33/46 (72%)		16/46 (35%)			
PVR			0.232		**0.010**	0.167	**0.005**
≥Grade B	21	13/21 (62%)		3/21 (14%)		(0.042–0.666)	
<Grade B	36	28/36 (78%)		18/36 (50%)			
Macula-off retinal detachment			0.752		**0.030**	0.165 (0.033–0.822)	**0.012**
Yes	16	11/16 (69%)		2/16 (13%)			
No	41	30/41 (73%)		19/41 (46%)			
Recurrent retinal detachment			0.763		**0.005**	0.149 (0.037–0.597)	**0.003**
Yes	22	15/22 (68%)		3/22 (14%)			
No	35	26/35 (74%)		18/35 (51%)			
Suprachoroidal hemorrhage			0.486		0.526	—	—
Present	2	1/2 (50%)		0/2 (0%)			
Absent	55	40/55 (73%)		21/55 (38%)			
Endophthalmitis			0.486		1.00	—	—
Yes	2	1/2 (50%)		1/2 (50%)			
No	55	40/55 (73%)		20/55 (36%)			

DCVA: distance-corrected visual acuity; PVR: proliferative vitreoretinopathy; OR: odds ratio; CI: confidence interval; chi-square exact test, two-tailed p value; *logistic regression p value.

patients had zone 1 trauma, 12 (21%) patients had zone 2 trauma, and 16 (28%) patients had zone 3 trauma ($p < 0.016$, chi-square test, two-tailed).

The most common cause of globe injury was an injury with a knife (Table 2). Injuries from a stone or a ball were also relatively common (Table 2). Associated ocular pathologies are presented in Table 3.

Anatomical success was achieved in 72% of the eyes by the final visit. Functional success (visual acuity ≥5/200) was achieved in 37% of the eyes. Preoperative and postoperative visual acuities are presented in Table 4. The association of several factors with postoperative anatomical and functional success is presented in Table 5. A multiple logistic regression

analysis was performed for variables which were significantly associated with functional success (Table 5).

The POTS was calculated for all patients. However, preoperative visual acuities were not present in the medical records of five patients (aged 2 to 3 years old). The OTS was not determined for these patients. In addition, the presence or absence of a relative afferent pupillary defect (RAPD) was not recorded in the medical records of most patients. As a result, a RAPD was not considered when determining OTS. When we compared the categorical distribution of final visual acuities for all categories, our results were significantly different than those suggested by the OTS and POTS (Tables 6 and 7).

TABLE 6: Comparison of final visual acuities and OTS categorical distributions between OTS study and our series.

Sum of raw points	OTS	NLP A/B	LP/HM A/B	1/200–19/200 A/B	20/200–20/50 A/B	≥20/40 A/B	p
0–44	1	74/0	15/60	7/20	3/20	1/0	<0.001
45–65	2	27/17	26/60	18/13	15/10	15/0	<0.001
66–80	3	2/0	11/9	15/46	31/27	41/18	<0.001
81–91	4	1/0	2/0	3/0	22/0	73/100	<0.001
92–100	5	0/0	1/0	1/0	57/0	94/0	N/A

OTS: Ocular Trauma Score; NLP: no light perception; LP: light perception; HM: hand motion; A: OTS study results (%); B: our study results (%); chi-square exact test, two-tailed p value.

TABLE 7: Comparison of final visual acuities and POTS categorical distributions between POTS study and our series.

Sum of raw points	POTS	NLP A/B	LP/HM A/B	CF A/B	0.1–0.5 A/B	≥0.6 A/B	p
0–44	1	26/0	11/60	11/20	26/20	26/0	<0.001
45–65	2	0/17	5/60	11/13	26/10	58/0	<0.001
66–80	3	0/0	0/9	0/46	33/27	67/18	<0.001
81–91	4	0/0	0/0	0/0	0/0	100/100	N/A
92–100	5	0/0	0/0	0/0	0/0	100/0	N/A

POTS: Pediatric Ocular Trauma Score; NLP: no light perception; LP: light perception; HM: hand motion; CF: counting fingers; A: OTS study results (%); B: our study results (%); chi-square exact test, two-tailed p value.

4. Discussion

In this study, we evaluated the clinical features and surgical outcomes after 23-G PPV in a group of consecutive pediatric patients suffering from traumatic retinal detachment associated with open- or closed-globe trauma. We divided patients into three age groups (0–6, 6–12, and 12–18 years). Although the 6–12-year age group had slightly more patients, the number of patients in each group was not statistically different. In agreement with the literature [2, 3], most of our patients were male (male-to-female ratio: 4.7 : 1), and open-globe trauma was more common (63% versus 37%). In pediatric cases involving retinal detachment, Sarazzin et al. [2] found that open-globe trauma was more common (62% versus 38%), and the male-to-female ratio was 5.2 : 1, which is very similar to our patient group.

The mechanism of traumatic open-globe injuries in adult and pediatric cases is usually well described [5, 9]. Acar et al. from Turkey reported in a series of pediatric open-globe traumas cases that the most common cause of injury was with a knife. Previous reports of pediatric traumatic retinal detachment have concentrated on clinical characteristics and surgical results. Thus, the mechanisms of injury in cases with traumatic retinal detachment are not well described. However, in this study, the mechanism of injury was recorded for all patients, and the most common cause of injury (30%) was with a knife. Also, it is noteworthy that although the mechanisms of injury were diverse, 59% of all injuries were caused either by a knife, a stone, or a ball (Table 2).

In this study, anatomical success was achieved in 72% of all eyes, and functional success (visual acuity ≥5/200) was achieved in 37% of all eyes by the final visit. Similar to previous reports in the literature, these outcomes are worse than those for retinal detachment in adults [2, 3, 5, 10]. The diversity of clinical features of trauma patients has led

several investigators to study the factors that influence final visual acuity. In the multivariate model, we found that better visual acuity (>HM) at the time of presentation was associated with a better (>5/200) postoperative visual acuity (OR: 4.073, 95% CI: 1.091–15.203). Macula-off retinal detachment (OR: 0.165, 95% CI: 0.033–0.822) and the presence of PVR at the time of presentation (OR: 0.167, 95% CI: 0.042–0.666) were associated with a worse (less than 5/200) postoperative visual acuity. In addition to these variables, the recurring retinal detachments during follow-up were also associated with a worse prognosis (OR: 0.149, 95% CI: 0.037–0.597). These findings are similar to the results of other studies of adult or pediatric retinal detachment [2, 3, 10, 11]. Although these variables are found to be predictors of a worse outcome after retinal detachment surgery, there is no scoring system that incorporates these variables. Furthermore, it was not surprising that patients with endophthalmitis or a suprachoroidal hemorrhage had worse anatomical and functional outcomes in this study. However, the numbers of patients were too limited to draw a statistically significant association for endophthalmitis and suprachoroidal hemorrhage.

The OTS is widely used after open- or closed-globe trauma in adult patients regardless of whether or not the patient presents with retinal detachment. Its prognostic value is well recognized. Some authors recently reported a good predictive value for OTS in pediatric globe injuries [12, 13]. Although RAPD often cannot be evaluated in traumatic children preoperatively, it has been suggested that an adapted OTS that does not consider RAPD has a high predictive value [6]. Initial visual acuity and the presence of RAPD are important factors used to determine the OTS. However, these two measurements are neither easy to obtain nor reliable in children after acute trauma. Thus, Acar et al. [5] suggested that the POTS could serve as an alternative to the OTS. However, when comparing the categorical distribution of final visual acuity in all categories, our results were significantly worse than those suggested by the OTS and POTS. The only study that evaluated the predictive value of the OTS in pediatric patients with retinal detachment was the study of Sarazzin et al. [2], and they reported that the visual acuity in these children was poorer when compared with the expected visual acuity based on the OTS. In agreement with Sarazzin et al. [2], and in contrast to other studies [5–8, 12, 13], we suggest that the OTS and POTS should be used with caution in pediatric patients suffering from retinal detachment.

Because of amblyopia risk, pediatric traumatic retinal detachments are considerably more morbid than adult traumatic retinal detachments. Associated traumatic pathologies, such as corneal lacerations and opacities, crystalline lens pathologies, and irregular astigmatism, also have amblyogenic potential. Accordingly, functional mismatch between anatomical and functional success may (at least partially) result from amblyopia. However, the associated pathologies reported in this study, as well as others like simultaneous traumatic optic neuropathy, may also be important in functional visual loss even in the absence of amblyopia.

In conclusion, this study shows that visual acuity, the presence of macula-off RD, and PVR at the time of presentation and recurrent retinal detachment during follow-up are all important predictors of final visual acuity. Some of the factors associated with a worse outcome are reported in this study and in the literature. However, there is currently no reliable *scoring system* to predict visual acuity in these patients. Although the OTS and POTS take into consideration the presence or absence of a retinal detachment and they are proposed to predict visual acuity after pediatric ocular trauma in patients with or without retinal detachment, they do not have a good predictive value if the patient presents with a retinal detachment.

Conflicts of Interest

The authors declare that there are no conflicts of interest regarding the publication of this article.

References

[1] M. Rahimi, M. Bagheri, and M. H. Nowroozzadeh, "Characteristics and outcomes of pediatric retinal detachment surgery at a tertiary referral center," *Journal of Ophthalmic and Vision Research*, vol. 9, no. 2, pp. 210–214, 2014.

[2] L. Sarrazin, E. Averbukh, M. Halpert, I. Hemo, and S. Rumelt, "Traumatic pediatric retinal detachment: a comparison between open and closed globe injuries," *American Journal of Ophthalmology*, vol. 137, no. 6, pp. 1042–1049, 2004.

[3] S. Sul, G. Gurelik, S. Korkmaz, S. Ozdek, and B. Hasanreisoglu, "Pediatric traumatic retinal detachments: clinical characteristics and outcomes," *Ophthalmic Surgery, Lasers and Imaging Retina*, vol. 48, no. 2, pp. 143–150, 2017.

[4] F. Kuhn, R. Maisiak, L. Mann, V. Mester, R. Morris, and C. D. Witherspoon, "The ocular trauma score (OTS)," *Ophthalmology Clinics of North America*, vol. 15, no. 2, pp. 163–165, 2002.

[5] U. Acar, O. Y. Tok, D. E. Acar, A. Burcu, and F. Ornek, "A new ocular trauma score in pediatric penetrating eye injuries," *Eye*, vol. 25, no. 3, pp. 370–374, 2011.

[6] M. M. Schörkhuber, W. Wackernagel, R. Riedl, M. R. Schneider, and A. Wedrich, "Ocular trauma scores in paediatric open globe injuries," *British Journal of Ophthalmology*, vol. 98, no. 5, pp. 664–668, 2014.

[7] L. Zhu, Z. Wu, F. Dong et al., "Two kinds of ocular trauma score for paediatric traumatic cataract in penetrating eye injuries," *Injury*, vol. 46, no. 9, pp. 1828–1833, 2015.

[8] Y. B. Unver, N. Acar, Z. Kapran, and T. Altan, "Visual predictive value of the ocular trauma score in children," *British Journal of Ophthalmology*, vol. 92, no. 8, pp. 1122–1124, 2008.

[9] R. Fu, S. Kancherla, A. W. Eller, and J. Y. Yu, "Characteristics and outcomes of open globe trauma in the urban versus rural population: a single center retrospective review," *Seminars in Ophthalmology*, vol. 33, no. 4, pp. 566–570, 2017.

[10] K. Nowomiejska, T. Choragiewicz, D. Borowicz et al., "Surgical management of traumatic retinal detachment with primary vitrectomy in adult patients," *Journal of Ophthalmology*, vol. 2017, Article ID 5084319, 4 pages, 2017.

[11] S. P. Read, H. A. Aziz, A. Kuriyan et al., "Retinal detachment surgery in a pediatric population: visual and anatomic outcomes," *Retina*, 2017, In press.

[12] S. P. Lesniak, A. Bauza, J. H. Son et al., "Twelve-year review of pediatric traumatic open globe injuries in an urban US population," *Journal of Pediatric Ophthalmology and Strabismus*, vol. 49, no. 2, pp. 73–79, 2012.

[13] H. Bunting, D. Stephens, and K. Mireskandari, "Prediction of visual outcomes after open globe injury in children: a 17-year Canadian experience," *Journal of American Association for Pediatric Ophthalmology and Strabismus*, vol. 17, no. 1, pp. 43–48, 2013.

26

Retrospective Comparison of 27-Gauge and 25-Gauge Microincision Vitrectomy Surgery with Silicone Oil for the Treatment of Primary Rhegmatogenous Retinal Detachment

Jie Li🅓, Bo Zhao, Sanmei Liu, Fang Li, Wentao Dong, and Jie Zhong🅓

Department of Ophthalmology, Sichuan Academy of Medical Science & Sichuan Provincial People's Hospital, School of Medicine, University of Electronic Science and Technology of China, Chengdu, China

Correspondence should be addressed to Jie Zhong; 13808063276@163.com

Academic Editor: Antonio Longo

Aim. To retrospectively compare the safety and effectiveness of 27-gauge (27G) microincision vitrectomy surgery (MIVS) with 25-guage (25G) MIVS for the treatment of primary rhegmatogenous retinal detachment (RRD) with silicone oil tamponade. *Methods.* Ninety-two patients with RRD who underwent MIVS from May 1, 2015, to June 30, 2017, were included in this study. Fifty-eight eyes underwent 25G MIVS and 34 eyes underwent 27G MIVS. We analyzed the characteristics of the patients, surgical time, main clinical outcomes, and rate of complications. *Results.* The mean surgical time was 56.7 ± 35.9 min for the 25G MIVS and 55.7 ± 36.1 min for the 27G MIVS, and there was no significant difference ($P = 0.894$) between the two groups. The primary anatomical success rate after a single operation was 94.8% for 25G MIVS and 91.2% for 27G MIVS ($P = 0.666$). Baseline and final visit best-corrected visual acuity (BCVA) were 1.9 ± 1.1 and 1.0 ± 0.8 in the 25G group, and 1.7 ± 1.0 and 1.1 ± 0.8 in the 27G group. Last visit BCVA increased significantly in both groups ($P < 0.001$). However, there were no significant differences in terms of visual improvement ratio (>0.2 logMAR) between the two groups ($P = 0.173$). No severe intraoperative complication was observed. Iatrogenic retinal breaks occurred in 2 eyes (3.4%) in the 25G group and 1 eye (2.9%) in the 27G group during the peripheral vitreous base shaving. The transient ocular hypertension (>25 mmHg) within postoperative week 1 was 25.9% in the 25G group and 11.8% in the 27G group ($P = 0.120$). *Conclusions.* This study found no significant anatomical or functional difference between 27G and 25G MIVS in the treatment of primary RRD. Therefore, 27G vitrectomy appears to be a safe and effective surgery for the treatment of primary RRD.

1. Introduction

Par plana vitrectomy (PPV), first introduced in 1971, has been widely used to treat posterior segment ocular diseases [1] and has evolved progressively driven by the desire for smaller instruments and greater functionality. More than a decade ago, 25- and 23-gauge microincision vitrectomy surgery (MIVS) instrument had dramatically simplified vitrectomy procedures [2–4]. In 2010, a 27G MIVS system was initially reported by Oshima et al. [5]. Recently, the feasibility of 27G MIVS has been demonstrated for various vitreoretinal diseases, including primary rhegmatogenous retinal detachment (RRD) [6–12]. However, there are only two prospective, comparative studies between 27G and 25G

MIVS for RRD in a relatively small number (30 to 40 eyes) of patients so far [10, 13]. The purpose of this study was to retrospectively compare the safety and effectiveness of 27G MIVS with 25G MIVS for the treatment of primary RRD in 92 patients. This study would expand our current knowledge of the safety and effectiveness of the 27G MIVS.

2. Subjects and Methods

2.1. Study Design and Patients. We retrospectively reviewed 92 eyes of 92 patients with RRD who underwent 25G and 27G transconjunctival sutureless vitrectomy at the Sichuan Provincial People's Hospital (SPPH, Chengdu, China) by two surgeons (Dr. Zhong and Dr. Liu) from May 1, 2015 to

June 30, 2017. This study has been proved by the Institutional Review Committee of SPPH and written informed consent was obtained from all patients before surgery. The procedures used conformed to the tenets of the Declaration of Helsinki. The inclusion criterion was primary RRD. The exclusion criteria were previous scleral buckling (SB) or vitrectomy, combined SB, trauma, proliferative vitreoretinopathy (PVR) of grade C, and significant ocular comorbidities such as uveitis, uncontrolled glaucoma, and severe or proliferative diabetic retinopathy. All patients underwent complete preoperative and postoperative ophthalmic examinations. The preoperative demographics of the patients are shown in Table 1.

2.2. Surgical Procedure. All surgeries were performed using a 25G or 27G MIVS (Constellation Vitrectomy system, Alcon Laboratories, Fort Worth, Texas, USA) and S88/OPMI Lumera T operation microscope with the RESIGHT wideangle viewing operation system (Carl Zeiss Meditec AG, Germany). Retrobulbar anesthesia was induced with 2% lidocaine and conjunctival disinfection with povidone-iodine. An infusion cannula was inserted through the inferotemporal sclera followed by the oblique insertion of 2 cannulas through superotemporal and superonasal sites at a position 3.5 to 4 mm posterior to limbus. The infusion cannula was connected to the inferotemporal cannula. When phacoemulsification and intraocular lens implantation were combined, all prepositioned 25G cannulas kept closed until the vitrectomy began (27G cannulas were self-closed due to valved-cannula design). All cataract surgeries were performed through a 2.4 mm clear-corneal incision. The surgical parameters of vitrectomy were 7500 cycles per minute (cpm) for 27G vitrectomy and 5000 cpm for 25G vitrectomy and a vacuum of 0 to 650 mmHg. After the vitreal core was resected, we created posterior vitreous detachment (PVD) in case there was no spontaneous PVD presented. The peripheral vitreous was shaved as much as possible with scleral indentation. Perfluorocarbon liquid (PFCL, Fluoron) was used to stabilize retina if needed. Fluid-air exchange and subretinal fluid drainage were performed, and endophotocoagulation was performed around all retinal tears. As sulfur hexafluoride (SF6) or perfluoropropane (C3F8) was not commercially available in Mainland China since June, 2015, we used silicone oil (5000 centistokes, Zeiss) for intraocular tamponade in all cases. Silicon oil injection was required in 27G MIVS, the 27-gauge cannula at 10 O'clock was removed, and 25-gauge cannula was placed at the same sclerotomy site. Silicon oil was injected through 25-gauge oil injection syringe. Peripheral retina was examined before the removal of cannulas and no sclerotomy site suture was placed. Patients were strictly instructed to comply with a certain position depending on the location of retinal breaks.

2.3. Main Outcome Measurements. All patients had a complete ophthalmological examination at each clinic visit after the surgery. We analyzed data including age, patients' gender, laterality of the procedure, refractive error, preoperative intraocular pressure (IOP), preoperative and postoperative

TABLE 1: Characteristics of patients.

	25G	27G	P value
Number of eyes (n)	58	34	
Gender			$0.239^{\dagger}$
Male (n, %)	26 (44.8%)	11 (32.4%)	
Female (n, %)	32 (55.2%)	23 (67.6%)	
Age (years)	58.5 ± 13.3	54.1 ± 12.5	$0.122^{\#}$
Lens status			0.105^{*}
Phakic	48 (82.8%)	31 (91.2%)	
Pseudophakic	10 (17.2%)	2 (5.9%)	
Aphakic	0 (0.0%)	1 (2.9%)	
Preoperative BCVA, logMAR	1.9 ± 1.1	1.7 ± 1.0	$0.322^{\ddagger}$
Preoperative IOP (mmHg)	9.8 ± 3.6	11.6 ± 2.9	$0.108^{\ddagger}$
Preoperative choroidal detachment	11 (19.0%)	3 (8.8%)	0.240^{*}
PVR (n, %)	4 (6.9%)	1 (2.9%)	0.648^{*}
Macular-off (n, %)	49 (84.5%)	30 (88.2%)	$0.761^{\dagger}$

BCVA: best correct visual acuity; IOP: intraocular pressure; PVR: proliferative vitreoretinopathy. $^{\#}$Independent T test; †Pearson's chi-squared test; ‡Wilcoxon signed-rank test; *Fisher's exact test.

decimal best-corrected visual acuity (BCVA), extent of retinal detachment, initial anatomical success rate, final anatomical success rate, intraoperative and postoperative complications, and duration of silicone oil filling. Intraoperative data included operative time, complications, sclerotomy site leakage, and suture rate of sclerotomy wounds.

2.4. Statistical Analysis. All data were tabulated and organized with Microsoft Excel (Microsoft Corp., Redmond, WA). All statistical analyses were performed using IBM SPSS Statistics 24.0 (IBM Corporation, New York, USA). BCVA was measured using the Chinese E standard logarithmic visual acuity chart, and the decimal acuities were converted to the logarithm of the minimal angle of resolution (logMAR) units. For statistical analyses, counting finger (CF) vision was defined as 2.0 logMAR and hand movements (HM) were defined as 3.0 logMAR [13, 14]. Pearson's chi-squared test was used for intergroup comparisons of patients' gender, rate of combined surgery including cataract surgery, and rate of postoperative visual improvement. Independent t-test was used for intergroup comparisons of patients' age, preoperative IOP, and surgical time. Wilcoxon signed-rank test was used for intergroup comparisons of difference in preoperative and postoperative BCVA. P value < 0.05 was considered as statistically significant.

3. Results

3.1. Preoperative Characteristics. The mean age of the patients was 58.5 ± 13.3 years (range: 19–79 years) in the 25G MIVS group and 54.1 ± 12.5 years (range: 27–76 years) in the

27G MIVS group. There were 26 (44.8%) men and 32 (55.2%) women in the 25G group, and 11 (32.4%) men and 23 (67.6%) women in the 27G group. Baseline logMAR BCVA (mean ± SD) was 1.9 ± 1.1 (range: 3.0 to 0) in the 25G group and 1.7 ± 1.0 (range: 3.0 to 0.1) in the 27G group. Clinical data of the patients including lens status, choroidal detachment, proliferative vitreoretinopathy, and macular on/off status are shown in Table 1. Overall, there were no statistically significant differences in the preoperative characteristics of the patients between the 25G and 27G MIVS groups.

3.2. Surgical Time and Results. Nine (16.4%) phakic eyes in the 25G group and three (8.8%) phakic eyes in the 27G group had simultaneous phacoemulsification with intraocular lens implantation ($P = 0.489$, Table 2). No complications occurred related to phacoemulsification such as posterior capsule rupture or zonular dialysis. The mean surgical time was 56.7 ± 35.9 min in the 25G group and 55.7 ± 36.1 min in the 27G group, and there was no significant difference ($P = 0.894$) between the two groups. The mean surgical time of 27G vitrectomy was gradually shortened, when the surgeon's surgical technique was more and more adept. The mean operative time used to treat the second half of the RRD cases in the 27G group was 42.6 ± 16.3 min, which was significantly shorter than that of the first half (68.8 ± 45.4 min, $n = 17$) ($P = 0.032$, Figure 1). All retinal breaks received endolaser, and no external cryoapplication was applied. In both groups, silicone oil tamponade was used in all the eyes. After the removal of the microcannulas, no sclerotomy site was sutured in both groups. Silicone oil was removed at 3 to 6 months after the primary vitrectomy (range from 81 days to 299 days, median 125 days).

3.3. Anatomical Results. The primary anatomical success rate after a single operation was 94.8% and 91.2% in the 25G and 27G groups ($P = 0.666$), respectively. In the 25G group, three (5.2%) eyes developed a recurrent retinal detachment during the follow-up period. In the 27G group, three (8.8%) cases of redetachment occurred during the follow-up period. The redetachment of the retina was due to PVR in four eyes (two eyes in the 25G group and two eyes in the 27G group) and new retinal breaks in two eyes (1 eye in the 25G group and 1 eyes in the 27G group). Three out of four eyes with PVR were reoperated using a novel two-port 27G vitrectomy technique without silicone oil removal as described in our previous study [15]. The other 3 cases were reoperated using conventional 25G PPV. Newly formed preretinal PVR membranes were peeled, subretinal fluid was drained, and all retinal breaks were sealed by endophotocoagulation with scleral depression. In the reoperated eyes, one eye underwent combined SB and one eye underwent silicon sponge placement. During the follow-up, one out of four PVR eyes developed a second recurrent retinal detachment and required relaxing retinotomy and long-term tamponade with SO.

3.3.1. Changes of BCVA and IOP. Baseline and final visit BCVA were 1.9 ± 1.1 and 1.0 ± 0.8 in 25G group and 1.7 ± 1.0 and 1.1 ± 0.8 in the 27G group, respectively ($P < 0.001$ for each intragroup comparison). Postoperative BCVA increased significantly in both groups at the one-month visit and the last visit postoperatively ($P < 0.001$, Figure 2(a)). No significant differences in terms of the visual improvement ratio at last visit (>0.2 logMAR) between the two groups ($P = 0.173$) were found. The mean IOP at baseline was 9.8 ± 3.6 mmHg in the 25G group and 11.6 ± 2.9 mmHg in the 27G group. When compared with the preoperative IOP, postoperative IOP was significantly higher at each time point ($P < 0.05$, Figure 2(b)).

3.4. Intraoperative Complications. No severe intraoperative complication was observed. However, one eye in the 25G group (1.7%) and four eyes in the 27G group (11.8%) developed the slight posterior capsule opacification due to the extruding of the cutter probe on the posterior lens capsule. The capsular opacification facilitated the formation of postoperative cataract which required phacoemulsification with intraocular lens implantation during the secondary SO removal surgery. Iatrogenic retinal breaks (IRBs) occurred in two eyes in the 25G group (3.4%) and one eye in the 27G group (2.9%) during the peripheral vitreous base shaving. All IRBs were sealed carefully by intraoperative endolaser photocoagulation, and none of them resulted in postoperative rhegmatogenous retinal detachment.

3.5. Postoperative Complications. A comparison of postoperative complications between the 25G and 27G groups is shown in Table 3. There was no case of endophthalmitis, intraocular bleeding, or choroidal detachment noted in the follow-up period in both groups. There were two eyes in the 25G group (3.4%) and three eyes in 27G group (8.8%) that had subconjunctiva oil leakage during the follow-up period ($P = 0.355$). Less than three eyes experienced severe hypotony (<6.5 mmHg) at each time point; there was no significant difference between the two groups. A few eyes encountered ocular hypertension (>25 mmHg) after both types of vitrectomy, but there was no significant difference between the two groups at each time point. The transient ocular hypertension within the first week postoperatively was 25.9% in 25G group, and 11.8% in 27G group ($P = 0.120$). Most of the elevated IOP occurred within 1 month postoperatively (95.7% in 25G group, 100% in 27G group). Most eyes from both groups with an elevated IOP were treated with antihypertensive eye drops, and the IOPs returned to normal levels without glaucoma surgery. Four eyes with persistent elevated IOP (two eyes in the 25G group and two eyes in the 27G group, respectively) underwent antiglaucoma surgery.

4. Discussion

Although the transconjunctival sutureless 27G MIVS was first introduced in 2010, its surgical indications have been expanded from macular surgery to vitreoretinal diseases in

TABLE 2: Comparison of surgical procedures and results between groups.

	25G	27G	P value
Combine cataract surgery, n (%)	9 (16.4)	3 (8.8)	0.489[†]
Surgical time (min)	56.7 ± 35.9	55.7 ± 36.1	0.894[*]
Postoperative IOP (mmHg)			
1 day	16.9 ± 8.6	15.2 ± 6.7	0.325[*]
1 week	15.3 ± 6.2	14.0 ± 4.6	0.317[*]
Last visit	14.3 ± 3.2	14.6 ± 2.7	0.600[*]
Postoperative BCVA, LogMAR at last visit	1.0 ± 0.8	1.1 ± 0.8	0.780[‡]
Visual improvement	−1.0 ± 1.0	−0.6 ± 0.8	0.082[‡]
Visual improvement (>0.2 logMAR)	39 (67.2%)	18 (52.9%)	0.173[†]
Follow-up period (days, range)	185.7 ± 140.2	186.4 ± 126.7	0.982[*]
Duration of silicone oil filling[#]	135.9.2 ± 39.8	132.6 ± 48.6	0.739[*]

BCVA: best correct visual acuity; IOP: intraocular pressure. [*]Independent T test; [†]Pearson's chi-squared test; [‡]Wilcoxon signed-rank test; [#]retinal redetachment excluded.

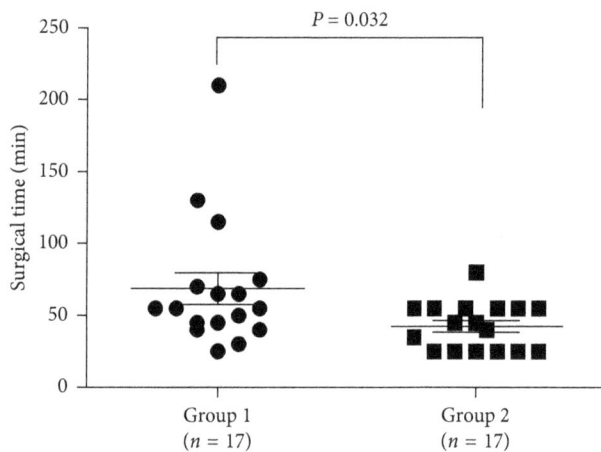

FIGURE 1: Surgical time used to treat RRD. Thirty-four eyes with RRD treated with 27G vitrectomy were equally divided into two groups. The mean operative time used to treat the first half (group 1, $n = 17$) cases was 68.8 ± 45.4 min, which was significantly shorter than that (42.6 ± 16.3 min) used to treat the second half (group 2, $n = 17$), $P = 0.032$.

the past few years. The safety and effectiveness of the 27G MIVS has been discussed and validated worldwide, the same as the evolution process of the previous 25G and 23G systems. Our aim was to further validate the safety and effectiveness of the 27G MIVS for the treatment of RRD. We focused on the surgical time, main clinical outcomes, visual improvement, and complications.

Operation effectiveness remains one of the most common concerns regarding 27G instrumentation, which has a smaller diameter probe (0.42 mm) than the 25G instrumentation (0.52 mm) [5]. Flow rate is the key factor for operation effectiveness. Theoretically, based on Poiseuille's law, a smaller vitrectomy probe would result in a greater flow resistance and slower flow rate. However, previous hydromechanics studies revealed that the 27G dual-pneumatic probes enable the control of duty cycles at an ultrahigh-speed cut rate (7500 cpm) and maintain an efficient vitreous flow rate [16, 17]. Mitsui et al. [6] found that the mean operative time for epiretinal membranes by 27G vitrectomy

was 20.2 min, which was not significantly different from that of the 25G vitrectomy. In several other studies, the mean operative time of 27G vitrectomy for more complicated surgical indications ranged from 32.0 min to 36.3 min [7, 8, 10], which was comparable with the initial experiences with 25G equivalents [2, 18]. Similar to Romano's finding [10], we found no significant difference regarding the surgical time in treating RRD using 25G and 27G MIVS ($P = 0.894$). When compared with the 25G group, the 27G group had a shorter surgical time, which might be due to the possibility that easier cases were chosen for 27G MIVS at the beginning of adoption of the 27G instrument. Furthermore, the surgical time for the 27G vitrectomy was gradually shortened when the surgeon became more skilled and got used to its flexibility. We found that the operative time used to treat the second half of the RRD cases in the 27G group was 42.6 ± 16.3 min, which was significantly shorter than that of the first half (Figure 1). Thus, although we cannot deny surgical effectiveness that could be affected by decreased flow rate within the smaller probe, our study suggested that surgical skill improvement and the high-speed cut rate of the 27G instrument could compensate for the reduced flow rate.

Similar to previous studies [10, 13, 19], last visit BCVA increased significantly in both the 25G and the 27G groups ($P < 0.001$). In terms of the visual improvement (>0.2 logMAR) ratio at last visit, there was no statistically significant differences between groups ($P = 0.177$). Hence, our study demonstrated that the 27G MIVS was an effective way to treat RRD.

In addition, the primary anatomical success rate after a single operation was comparable in both groups (94.8% in the 25G group and 91.2% in the 27G group, $P = 0.666$). The primary anatomical success rate using 27G MIVS was similar to earlier reports which ranged from 90% to 93% [10, 13]. These primary anatomical success rates using 27G MIVS are as good as, or even better than, that of the 25G MIVS which ranged from 74.0% to 95.45% [14, 20–22]. All patients in our study were treated with SO tamponade, and the primary anatomical success rates were similar to the previous study (93.5%) of patients with primary RRD operated on with vitrectomy and tamponated with silicone oil

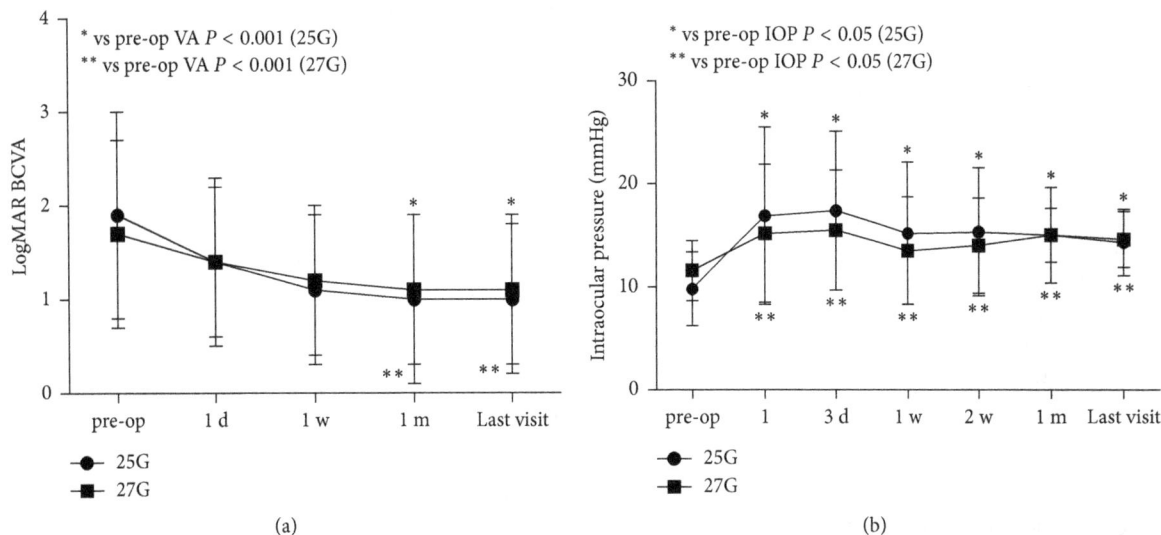

(a)   (b)

FIGURE 2: Time course of logMAR BCVA and IOP. (a) The mean logMAR BCVA at preoperative, postoperative day 1, week 1, month 1, and last visit was 1.9 ± 1.1, 1.4 ± 0.9, 1.1 ± 0.8, 1.0 ± 0.9, and 1.0 ± 0.8 in the 25G group, and 1.7 ± 1.0, 1.4 ± 0.8, 1.2 ± 0.8, 1.1 ± 0.8, and 1.1 ± 0.8 in the 27G group. When compared with the preoperative BCVA, postoperative BCVA at 1 month and the last visit increased significantly in both groups (P < 0.001). BCVA, best-corrected visual acuity, logMAR, logarithm of the minimal angle; (b) The mean IOP at baseline was 9.8 ± 3.6 mmHg in the 25G group and 11.6 ± 2.9 mmHg in the 27G group. At postoperative1 day, 3 day, 1 week, 2 weeks, 1 month, and last visit, IOP was 16.9 ± 8.6, 17.4 ± 7.7, 15.2 ± 6.9, 15.3 ± 6.2, 15.0 ± 4.6, and 14.3 ± 3.2 mmHg, in the 25G group, and 15.2 ± 6.7, 15.5 ± 5.8, 13.5 ± 5.2, 14.0 ± 4.6, 15.0 ± 2.6, and 14.6 ± 2.7 mmHg in the 27G group. No significant differences in IOP between the two groups were observed during the follow-up. However, When compared with the preoperative IOP, postoperative IOP was significantly higher at each time point (P < 0.05) in both the 25G and 27G groups; IOP, intraocular pressure.

TABLE 3: Comparison of intraoperative and postoperative complications between groups.

	25G, n (%)	27G, n (%)	P value
Intraoperative complications			
Iatrogenic retinal breaks	2 (3.4)	1 (2.9)	1.000[‡]
Posterior capsule injuries	1 (1.7)	4 (11.8)	0.060[‡]
Intraocular bleeding	0	0	
Choroidal detachment	0	0	
Postoperative complications			
Endophthalmitis	0	0	
Redetachment	3 (5.2)	3 (8.8)	0.666[‡]
Subconjunctiva SO leakage	2 (3.4)	3 (8.8)	0.355[‡]
Severe hypotony (<6.5 mmHg)			
1 to 7 days postoperative	3 (5.2)	1 (2.9)	1.000[‡]
2 weeks to 1 month	1 (1.7)	0 (0.0)	1.000[‡]
Last visit	1 (1.7)	0 (0.0)	1.000[‡]
Elevated IOP (>25 mmHg)			
1 to 7 days postoperative	15 (25.9)	4 (11.8)	0.120[†]
2 weeks to 1 month	7 (12.1)	6 (17.6)	0.540[#]
Last visit	1 (1.7)	0 (0.0)	1.000[‡]

SO: silicone oil; IOP: intraocular pressure. [†]Pearson's chi-squared test; [‡]Fisher's exact test; [#]chi-square test (continuity correction).

[23]. Meanwhile, SO tamponade may result in a lower rate of retinal displacement postoperatively [24]. Therefore, although definitive comparisons between studies are usually difficult, as they differ in many parameters, our results showed that the 27G PPV was as effective as the 25G in reattaching the retina after initial surgery.

Postoperative hypotony remains a major concern after sutureless vitrectomy, especially in 25G and 23G vitrectomy. With smaller wounds, 27G MIVS resulted in much lower rate of postoperative hypotony, ranging from 0 to 9.2% [6, 7, 10, 19]. Romano et al. used oblique incisions and displacement of the conjunctiva to reduce the severe hypotony postoperatively [10]. In our study, oblique incision was also implied and only 2.9% eyes experienced severe hypotony (<6.5 mmHg) in the 27G group. Since we had a higher rate of silicone oil tamponade than previous reports, this may contribute to lower the hypotony rate. On the contrary, in our study, the rates of transient ocular hypertension (>25 mmHg) in both groups (25.9% in the 25G group and 11.8% in the 27G group) within the first postoperative week were much higher than that of the previous reports with lower rate of SO tamponade, which ranged from 0 to 5% [7, 10, 13]. Similarly, Antoun et al. reported an incidence of ocular hypertension (defined as IOP > 21 mmHg) of 55% after vitrectomy surgery with SO tamponade [23]. This result suggested that a higher silicone oil infusion rate may result in a higher postoperative IOP.

Intra- and postoperative complications were similar in both the 27G and 25G groups. Postoperative endophthalmitis, intraocular bleeding, and choroidal detachment were not observed in both groups. IRBs and postoperative subconjunctival SO leakage rate were comparable between the 27G and 25G MIVS. It is worth noting that in the 27G group, there was a higher rate of posterior capsular injuries than that of the 25G group, although statistically significant difference was not reached (P = 0.060). The capsular injuries were induced by cutter probe extruding on posterior capsular when performing the peripheral vitreous shaving. The reason why the 27G probe is more likely touch the posterior capsular may be because the 27G vitrectomy probe was more flexible and likely to be bent than the 25G instruments. Thus, we suggested that at the beginning of use of the 27G instruments for more challenging cases such as RRD, surgeons should keep in mind its property of flexibility, especially when performing the peripheral vitreous shaving. Nevertheless, this aspect did not affect the performance of the vitrectomy surgery. With the help of scleral indentation by a surgical assistant, there was no eye in the 27G group requiring conversion to larger-gauge instrumentation during peripheral vitreous shaving.

Similar to other surgeons, we found that the 27G instrumentation had several advantages [7, 13]. For example, using "3D" mode in constellation vitrectomy system, we could set a high cut rate with a low aspiration rate to reduce vitreoretinal traction from the probe tip, which would benefit peripheral shaving and possibly reduce iatrogenic retinal breaks. When performing the core vitrectomy, we can move to a more powerful aspiration rate to increase surgical efficiency. With its smaller diameter, the 27G probe can be more easily inserted into a tiny space such as subretinal membrane area. In addition, the current 27G vitrectomy probe featured a port placed 0.2 mm from the end of the probe. This feature could be used for BSS removal in the fluid-air exchange procedure and the removal of subretinal fluid. Therefore, the small, delicate, controlled, multifunctional 27G cutter saved time which was needed for the change of instruments. However, shorter effective work length of the 27G instrument restricts its application in the case with high myopia.

Our present study had several limitations. First, it was a retrospective, uncontrolled, noncomparative study from one center. Second, as the commercialized medical gas was recalled by China's State Food and Drug Administration in 2015 due to reported adverse events, we could not include gas tamponade data. Third, to perform silicone oil injection, we had to convert to a 25G oil injection syringe, which might also introduce potential bias and influence the data with respect to IOP, wound healing, and operative time. Nevertheless, our study suggested that the 27G vitrectomy with a high-speed cutting rate appeared to be as safe and effective as 25G vitrectomy in RRD surgery. Future randomized and controlled study with more patients is required to validate the advantages and disadvantage of 27G vitrectomy.

Disclosure

Content related to this study has been accepted as a poster (no. 4239-C0081) in ARVO Annual Meeting 2018. Jie Li and Bo Zhao have contributed equally to this work.

Conflicts of Interest

The authors declare that there are no conflicts of interest regarding the publication of this paper.

Acknowledgments

This study was financially supported by the National Natural Science Fund of China (81700841) and the Fundamental Research Funds for the Central Universities, University of Electronic Science and Technology of China (ZYGX2015J126).

References

[1] R. Machemer, H. Buettner, E. W. Norton, and J. M. Parel, "Vitrectomy: a pars plana approach," *Transactions-American Academy of Ophthalmology and Otolaryngology*, vol. 75, no. 4, pp. 813–820, 1971.

[2] G. Y. Fujii, E. De Juan, M. S. Humayun et al., "A new 25-gauge instrument system for transconjunctival sutureless vitrectomy surgery," *Ophthalmology*, vol. 109, no. 10, pp. 1807–1812, 2002.

[3] C. Eckardt, "Transconjunctival sutureless 23-gauge vitrectomy," *Retina*, vol. 25, no. 2, pp. 208–211, 2005.

[4] S. Rizzo, F. Genovesi-Ebert, S. Murri et al., "25-gauge, sutureless vitrectomy and standard 20-gauge pars plana vitrectomy in idiopathic epiretinal membrane surgery: a comparative pilot study," *Graefe's Archive for Clinical and Experimental Ophthalmology*, vol. 244, no. 4, pp. 472–479, 2006.

[5] Y. Oshima, T. Wakabayashi, T. Sato, M. Ohji, and Y. Tano, "A 27-gauge instrument system for transconjunctival sutureless microincision vitrectomy surgery," *Ophthalmology*, vol. 117, no. 1, pp. 93.e102–102.e102, 2010.

[6] K. Mitsui, J. Kogo, H. Takeda et al., "Comparative study of 27-gauge vs 25-gauge vitrectomy for epiretinal membrane," *Eye*, vol. 30, no. 4, pp. 538–544, 2016.

[7] M. A. Khan, A. Shahlaee, B. Toussaint et al., "Outcomes of 27 gauge microincision vitrectomy surgery for posterior segment disease," *American Journal of Ophthalmology*, vol. 161, pp. 36.e2–43.e2, 2016.

[8] S. Rizzo, F. Barca, T. Caporossi, and C. Mariotti, "Twenty-seven-gauge vitrectomy for various vitreoretinal diseases," *Retina*, vol. 35, no. 6, pp. 1273–1278, 2015.

[9] O. Toygar, C. W. Mi, D. M. Miller, and C. D. Riemann, "Outcomes of transconjunctival sutureless 27-gauge vitrectomy with silicone oil infusion," *Graefe's Archive for Clinical and Experimental Ophthalmology*, vol. 254, no. 11, pp. 2111–2118, 2016.

[10] M. R. Romano, G. Cennamo, M. Ferrara, M. Cennamo, and G. Cennamo, "Twenty-seven-gauge versus 25-gauge vitrectomy for primary rhegmatogenous retinal detachment," *Retina*, vol. 37, no. 4, pp. 637–642, 2016.

[11] B. Shahzadi, S. F. Rizwi, F. M. Qureshi, K. Latif, and S. A. Mahmood, "Outcomes of transconjunctival sutureless 27-gauge micro-incision vitrectomy surgery in diabetic vitreous haemorrhage," *Pakistan Journal of Medical Sciences*, vol. 33, no. 1, pp. 86–89, 2017.

[12] Z. Zhang, Y. Wei, X. Jiang, and S. Zhang, "Surgical outcomes of 27-gauge pars plana vitrectomy with short-term postoperative tamponade of perfluorocarbon liquid for repair of

giant retinal tears," *International Ophthalmology*, vol. 38, no. 4, pp. 1505–1513, 2017.

[13] S. Rizzo, S. Polizzi, F. Barca, T. Caporossi, and G. Virgili, "Comparative study of 27-gauge versus 25-gauge vitrectomy for the treatment of primary rhegmatogenous retinal detachment," *Journal of Ophthalmology*, vol. 2017, Article ID 6384985, 5 pages, 2017.

[14] H. Kunikata and K. Nishida, "Visual outcome and complications of 25-gauge vitrectomy for rhegmatogenous retinal detachment; 84 consecutive cases," *Eye*, vol. 24, no. 6, pp. 1071–1077, 2010.

[15] S. Liu, J. Li, W. Dong et al., "Recurrent retinal detachment in silicone oil-filled eyes treated with two-port 27-gauge pars plana vitrectomy," *Guoji Yanke Zazhi*, vol. 17, no. 9, pp. 1620–1624, 2017.

[16] D. J. K. Abulon and D. C. Buboltz, "Performance comparison of high-speed dual-pneumatic vitrectomy cutters during simulated vitrectomy with balanced salt solution," *Translational Vision Science and Technology*, vol. 4, no. 1, p. 6, 2015.

[17] S. Osawa and Y. Oshima, "27-gauge vitrectomy," in *Developments in Ophthalmology*, pp. 54–62, Karger, Basel, Switzerland, 2014.

[18] R. R. Lakhanpal, M. S. Humayun, E. de Juan Jr. et al., "Outcomes of 140 consecutive cases of 25-gauge transconjunctival surgery for posterior segment disease," *Ophthalmology*, vol. 112, no. 5, pp. 817–824, 2005.

[19] K. Yoneda, K. Morikawa, Y. Oshima, S. Kinoshita, and C. Sotozono, "Surgical outcomes of 27-gauge vitrectomy for a consecutive series of 163 eyes with various vitreous diseases," *Retina*, vol. 36, no. 11, pp. 2130–2137, 2017.

[20] M. M. Lai, A. J. Ruby, R. Sarrafizadeh et al., "Repair of primary rhegmatogenous retinal detachment using 25-gauge transconjunctival sutureless vitrectomy," *Retina*, vol. 28, no. 5, pp. 729–734, 2008.

[21] Z. Kapran, N. Acar, T. Altan, Y. B. Unver, and S. Yurttaser, "25-Gauge sutureless vitrectomy with oblique sclerotomies for the management of retinal detachment in pseudophakic and phakic eyes," *European Journal of Ophthalmology*, vol. 19, no. 5, pp. 853–860, 2009.

[22] N. Acar, Z. Kapran, T. Altan, Y. B. Unver, S. Yurtsever, and Y. Kucuksumer, "Primary 25-gauge sutureless vitrectomy with oblique sclerotomies in pseudophakic retinal detachment," *Retina*, vol. 28, no. 8, pp. 1068–1074, 2008.

[23] J. Antoun, G. Azar, E. Jabbour et al., "Vitreoretinal surgery with silicone oil tamponade in primary uncomplicated rhegmatogenous retinal detachment: clinical outcomes and complications," *Retina*, vol. 36, no. 10, pp. 1906–1912, 2016.

[24] R. dell'Omo, A. Scupola, D. Viggiano et al., "Incidence and factors influencing retinal displacement in eyes treated for rhegmatogenous retinal detachment with vitrectomy and gas or silicone oil," *Investigative Opthalmology and Visual Science*, vol. 58, no. 6, pp. 191–199, 2017.

27

Prevalence of Keratoconus in a Refractive Surgery Population

Abdulrahman Mohammed Al-Amri ⓘ

College of Medicine, King Khalid University, Abha, Saudi Arabia

Correspondence should be addressed to Abdulrahman Mohammed Al-Amri; amaamri@gmail.com

Academic Editor: Antonio Queiros

Objective. This study examined the prevalence of keratoconus among patients who were interested in undergoing refractive surgery. Corneal tomography measurements were used to help detect keratoconus. *Methods.* Adult subjects who presented to the private hospital Cataract and Refractive Surgery Unit (Abha, Saudi Arabia) for refractive surgery evaluation were considered for inclusion in this cross-sectional, retrospective study. All subjects were from the Aseer province, a southern, high-altitude region in Saudi Arabia, and presented between January and December 2017. The incidence of keratoconus and other refractive surgery contraindications were examined. *Results.* A total of 2931 patients were considered for inclusion in analyses. Of these, 2280 patients (77.8%) were not candidates for refractive surgery. These 2280 patients had a mean age of 24.1 ± 6.6 years and 1231 patients (54.0%) were male. Of the subjects who did not undergo refractive surgery, 548 (24%) had keratoconus, 400 (17.5%) were keratoconus suspects, 344 (15.1%) had thin corneas, 321 (14.1%) had high myopia, and 52 (2.3%) had a high astigmatism. An additional 479 subjects (21%) were candidates for refractive surgery, but chose not to undergo a procedure. *Conclusion.* The incidence of keratoconus in Saudi Arabian refractive surgery prospects was 18.7%. Keratoconus was the most common reason for not performing refractive surgery and accounted for 24.0% of cases in which surgery was not performed.

1. Introduction

Keratoconus is a cone-shaped protrusion of the cornea that was named using the Greek terms "kerato" and "konos," which mean "cornea" and "cone," respectively. Keratoconus begins as a corneal thinning and results in a corneal bulge. As a result, light is irregularly refracted through the cornea (astigmatism), which is apparent during retinoscopy. As the cornea progressively steepens, astigmatism becomes more severe and visual acuity subsequently decreases [1, 2]. Keratoconus can be treated in several ways, depending upon disease stage. Contact lenses can be used to correct vision in early disease stages, but this solution often becomes inadequate and some patients cannot wear contact lenses. Therefore, some treating physicians choose to implant intrastromal corneal ring segments to flatten and stabilize the cornea, to improve vision, and, in some cases, enable the use of contact lenses [3]. However, in advanced cases, corneal transplantation (full or partial thickness) is often needed. In recent years, collagen cross-linking procedures have been used to successfully stabilize and reshape the cornea, resulting in long-term vision improvements [4–7]. Additionally, successfully treated patients may avoid corneal transplantation.

Keratoconus is of particular significance in refractive surgery candidates because operating on an eye with undetected keratoconus is a major cause of postoperative corneal ectasia [8–11]. The underlying cause of this progressive, bilateral, ectatic condition remains unknown. However, genetics are believed to play a role because up to 20% of patients with keratoconus have a positive family history for condition [12, 13] and a family history of keratoconus is a risk factor for developing the condition [14–18]. Allergy-induced mechanisms may also play a role because the risks of developing keratoconus are higher [19–21] and age of onset is lower [22] in patients with allergic or atopic disease.

Many studies have been performed around the globe to assess the incidence of keratoconus. The overall incidence of keratoconus is estimated at 50 cases per 100,000 people (0.05%) [23]. However, this widely varies by geographical region, as summarized in Table 1. For example, a study on

Table 1: Epidemiology of keratoconus in various countries around the world.

Study	Country	Prevalence (cases/100,000)	Incidence (cases/100,000)	Age at onset (years)	Keratoconus family history (%)
Assiri et al. [13]	Saudi Arabia	—	20	18.5	16
Hashemi et al. [16]	Iran	4000	—	—	—
Ziaei et al. [29]	Iran	2500	22.3–24.9	—	15
Waked et al. [30]	Lebanon	3330	—	—	12.1
Millodot et al. 2011 [21]	Israel	2340	—	—	22
Shneor et al. [43]*	Israel	3180	—	—	0
Shehadeh et al. [31]	Palestine	1451.6	—	—	—
Jonas et al. [25]	India	2300	—	—	—
Godefrooij et al. [32]	The Netherlands	265	13.3	28.3	—
Nielsen et al. [33]	Denmark	86	1.3	—	—
Pearson et al. [34]**	United Kingdom	57, 229	4.5, 19.6	26.5, 22.3	—
Kennedy et al. [17]	United States	54.5	2.0	—	—

*$n = 10$ subjects with keratoconus. **Data reported for white and Asian populations, respectively.

a Russian population reported an incidence of 0.2 cases per 100,000 people (0.0002%) [24], while a study on a central Indian population reported an incidence of 2300 cases per 100,000 people (2.3%) [25]. The incidence of keratoconus in the United States has been estimated to be 54.5 cases per 100,000 people (0.06%) [17]. However, keratoconus detection rates can vary based on investigative method used and sample size examined [26, 27]. Corneal topography is the gold standard for detecting keratoconus. Therefore, prior studies that investigated keratoconus incidence in refractive surgery prospects, all of whom undergo corneal topography studies, are of particular importance. These studies found an incidence of 3.0% and 5.5% for keratoconus and suspected keratoconus in a Caucasian population, respectively [10]. In another study on a Yemenite population, the incidences for keratoconus and suspected keratoconus were 18% and 10%, respectively [28]. The current study also used a topography-based approach to examine the incidence of keratoconus in patients presenting to our clinic seeking refractive surgery. It should be noted that all included subjects were from a high altitude region of Saudi Arabia.

2. Materials and Methods

This study was reviewed and approved by the private hospital human research Ethics Committee (EC). Written informed consent was obtained from all patients. All study conduct adhered to the tenets of the Declaration of Helsinki.

2.1. Study Subjects. This cross-sectional study examined data that were retrospectively obtained from patient files. All subjects presented to the private hospital Cornea and Refractive Surgery Unit (Abha, Saudi Arabia) between January and December 2017 seeking refractive surgery. All subjects had undergone standard ophthalmologic examination and corneal tomographic assessment with the Pentacam HR system (Oculus, GmbH, Wetzlar, Germany). Additionally, contact lens users had not worn their lenses for at least 3 weeks prior to examination. Patients were excluded from the study if they were younger than 18 years of age or if they had

a history of ocular surgery or trauma. Patients were also excluded if they had incomplete medical records.

2.2. Data Collection. Patient demographic, corneal topographic, and medical data were collected from standard examinations performed to determine refractive surgery eligibility. Reasons for not undergoing refractive surgery were identified, with specific focus on the presence/absence of keratoconus. Subjects were classified as having keratoconus if at least two of the following criteria were met: corneal thickness $<500\,\mu m$, asymmetric bowtie on corneal topography map, corneal steepening $\geq 47\,D$, skewed radial axis $>21°$, posterior elevation $>20\,\mu m$, and inferior-superior (I-S) asymmetry $>1.4\,D$. Subjects were classified as keratoconus suspects if one of the following criteria was met: corneal thickness $<450\,\mu m$, asymmetric bowtie on corneal topography map, corneal steepening $\geq 48\,D$, posterior elevation $>25\,\mu m$, or I-S asymmetry $>1.6\,D$.

2.3. Data Analyses. Continuous data are presented as mean ± standard deviation. Frequency and prevalence data are presented as n (%). Data normality was verified using a standard normality test, continuous data were compared using unpaired Student's t-tests and categorical data were compared using chi-square tests. Correlations between subject characteristics and keratoconus frequency were examined using Pearson's correlation analyses. All statistical analyses were performed using the Statistical Package for Social Sciences (SPSS) software (ver. 20, SPSS, Inc., Chicago, IL). Statistical significance was defined as $p < 0.05$.

3. Results

A total of 2931 patients were included in this study. Of these, 2280 patients (77.8%) were not candidates for refractive surgery. These subjects had a mean age of 24.1 ± 6.6 years (range: 18–52 years) and 1231 (54.0%) were female. As summarized in Table 2, the most common reasons for not undergoing surgery were keratoconus (548 patients [24.0%]), keratoconus suspect (400 patients [17.5%]), thin corneas (344 patients [15.1%]), and high myopia (321 patients [14.1%]). An

TABLE 2: Reasons for not performing a procedure in refractive surgery candidates (n = 2280 patients).

Reason	n (patients)	%
Keratoconus	548	24.0
Chose not to undergo a procedure	479	21.0
Keratoconus suspect	400	17.5
Thin corneas (<450 μm)	344	15.1
High myopia	321	14.1
High astigmatism	52	2.3
Dry eyes	39	1.7
Amblyopia	27	1.2
Unstable refraction	25	1.1
Retinal disorder	22	1.0
Large pupil	13	0.6
History of radial keratotomy	8	0.4
Cataract	2	0.1

additional 479 patients (21.0%) were refractive surgery candidates, but chose not to undergo a procedure.

The overall prevalence of keratoconus in our study sample was 18.7% in all patients and 24.0% in patients who did not undergo refractive surgery. Slightly more than half of the patients with keratoconus were female (284 of 548 patients [52.0%]) and 22.4% of patients had a family history that was positive for keratoconus. The gender distribution was not significantly different between patients with and without keratoconus (1196 of 2384 patients [50.1%]). However, the proportion of female patients was significantly higher in patients with keratoconus (52.0%) than in those who did not have keratoconus (765 of 1733 patients [44.1%], p = 0.001). Patients with keratoconus were distributed across age groups as follows: 142 patients (26.0%) between 18 and 20 years of age, 182 (33.3%) patients between 21 and 31 years of age, 168 (30.7%) patients between 32 and 42 years of age, and 65 patients (11.9%) between 43 and 53 years of age. This age distribution was not significantly different than in patients without keratoconus (p = 0.001). However, there was a moderate negative correlation between keratoconus presence and patient age (r = −0.612, p = 0.01).

Similarities and differences between normal, keratoconus suspects, and keratoconus subjects were examined (Table 3). Keratoconus was not found in 1130 subjects (651 procedures plus 479 patients who were refractive surgery candidates and did not undergo a procedure). A total of 400 subjects (17.5%) were keratoconus suspects and 548 subjects (24.0%) had keratoconus. Keratoconus subjects (29.3 ± 5.1 years) were significantly older than both keratoconus suspects (24.9 ± 3.8 years) and normal subjects (18.6 ± 4.1 years), and keratoconus suspects were significantly older than normal subjects (all p < 0.001). Additionally, both the keratoconus suspect (29.3%) and keratoconus suspect (23.2%) groups had a higher percentage of patients with a family history of keratoconus than the normal group (17.4%, p < 0.001 and p = 0.009, resp.). Family history was not significantly different between the keratoconus suspect and keratoconus suspect groups (p = 0.174). All examined corneal abnormalities were observed more often in subjects with keratoconus than in subjects suspected of having keratoconus (all p < 0.001).

4. Discussion

The current study assessed keratoconus prevalence among refractive surgery prospects in the Aseer (Asir) province of Saudi Arabia. We found an overall keratoconus incidence of 18.7% (18700 cases/100,000 people), which was higher than the historical range of 0.03–3.18% [13, 16, 17, 22–24, 29–35]. A total of 547 of 2280 patients (24.0%) who did not undergo refractive surgery had keratoconus, making it the most common reason for not undergoing a procedure. Another 399 patients (17.5%) were keratoconus suspects.

Keratoconus is influenced by family history [14–18] and ethnicity [36, 37]. Therefore, we compared our findings to those previously obtained in the Middle East. The keratoconus incidence observed in the current study is higher than that previously reported in the Middle East and other regions. A 2005 Saudi Arabian study [13] found a keratoconus incidence of only 20 cases/100,000 people (0.02%). However, that study relied upon keratometry data to detect keratoconus and only included patients referred to a provincial tertiary ophthalmology department. Because corneal tomography is the gold standard for detecting keratoconus [13, 18, 38], it is possible that this 2005 incidence was artificially low. Our findings (24.0% prevalence) are somewhat in agreement with a recent study that found a 17.5% prevalence of keratoconus among college-age refractive surgery prospects in northern Egypt [39]. It may have been that our methods were more sensitive for detecting keratoconus because our incidence of keratoconus suspects was also higher than that in a college-age Palestinian population (17.5% vs. 8.4%). It is puzzling why presumably healthy, young refractive surgery candidates would have such a high prevalence of keratoconus. Therefore, the findings of the current study and the prior Egyptian study may indicate that keratoconus is more prevalent than believed in some regions. Further study is needed in these populations to confirm and better understand our findings.

Slightly fewer men than women had keratoconus in the current study (48% men). This gender distribution does not agree with prior studies, which found that 55–75% of patients with keratoconus were male [17, 24, 32, 34, 40, 41]. Furthermore, men are at a significantly higher risk for developing keratoconus (odds ratio: 2.3–5.4 [16, 21]) and often develop the condition at a younger age [41, 42] than women. Perhaps our relatively small sample size contributed to our findings regarding gender. However, it should be noted that one Iraqi keratoconus patient study populations was made up of 61.1% women [43].

Patients with keratoconus were evenly distributed across age groups, with the exception of the oldest group (43–53 years of age). This is in agreement with prior studies, which found that most keratoconus patients are diagnosed between 21 and 40 years of age [40]. We also found that patient age was significantly and negatively correlated with keratoconus frequency, which may be related to negative correlation between age and severity that was previously reported [34, 37]. Additionally, 22.4% of our patients with keratoconus had a positive family history for the condition, which is in agreement with prior studies [34, 37].

TABLE 3: Subject and ocular parameters of normal (LASIK candidate), keratoconus suspects, and keratoconus subjects.

	No KC	KC suspect	KC	p (N vs KCS)	p (N vs KC)	p (KCS vs KC)
n (subjects)	1130	400	548			
Subject age (years)	18.6 ± 4.1	24.9 ± 3.8	29.3 ± 5.1	<0.001	<0.001	<0.001
Family history of KC	197 (17.4%)	93 (23.2%)	149 (27.1%)	0.009	<0.001	0.174
Corneal thickness < 500 μm	—	321 (80.25%)	520 (94.8%)	—	—	<0.001
Asymmetric bowtie	—	278 (69.5%)	493 (89.9%)	—	—	<0.001
Corneal steepening $\geq$ 47 D	—	356 (89%)	531 (96.9%)	—	—	<0.001
Skewed radial axis > 21°	—	160 (40%)	372 (67.9%)	—	—	<0.001
Posterior elevation	—	276 (69%)	487 (88.9%)	—	—	<0.001
I-S asymmetry	—	324 (81%)	504 (91.9%)	—	—	<0.001

N = no KC; KC = keratoconus; KCS = KC suspect; I-S = inferior-superior.

Our study had several limitations related to its retrospective study design and a relatively small sample size. Further prospective studies with a larger number of patients are needed to confirm and better understand our results. In summary, our population had a very high incidence of keratoconus, which was the cause for not undergoing refractive surgery in 24.0% of patients who were not candidates. Age and gender did not heavily influence keratoconus rates in our study population.

Conflicts of Interest

The author declares that there are no conflicts of interest.

References

[1] Z. Hassan, E. Szalai, L. Módis, A. Berta, and G. Németh, "Assessment of corneal topography indices after collagen crosslinking for keratoconus," European Journal of Ophthalmology, vol. 23, pp. 635–640, 2013.

[2] M. Poli, P. L. Cornut, T. Balmitgere, F. Aptel, H. Janin, and C. Burillon, "Prospective study of corneal collagen cross-linking efficacy and tolerance in the treatment of keratoconus and corneal ectasia: 3-year results," Cornea, vol. 32, pp. 583–590, 2013.

[3] A. Ertan and J. Colin, "Intracorneal rings for keratoconus and keratectasia," Journal of Cataract & Refractive Surgery, vol. 33, pp. 1303–1314, 2007.

[4] A. Caporossi, C. Mazotta, S. Baiocchi, and T. Caporossi, "Long-term results of riboflavin ultraviolet corneal collagen cross-linking for keratoconus in Italy: the Siena eye cross study," American Journal of Ophthalmology, vol. 149, pp. 585–593, 2010.

[5] F. Raiskup, A. Theuring, L. E. Pillunat, and E. Spoerl, "Corneal collagen cross-linking with riboflavin and ultraviolet—a light in progressive keratoconus: ten-year results," Journal of Cataract & Refractive Surgery, vol. 41, pp. 41–46, 2015.

[6] D. P. O'Brart, P. Patel, G. Lascaratos et al., "Corneal cross-linking to halt the progression of keratoconus and corneal ectasia: seven-year follow-up," American Journal of Ophthalmology, vol. 160, pp. 1154–1163, 2015.

[7] G. D. Kymionis, M. A. Grentzelos, D. A. Liakopoulos et al., "Long-term follow-up of corneal collagen cross-linking for keratoconus-the Cretan study," Cornea, vol. 33, pp. 1071–1079, 2014.

[8] S. Feizi, B. Einollahi, A. Raminkhoo, and S. Salehirad, "Correlation between corneal topographic indices and higher-order aberrations in keratoconus," Journal of Ophthalmic & Vision Research, vol. 8, pp. 113–118, 2013.

[9] J. L. Alió, J. I. Belda, A. Artola et al., "Contact lens fitting to correct irregular astigmatism after corneal refractive surgery," Journal of Cataract & Refractive Surgery, vol. 28, pp. 1750–1757, 2002.

[10] D. Varssano, I. Kaiserman, and R. Hazarbassanov, "Topographic patterns in refractive surgery candidates," Cornea, vol. 23, pp. 602–607, 2004.

[11] T. Seiler and A. W. Quurke, "Iatrogenic keratectasia after LASIK in a case of forme fruste keratoconus," Journal of Cataract & Refractive Surgery, vol. 24, pp. 1007–1009, 1998.

[12] M. Naderan, M. T. Rajabi, P. Zarrinbakhsh, M. Naderan, and A. Bakhshi, "Association between family history and keratoconus severity," Current Eye Research, vol. 41, pp. 1414–1418, 2016.

[13] A. A. Assiri, B. I. Yousuf, A. J. Quantock, and P. J. Murphy, "Incidence and severity of keratoconus in Asir province, Saudi Arabia," British Journal of Ophthalmology, vol. 89, pp. 1403–1406, 2005.

[14] A. Gordon-Shaag, A. Millodot, M. Essa, J. Garth, M. Ghara, and E. Shneor, "Is consanguinity a risk factor for keratoconus?," Optometry and Vision Science, vol. 90, pp. 448–454, 2013.

[15] A. Gordon-Shaag, M. Millodot, I. Kaiserman et al., "Risk factors or keratoconus in Israel: a case-control study," Ophthalmic and Physiological Optics, vol. 35, pp. 673–681, 2015.

[16] H. Hashemi, S. Heydarian, A. Yekta et al., "High prevalence and familial aggregation of keratoconus in an Iranian rural population: a population-based study," Ophthalmic and Physiological Optics, vol. 38, pp. 447–455, 2018.

[17] R. H. Kennedy, W. M. Bourne, and J. A. Dyer, "A 48-year clinical and epidemiologic study of keratoconus," American Journal of Ophthalmology, vol. 101, pp. 267–273, 1986.

[18] M. Edwards, C. N. McGhee, and S. Dean, "The genetics of keratoconus," Clinical and Experimental Ophthalmology, vol. 29, pp. 345–351, 2001.

[19] J. P. Thyssen, P. B. Toft, A. S. Halling-Overgaard, G. H. Gislason, L. Skov, and A. Egeberg, "Incidence, prevalence, and risk of selected ocular disease in adults with atopic dermatitis," Journal of the American Academy of Dermatology, vol. 77, pp. 280–286, 2017.

[20] I. Merdler, A. Hassadim, N. Sorkin, S. Shapira, Y. Gronovich, and Z. Korach, "Keratoconus and allergic diseases among Israeli adolescents between 2005 and 2013," Cornea, vol. 34, pp. 525–529, 2015.

[21] M. Millodot, E. Schneor, S. Albou, E. Atlani, and A. Gordon-Shaag, "Prevalence and associated factors of keratoconus in Jerusalem: a cross-sectional study," *Ophthalmic Epidemiology*, vol. 18, pp. 91–97, 2011.

[22] M. Naderan, M. T. Rajabi, P. Zarrinbakhsh, and A. Bakhshi, "Effect of allergic disease on keratoconus severity," *Ocular Immunology and Inflammation*, vol. 25, pp. 418–423, 2017.

[23] Y. S. Rabinowitz, "Keratoconus," *Survey of Ophthalmology*, vol. 42, pp. 297–319, 1998.

[24] E. N. Gorskova and E. N. Sevost'ianov, "Epidemiology of keratoconus in the Urals," *Vestnik Oftalmologii*, vol. 114, pp. 38–40, 1998, in Russian.

[25] J. B. Jonas, V. Nangia, A. Matin et al., "Prevalence and associations of keratoconus in rural Maharashtra in central India: the central India eye and medical study," *American Journal of Ophthalmology*, vol. 148, pp. 760–765, 2009.

[26] A. Gordon-Shaag, A. Millodot, E. Shneor, and Y. Liu, "The genetic and environmental factors for keratoconus," *BioMed Research International*, vol. 2015, Article ID 795738, 19 pages, 2015.

[27] N. K. Dutta and L. C. Dutta, "Applied and functional anatomy of the cornea," *Modern Ophthalmology*, p. 131, Jaypee Brothers, New Delhi, India, 3rd edition, 2005.

[28] M. A. Bamashmus, M. F. Saleh, and M. A. Awadalla, "Reasons for not performing keratorefractive surgery in patients seeking refractive surgery in a hospital-based cohort in "Yemen"," *Middle East African Journal of Ophthalmology*, vol. 17, pp. 349–353, 2010.

[29] H. Ziaei, M. R. Jafarinasab, M. A. Javadi et al., "Epidemiology of keratoconus in an Iranian population," *Cornea*, vol. 31, pp. 1044–1047, 2012.

[30] N. Waked, A. M. Fayad, A. Fadlallah, and H. El Rami, "Keratoconus screening in a Lebanese students' population," *Journal Français d'Ophtalmologie*, vol. 35, pp. 23–29, 2012, in French.

[31] M. M. Shehadeh, V. F. Diakonis, S. A. Jalil et al., "Prevalence of keratoconus among a Palestinian tertiary student population," *Open Ophthalmology Journal*, vol. 9, pp. 172–176, 2015.

[32] D. A. Godefrooij, G. A. de Wit, C. S. Uiterwaal, S. M. Imhof, and R. P. L. Wisse, "Age-specific incidence and prevalence of keratoconus: a nationwide registration study," *American Journal of Ophthalmology*, vol. 175, pp. 169–172, 2017.

[33] K. Nielsen, J. Hjortdal, E. Asgaard Nohr, and N. Ehlers, "Incidence and prevalence of keratoconus in Denmark," *Acta Ophthalmologica Scandinavica*, vol. 85, pp. 890–892, 2007.

[34] A. R. Pearson, B. Soneji, N. Sarvananthan, and J. H. Sandford-Simtih, "Does ethnic origin influence the incidence or severity of keratoconus?," *Eye (London)*, vol. 14, no. 4, pp. 625–628, 2000.

[35] E. Shneor, M. Millodot, A. Gordon-Shaag et al., "Prevalence of keratoconus among young Arab students in Israel," *International Journal of Keratoconus and Ectatic Corneal Diseases*, vol. 3, pp. 9–14, 2014.

[36] M. A. Woodward, T. S. Blachley, and J. D. Stein, "The association between sociodemographic factors, common systemic diseases, and keratoconus: an analysis of a nationwide healthcare claims database," *Ophthalmology*, vol. 123, pp. 457–465, 2016.

[37] T. Georgiou, C. L. Funnell, A. Cassels-Brown, and R. O'Conor, "Influence of ethnic origin on the incidence of keratoconus and associated atopic disease in Asians and white patients," *Eye*, vol. 18, pp. 379–383, 2004.

[38] D. Patel and C. McGhee, "Understanding keratoconus: what have we learned from the New Zealand perspective?," *Clinical and Experimental Optometry*, vol. 96, pp. 183–187, 2013.

[39] A. S. Saro, G. A. Radwan, U. A. Mohammed, and M. A. Abozaid, "Screening for keratoconus in a refractive surgery population of Upper Egypt," *Delta Journal of Ophthalmology*, vol. 19, pp. 19–23, 2018.

[40] A. Ertan and O. Muftuoglu, "Keratoconus clinical findings according to different age and gender groups," *Cornea*, vol. 27, pp. 1109–1113, 2008.

[41] H. Owens and G. Gamble, "A profile of keratoconus in New Zealand," *Cornea*, vol. 22, pp. 122–125, 2003.

[42] B. A. Fink, H. Wagner, K. Steger-May et al., "Differences in keratoconus as a function of gender," *American Journal of Ophthalmology*, vol. 140, pp. 459–468, 2005.

[43] K. F. Kasim and A. Shahad, "Prevalence of refractive errors in patients with keratoconus among sample of Iraqi population," *Open Access Journal of Ophthalmology*, vol. 2, article 000134, 2017.

28

Evaluation of Vitrectomy with Planned Foveal Detachment as Surgical Treatment for Refractory Diabetic Macular Edema with or without Vitreomacular Interface Abnormality

Ahmed M. Abdel Hadi ⓘ

Ophthalmology, Faculty of Medicine, Alexandria University, Alexandria, Egypt

Correspondence should be addressed to Ahmed M. Abdel Hadi; aabdelhadi2010@gmail.com

Academic Editor: Toshinori Murata

Purpose. To evaluate the therapeutic efficacy of subretinal BSS injections done during vitrectomy for refractory diabetic macular edema (DME) resistant to other modes of treatment including previous vitrectomy. *Materials and Methods.* A prospective, interventional noncomparative case series in which cases had refractory DME with a central macular thickness (CMT) $\geq 300\,\mu$m, despite previous anti-VEGF therapy (ranibizumab or bevacizumab with shifting to aflibercept). Some cases even received intravitreal triamcinolone acetonide injection, before attempting this solution. The study included group 1, surgically naïve eyes, and group 2, cases with persistent edema despite a previous vitrectomy (7 eyes (25%)). The cases were also divided into group a, eyes with normal vitreomacular interface, and group b, with abnormal vitreomacular attachment (VMA) (6 (21.4%)). The 1ry endpoint for this study was the change in CMT after 9–12 months from surgery. The 2ry endpoints were change in BCVA, recurrence of DME, and surgical complications. *Results.* The study included 28 eyes, 6 (21.4%) of which suffered from edema recurrence. The mean recorded CMT was $496 \pm 88.7\,\mu$m and $274.1 \pm 31.6\,\mu$m preoperatively and postoperatively, respectively. In all eyes, the preoperative mean BCVA in decimal form was 0.2 ± 0.11, which improved significantly to 0.45 ± 0.2. In the end, the CMT of groups 1 and 2 measured $239\,\mu$m and $170.8\,\mu$m, respectively ($p = 0.019$). The preoperative BCVA in groups 1 and 2 was 0.16 ± 0.07 and 0.37 ± 0.14, respectively, which improved to a mean of 0.34 ± 0.09 and 0.7 ± 0.16 postoperatively, respectively ($p = 0.185$). *Conclusion.* Vitrectomy with a planned foveal detachment technique was shown to be a promising solution for refractory DME cases with rapid edema resolution. CMT was shown to improve more in eyes where conventional vitrectomy was not attempted. Moreover, cases with VMA resistant to pharmacotherapy was shown to respond well to this technique. The study has been registered in Contact ClinicalTrials.gov PRS Identifier: NCT03345056.

1. Introduction

Many therapeutic options exist for diabetic macular edema (DME)—the leading cause of visual diminution in patients with diabetic retinopathy (DR). Since 2010, antivascular endothelial growth factors (anti-VEGF) have become the gold standard for DME treatment, replacing macular laser photocoagulation [1, 2].

Many eyes respond favorably to anti-VEGF agents; nevertheless, some do not achieve optimal edema control, and this group is referred to as refractory DME. The prevalence of refractory DME is estimated to be up to 50% [1],

constituting a large unmet defect in DME management. Switching from one anti-VEGF agent to another is a viable first step for resistant DME management [3]. In addition, corticosteroids are considered by many researchers as the main therapy for DME refractory to anti-VEGF treatment, due to their multimodal actions [4]. Despite these strategies, resistant DME cases still exist.

Surgery is thought to play a role in nontractional cases, allowing a more efficient clearance of VEGF and other cytokines from the retina and allowing a better oxygen access from the anterior segment to the retina, thereby reducing DME [5]. In addition, the presence of a vitreoretinal interface abnormality (VRA) reduces the therapeutic effect of anti-VEGF agents in patients with DME. These agents may alter the balance between angiogenic and fibrotic growth factors in patients with diabetic retinopathy, termed the angiofibrotic switch, which can result in increased retinal traction in some patients with proliferative diabetic retinopathy (PDR) prior to surgery [6]. Vitrectomy can relieve this tractional component and can result in resolution of the edema [7].

Improvement of the condition of the retina after vitrectomy takes time, and during that time, the photoreceptor cells may become permanently damaged [8–11] by the chronic macular edema leading to poor visual prognosis [12]. Furthermore, recent optical coherence tomography (OCT) observations show that a shorter time from the onset of DME to its resolution is the major factor affecting the integrity of the ellipsoid zone and a good visual outcome [13, 14], indicating the importance of rapid resolution of DME after vitrectomy.

Morizane et al. evaluated the therapeutic efficacy of subretinal balanced salt solution (BSS) injections in conjunction with conventional vitrectomy for treating diffuse DME. They demonstrated that this technique is effective for rapid resolution of diffuse DME resistant to anti-VEGF therapy and for the improvement of visual acuity [15]. Their study did not evaluate the usefulness of this technique in cases with vitreomacular interface abnormality resistant to intravitreal pharmacotherapy. Intravitreal corticosteroids were also not tried in their cohort of resistant cases, because various methods for administering steroids, including dexamethasone intravitreal implants, were not approved in Japan at the time. Therefore, they used sub-Tenon injection of triamcinolone acetonide in their study [16].

The present study is aimed at evaluating the therapeutic efficacy of subretinal BSS injections in conjunction with conventional vitrectomy for refractory DME resistant to more than one anti-VEGF agent, intravitreal corticosteroids, and to previous vitrectomy.

2. Materials and Methods

This study was a prospective, interventional noncomparative case series. The author adhered to the tenets of the Declaration of Helsinki. All patients were informed about the risks and benefits of the surgery, and written consent was obtained after thorough explanation of the procedure in clear simple words. The study was approved by the Institutional Review Board and the Ethics Committee at the Faculty of Medicine, Alexandria University.

Twenty-eight eyes of 28 patients with DME resistant to anti-VEGF and corticosteroid (Cst) therapy were included in this study. Some had already undergone pars plana vitrectomy for refractory DME. In all cases, vitrectomy was performed with subretinal injection of BSS between November 2015 and November 2017.

The inclusion criterion for eyes with refractory DME was a central macular thickness (CMT) of more than 300 μm despite undergoing anti-VEGF therapy (5-6 monthly injections of ranibizumab (IVR) or bevacizumab (IVB) with

shifting to aflibercept (IVA) for additional three injections). Some cases received Cst injection as well, before attempting this surgical solution in the form of intravitreal triamcinolone acetonide (1 or 2 injections) three months apart. All cases were psuedophakic. Cases subjected to conventional vitrectomy with internal limiting membrane (ILM) peeling were also enrolled in the study.

They were analysed after subdivision into group 1, including cases in which vitrectomy was not attempted, and group 2, including cases with persistent edema despite a previous vitrectomy (performed at least 6 months before the intervention). The cases were also divided into two groups: group a with normal vitreomacular interface (VMI) (defined as the absence of either perifoveal vitreoretinal attachment within 2500 μm of the foveal center or hyperreflective inner retinal band), group b with vitreomacular abnormality (VMA) in the form of ERM (defined as a hyperreflective inner retinal band with or without associated retinal inner surface plication).

The major exclusion criteria were (1) the presence of apparent retinal pigment epithelium (RPE) atrophy at or near the macula; (2) the presence of proliferative diabetic fibrovascular membranes threatening or at the macula; (3) the presence of diabetic optic atrophy; and (4) the presence of neovascular glaucoma.

All patients underwent complete ophthalmologic examinations with special emphasis on best-corrected visual acuity (BCVA) using the 6 m Landolt C acuity chart (converted to decimal) and indirect and contact lens slit lamp biomicroscopy. Spectral domain or swept source OCT (Cirrus; Carl Zeiss Meditec Inc., Dublin, CA; Spectralis; Heidelberg Engineering GmbH, Heidelberg, Germany) was used to examine all eyes before surgery and at 1 month and at the final visit after surgery. Central retinal thickness was defined as the distance between the inner surface of the RPE and the inner surface of the neurosensory retina at the macula. All patients were followed up for at least 10 months.

2.1. Data Analysis. To evaluate the surgical outcomes, preoperative and postoperative CMT and BCVAs of both groups (1, 2) and (a, b) were compared using paired tests. Significance was considered starting at a cut-off p value of 0.05. All statistical analyses were performed using SPSS for Windows, version 22.0 (SPSS Inc., Chicago, IL). Quantitative data are presented as mean $\pm$ standard deviation, while qualitative data are represented in number and percentage.

2.2. Surgical Technique. The surgery was performed using a 23-gauge, transconjunctival, microincision vitrectomy system. After core vitrectomy, posterior hyaloid detachment was attempted with the vitrectomy cutter in the suction mode. We then stained the ILM with dual stain (Membrane-Blue-Dual, DORC International), which contains a combination of 0.15% trypan blue, 0.025% Brilliant Blue G (BBG), and 4.00% polyethylene glycol (PEG). It was injected under air and left there for 30 seconds. Subsequently, the ILM peeling was attempted and peripheral vitrectomy was carried out as the peripheral residual vitreous was more evident after the dual stain application. We then injected 0.3–0.5 ml of BSS into the subretinal space to detach the fovea, ensuring that the foveal detachment covered the entire area with DME. This injection of BSS was performed at the site where the ILM had been removed using a 38-gauge cannula (MedOne Surgical Inc., Sarasota, FL) with a pressure of 4 to 6 psi (viscous fluid control system, Alcon Laboratories, Fort Worth, TX) [17] (Video 1).

In cases with VMI abnormality, the EMM was peeled using an end-gripping 23-gauge forceps after staining with dual stain, which stains both the ILM and the ERM. Then, ILM peeling was attempted with the 23-gauge end-grasping forceps (Rumex International Co., USA). Subretinal injection of BSS was done as mentioned above (Video 2).

In eyes with persistent DME despite previous vitrectomy, staining was also done under air to ensure ILM removal above the entire area involved in the edema process and proper peripheral vitreous trimming before attempting subretinal BSS injection (Video 3).

2.3. Endpoints. The primary endpoint for this study was the change in CMT at the final visit (from 9–12 months after surgery). The secondary endpoints were change in BCVA at the final visit after surgery, recurrence of DME, and surgical complications. The state of the ellipsoid zone and the ELM (as shown by the preoperative OCT) was also compared to its appearance in the OCT taken during the final visit. Recurrence of DME was defined as an increase in CMT $\geq 10\%$ of the least thickness attained during the period of follow-up, with concomitant drop of at least one line of BCVA.

3. Results

3.1. Preoperative Characteristics. The study included 28 eyes of 28 patients with a mean age of 53.1 ± 7.2 years. All eyes had CME, with 13 eyes (46.4%) suffering from neurosensory detachment (NSD), while only 6 eyes (21.4%) had vitreomacular interface abnormality (VMA) in the form of a fine epimacular membrane. Thirteen eyes (46.4%) received IVB followed by 3 IVA injections before including them in this study, while 16 eyes (57.1%) received preoperative IVR followed by 3 IVA before rendering them refractory and including them in the study. CST was given in 12 eyes (42.9%) after failure of either protocol of anti-VEGF to decrease CMT.

As regards the preoperative OCT finding, preoperative ellipsoid zone was intact in 13 eyes (46.4%) and disrupted in the rest of the included eyes. The preoperative ELM was intact in 12 eyes (42.9%) preoperatively. In 7 eyes (25%), a vitrectomy with ILM peeling was carried out for refractory DME 6 months prior to their inclusion in this study.

3.2. Operative Complications. Intraoperative complications were identified in three eyes. An iatrogenic macular hole occurred in two eyes (7.1%) during subretinal BSS injection, but postoperatively, the hole was found to be closed with improvement of BCVA (Video 1). In another case, an iatrogenic break occurred in the nasal retina during injection of the dual stain. Endolaser was applied, and the patient was instructed to attain a prone position for two days.

3.3. Postoperative Findings. The cases had a mean follow-up period of 10.6 ± 1.1 months postoperatively. The mean preoperative CMT was $496.07 \pm 88.7 \mu m$, while the postoperative mean CMT decreased to $335 \pm 67 \mu m$, when measured 4 weeks postoperatively. The mean CMT further dropped with subsequent OCT measurements and reached a mean of $274.1 \pm 31.6 \mu m$ at the final follow-up visit for all included eyes ($p = 0.029$).

Six eyes (21.4%) suffered from recurrence of their edema defined as increase in CMT by more than 10% of the least thickness attained during the period of follow-up, with concomitant drop of at least one line of BCVA. Intravitreal triamcinolone (IVTA) (once in 2 eyes and twice in 4 eyes) was given to treat these recurrences. All these eyes showed improvement of CMT and BCVA after IVTA and regained the postintervention parameters (Figure 1).

In all operated 28 eyes, the preoperative mean ± SD BCVA in decimal form was 0.2 ± 0.11, while at the final follow-up visit, the mean ± SD BCVA improved to 0.45 ± 0.2 ($p = 0.000019$). No improvement occurred postoperatively in the ellipsoid zone integrity in all eyes even in those with complete resolution of edema. Despite this finding, BCVA did improve in eyes with edema resolution to different extents. As for the ELM, postoperative 16 eyes (57.1%) showed continuous ELM with resolution of edema.

3.4. Subgroup Analysis. Cases were divided into group 1 which included eyes where vitrectomy was not attempted as a solution for refractory DME (Figure 2) and group 2 which included eyes with a history of vitrectomy for more than 6 months (Figure 3). Table 1 shows the pre- or postoperative characteristics of the two groups.

Eyes included were also divided into group a (with normal vitreomacular interface) and group b (vitreoretinal abnormalities present in the form of ERM, Figures 3 and 4). Table 2 shows a comparison between groups a and b.

4. Discussion

Despite all the pharmacological and surgical interventions currently utilized for refractory DME, the results for many cases are disappointing. This led to the introduction of the planned foveal separation with submacular BSS injection with favorable results [15]. In addition to its success in cases in which all other treatment protocols failed, a rapid edema resolution was noticed. The technique was associated with intact ELM and ellipsoid zone on OCT and better visual outcomes which was clearly depicted in previous studies tackling this point [13, 14, 18–20]. Yet, this technique had not been previously attempted in vitrectomized eyes and in those with ERM.

The refractory edema responded better with this technique than with conventional vitrectomy with or without ILM peeling. This was shown by Ulrich et al., who found that there was no significant change in CMT at 1 and 3 months after conventional vitrectomy, ($p = 0.91$, 0.29) or in visual acuity ($p = 0.69$, 0.21). However, it was not until 6 months postoperatively that the CMT had significantly decreased ($p = 0.03$) and the visual acuity showed

(a)   (b)

(c)   (d)

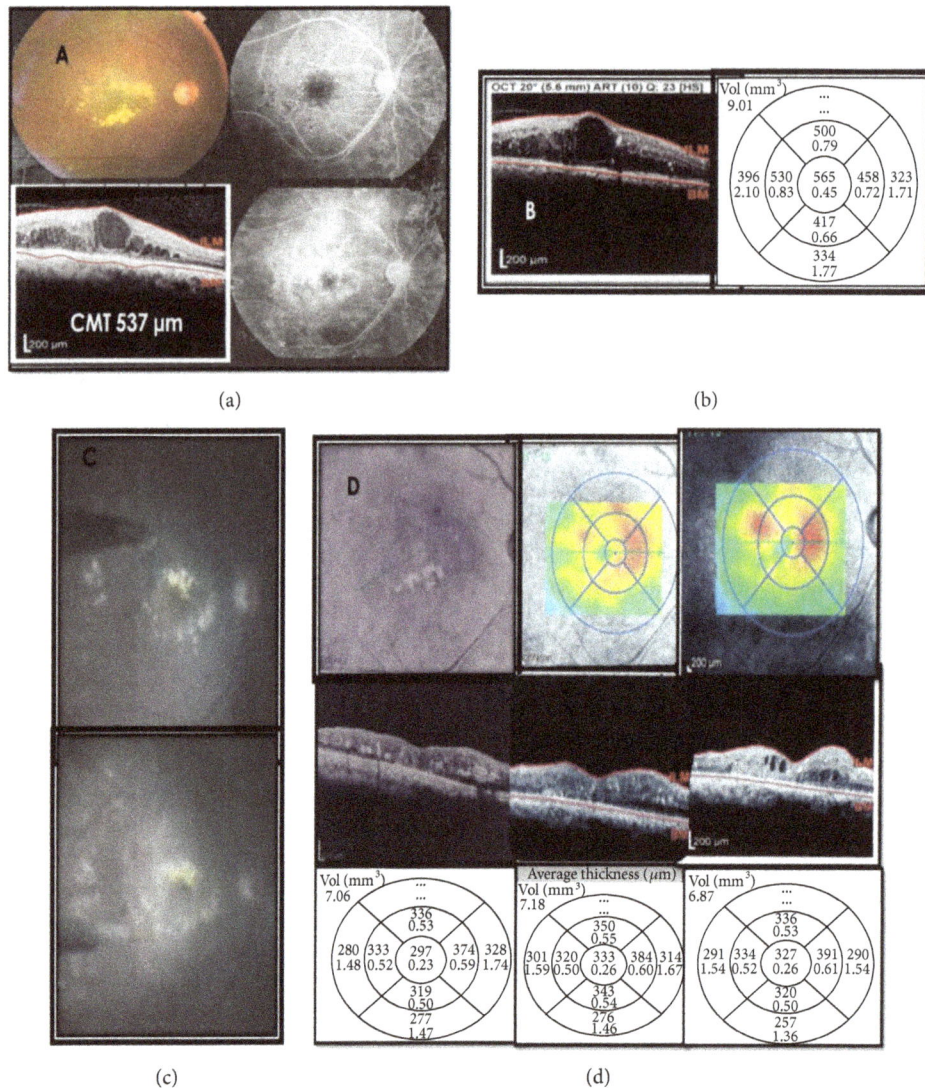

Figure 1: (a) Preoperative color fundus photo and FA showing diffuse DME with foveal hard exudate accumulation, CMT by OCT measuring 537 microns after 9 IVB injections over 1 year, BCVA measuring 0.1. (b) OCT after 3 IV triamcinolone (TA) injections 3 months apart with CMT measuring 565 microns and no improvement in BCVA. (c) Upper photo showing ILM peeling after dual stain application, while lower phot showing submacular BSS injection. (d) Red free showing significant decrease in amount of hard exudates 1 month postoperation, with drop of CMT to 297 microns and BCVA improvement to 0.3. Middle OCT with the thickness map showing recurrence of DME measuring 333 microns 6 months postoperation. The right-hand side OCT image and thickness map after 2 IVTA injections 2 months apart with slight CMT improvement of 327 microns while regaining a BCVA of 0.3 which was measured 10 months postoperation.

improvement ($p = 0.0$) [19]. Similarly, the Diabetic Retinopathy Clinical Research Network reported that 3 months after vitrectomy, the decrement in CMT was only 160 μm [7]. Likewise, Yamamoto et al. observed that although the CMT decreased by 140 μm 1 week after surgery, it took 4 months for the CMT to drop below 300 μm [9].

The current study demonstrated a more rapid and significant decrease in CMT: by $163.9 \pm 32.6\,\mu$m after 4 weeks and $227.01 \pm 80.01\,\mu$m at the final visit (10.6 ± 1.2 months) in group a and by $147.97 \pm 16.2\,\mu$m after 4 weeks and $203.17 \pm 70.4\,\mu$m at the final visit (10.5 ± 0.5 months) in group b, but this difference was not statistically significant ($p = 0.645$). Likewise, BCVA improved in group a from a mean of 0.2 ± 0.11 preoperatively to a mean of 0.44 ± 0.2 postoperatively

and from a mean of 0.217 ± 0.11 preoperatively to 0.5 ± 0.22 postoperatively in group b. These values were again not statistically significant. These results indicate that the planned foveal detachment technique works like an adjunctive step to conventional vitrectomy to speed up the resolution of DME and improve BCVA, regardless of the vitreomacular interface state before the surgery.

The rapid resolution of macular edema by the planned foveal detachment technique was noticed to be more in surgically naïve DME patients (group1) measuring 239 μm at the final follow-up visit than in group 2 eyes, subjected previously to both anti-VEGF and conventional vitrectomy, reaching 170.8 μm at the final follow-up visit. This difference in outcome was statistically significant ($p = 0.019$).

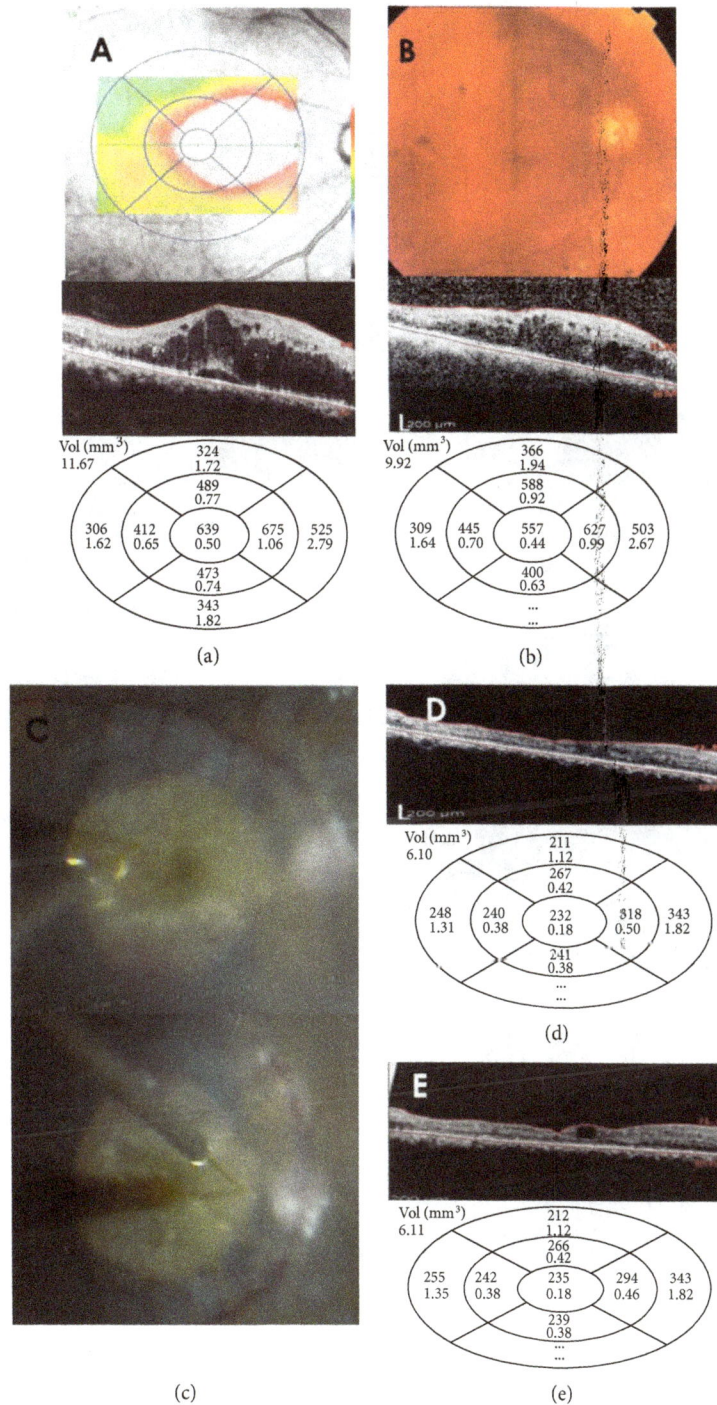

FIGURE 2: (a) Right eye: preoperative red free color-coded map showing marked DME with cystoid and neurosensory detachment shown in the OCT image, disruption of both ellipsoid zone, and ELM, with CMT measuring 639 microns after 8 IVR injections and 3 IVA injections over 1 year with BCVA equals 0.06. (b) Color fundus photo and OCT image of the same eye after two IVTA injections with CMT improving to 557 microns, but BCVA remained at 0.06. (c) Subretinal BSS injection after ILM peeling done at 2 different sites to cover the entire area of edema. (d) OCT image showing complete resolution of edema 4 weeks postoperatively with a CMT of 232 microns and BCVA of 0.16. The ellipsoid zone and ELM integrity were not regained. (e) CMT measured 10.2 months later equals 235 microns with stable BCVA.

As regards the visual acuity, the preoperative BCVA in group 1 (surgically naïve eyes) was 0.16 ± 0.07, which improved to a mean of 0.34 ± 0.09, while in group 2 (eyes with previous vitrectomy), the preoperative BCVA was 0.37 ± 0.14, which improved to a mean of 0.7 ± 0.16 postoperatively. This was not statistically significant ($p = 0.185$). So, although there was a significant difference in the mean CMT between the two groups (1 and 2), the mean BCVA postoperatively did not differ significantly. This might be explained by the fact that the chronicity of the edema in

(a)

(b)

(c)

(d)

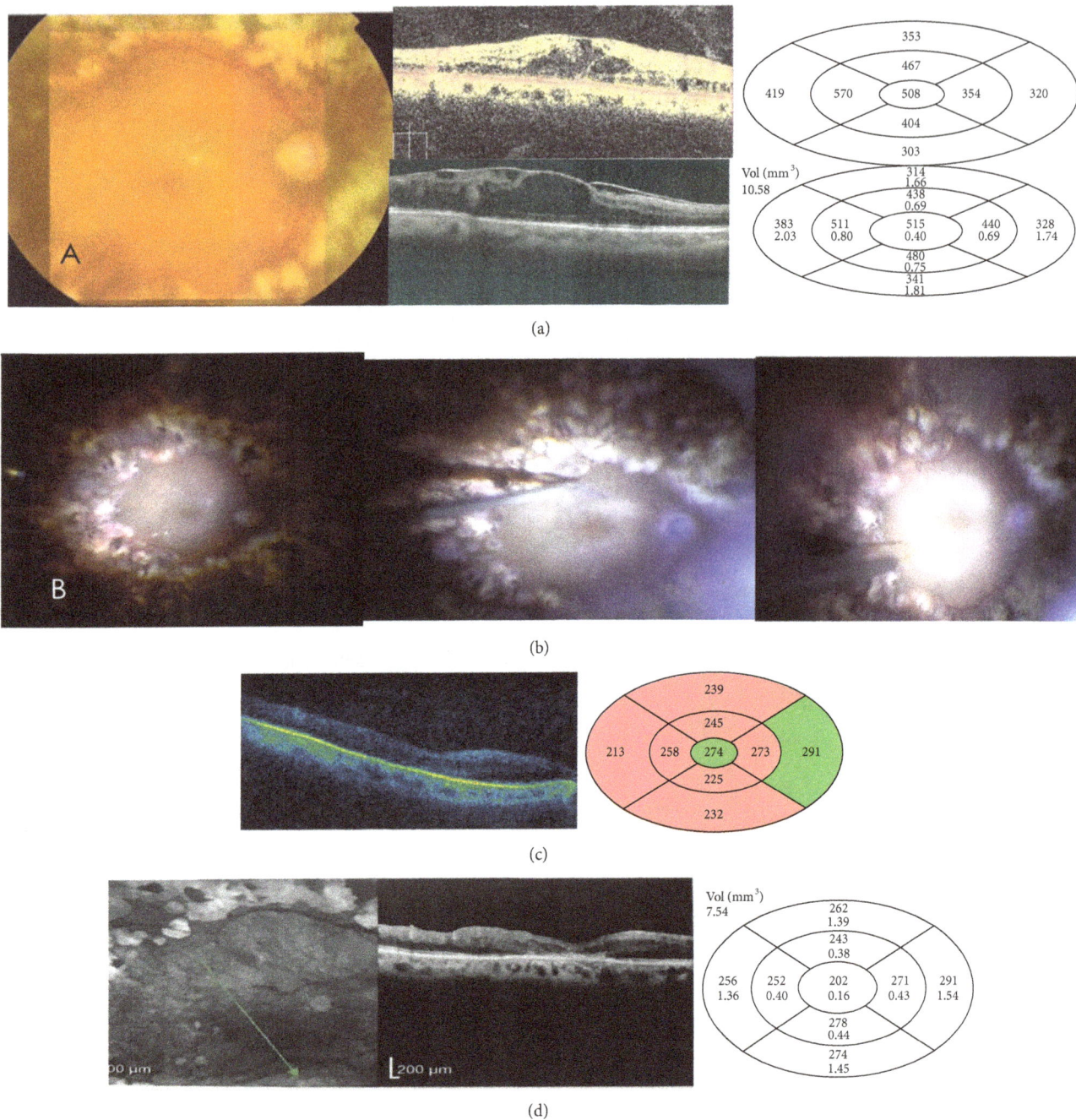

FIGURE 3: (a) Color fundus photo of a 59-year-old female who had vitrectomy done for refractory DME after failure of anti-VEGF (10 IVB and 3 IVA) to improve the edema. Upper OCT image and map showing CMT of 508 microns a year after the vitrectomy with BCVA of 0.05, totally disrupted ellipsoid zone and ELM. Lower OCT image and thickness map after 3 IVTA injections 3 months apart as a trial to improve the edema, CMT measuring 515 microns without VA gain and appearance of an ERM. (b) During surgery, ILM peeling was reattempted, and submacular BSS was injected to cover the whole area of the edema. (c) OCT of the macula 1 month postoperatively shows resolution of the edema with CMT 274 microns and BCVA of 0.1. (d) Red free photo 9.5 months postop. with thickness dropped further to 202 microns and BCVA still 0.1, probably due to the marked ELM and ellipsoid zone disruption.

both groups was a limiting factor against marked BCVA improvement despite the greater improvement in CMT. This was obvious in group 1 where similar improvement in postoperative BCVA occurred despite a marked drop of CMT in relation to group 2.

The superiority of planned foveal detachment may be explained by multiple factors according to Morizane et al.

These include facilitation of egress of edema fluid from the retina to the choroid by reducing both the oncotic pressure and viscosity of the subretinal fluid as well as the wash out of inflammatory cytokines and migratory cells above the RPE. Both mechanisms might be responsible for activation of the RPE to pump fluid from the retina to the choroid. Since these mechanisms could be effective within hours or days of surgery,

TABLE 1: Pre- and postoperative characteristics of groups 1 and 2.

Variable studied	Group 1	Group 2	p value
Number of eyes in each group	21	7	
Age mean ± SD (years)	53.38 ± 8.2	52.7 ± 3.4	
OCT findings			
Presence of neurosensory detachment preoperatively	9 (42.9%)	4 (57.1%)	0.51
Presence of VMA preoperatively	3 (14.3%)	3 (42.9%)	0.11
Intact ellipsoid zone	10 (47.6%)	3 (42.9%)	0.827
Preop. continuous ELM	9 (42.9%)	3 (42.9%)	1.0
Postop. continuous ELM	13 (69.9%)	3 (42.9%)	0.3
Preoperative CMT mean ± SD (μm)	521.3 ± 83.6	420.2 ± 56.3	
Postoperative CMT (final visit) mean ± SD (μm)	282.3 ± 20.8	249.4 ± 45.7	0.019*
Preoperative injection history			
Bevacizumab + aflibercept	10 (47.6%)	3 (42.9%)	0.11
Ranibizumab + aflibercept	12 (57.1%)	4 (57.1%)	1.0
CST after anti-VEGF failure	8 (38.1%)	4 (57.1%)	
BCVA (decimal form)			
Preoperative	0.16 ± 0.07	0.34 ± 0.09	
Postoperative (final visit)	0.37 ± 0.14	0.7 ± 0.16	0.185*
Recurrence of edema within FU period	6 (28.6%)	0 (0.0%)	0.1
Follow-up period in months	10.57 ± 1.1	10.86 ± 1.2	

*Mann–Whitney test.

TABLE 2: Characteristics of group a (normal vitreomacular interface) and group b (vitreoretinal abnormalities present).

Variable studied	Group a	Group b	Significance (2-tailed)
Number of eyes in each group	22	6	
Age	52.82 ± 7.6	54.5 ± 6.3	
Previous vitrectomy attempted	4 (18.2%)	3 (50.0%)	0.288
Follow-up in months	10.68 ± 1.2	10.5 ± 0.5	
OCT characteristics of the 2 groups			
Preoperative mean ± SD CMT (μm)	497.6 ± 93.1	490.3 ± 77.3	
CMT at 4 weeks	333.7 ± 69.7	342.33 ± 61.1	
Final CMT	270.5 ± 33.9	287.1 ± 16.6	
CMT improvement	227.01 ± 80.01	203.17 ± 70.4	0.645*
Intact ELM at final visit	14 (63.6%)	2 (33.3%)	0.354
BCVA in decimal form			
Preoperative	0.2 ± 0.11	0.217 ± 0.11	
Final	0.44 ± 0.2	0.5 ± 0.22	
Lines of improvement	3.82 ± 29	3.67 ± 1.21	0.883*
Recurrence of macular edema	6 (27.3%)	0	0.289
Complications			
Macular hole	1 (4.5%)	1 (4.5%)	0.529
Iatrogenic break	1 (16.7%)	0 (0.0%)	0.435

*Mann–Whitney.

they were consistent with their observations of rapid complete resolution of the macular edema after surgery [15].

In the present study, it is also notable that the resolution of DME continued for at least 10 months without additional treatment in most cases (22 eyes, 78.6%). This long-term effect may be explained by the fact that marked and rapid improvement in the retinal environment, due to drainage of the edema fluid, breaks the vicious cycle of ischemia-vascular hyperpermeability-chronic inflammation-ischemia seen in diabetic patients [15].

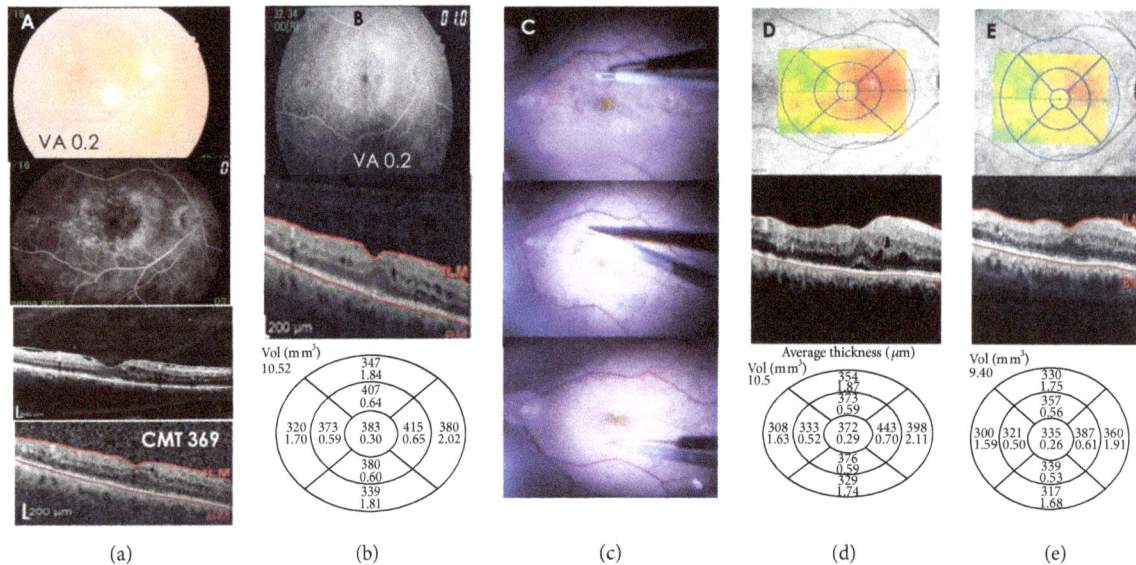

| (a) | (b) | (c) | (d) | (e) |

FIGURE 4: (a) Color fundus photo and late FA image of a male 53 years of age with type 2 DM, suffering from refractory DME with VMA with a CMT of 369 microns after 8 IVR injections over the past 9 months. BCVA recorded was 0.2. (b) Diffuse DME shown in a late FA image with CMT of 383 after shifting to IVA for three consecutive injections. (c) Upper snap shot during removal of the fine ERM stained with the dual stain, middle image showing ILM peeling, while the lower photo was taken during submacular BSS injection. (d) Red free with color-coded map showing slight CMT improvement 4 weeks postoperatively reaching 372 microns. (e) Eight months postoperation with edema reaching 335 without additional treatment and BCVA improved to 0.8.

During the surgical procedure for the planned foveal detachment technique, special attention is needed to avoid an iatrogenic macular hole or injuries to Bruch's membrane during the subretinal injection of BSS. Therefore, Morizane et al. used a viscous fluid-control system (Alcon Laboratories, Fort Worth, TX, USA) with a low injection pressure to regulate the speed of subretinal injection [15].

In the present study, a similar maneuver was used for subretinal fluid injection. Still, 2 cases (7.1%) suffered iatrogenic holes during injection. However, the postoperative follow-up revealed closure of the macular holes with improvement of the final visual acuity in these cases. Even without submacular saline injection, the risk of macular hole induction exists, as Grigorian et al. reported an incidence of 2% with conventional vitrectomy for DME [21].

Most of the cases included in the current study have had DME for more than a year, with significant ellipsoid zone (EZ)—previously called the photoreceptor inner segment/outer segment (IS/OS) junction—disruption in 15 eyes (53.6%). In these cases, ellipsoid zone disruption neither improved nor worsened postoperatively. Despite this, the CMT, BCVA and, to a certain extent, the ELM continuity improved after resolution of edema postoperatively. A similar conclusion was drawn by Chhablani et al., where the strongest clue for vision improvement was preoperative damage to the ELM ($p = 0.0277$) compared to the IS/OS junction ($p = 0.03$) [22].

In conclusion, vitrectomy with planned foveal detachment technique appears to be a promising solution for DME cases that is resistant to all other forms of treatment (repeated anti-VEGF, Cst injections, and even conventional vitrectomy with ILM peeling) with rapid and efficient edema

resolution in those resistant eyes. CMT was better in eyes where conventional vitrectomy was not attempted. Moreover, cases with VMA resistant to pharmacotherapy was shown to respond well to this technique.

The current study is limited by its uncontrolled design and small sample size. Further randomized controlled clinical studies involving a larger number of patients with longer duration of follow-up are needed to define the exact role of this procedure in the management of DME.

Conflicts of Interest

The author declares that there is no conflict of interest regarding the publication of this paper.

Supplementary Materials

Video 1: edited video showing the ILM peeling in a surgically naïve case with a refractory DME in spite of 9 IVB injections during the course of 1 year and 3 IV triamcinolone (TA) injections 3 months apart, BCVA measuring 0.1. Secondary iatrogenic macular hole occurred during submacular BSS injection. Fluid-air exchange at the end of the surgery. Video 2: edited video showing a case with fine EMM and refractory DME in spite of repeated ranibizumab injections and 3 aflibercept injections along the course of 8 months, the EMM that was peeled using an end-gripping 23-gauge forceps after staining with dual stain, subretinal injection of BSS was attempted as mentioned above. Fluid air exchange was then done. Video 3: edited movie for an eye with persistent DME despite previous vitrectomy, staining was also done under air to ensure ILM removal above the entire area involved in the edema process and proper peripheral vitreous trimming before attempting subretinal BSS injection was done. Air was left as a tamponade at the conclusion of surgery. *(Supplementary Material)*

References

[1] M. J. Elman, N. M. Bressler, H. Qin et al., "Expanded 2-year follow-up of ranibizumab plus prompt or deferred laser or triamcinolone plus prompt laser for diabetic macular edema," *Ophthalmology*, vol. 118, no. 4, pp. 609–614, 2011.

[2] D. M. Brown, Q. D. Nguyen, D. M. Marcus et al., "Long-term outcomes of ranibizumab therapy for diabetic macular edema: the 36-month results from two phase III trials: RISE and RIDE," *Ophthalmology*, vol. 120, no. 10, pp. 2013–2022, 2013.

[3] E. Rahimy, A. Shahlaee, M. A. Khan et al., "Conversion to aflibercept after prior anti-VEGF therapy for persistent diabetic macular edema," *American Journal of Ophthalmology*, vol. 164, pp. 118–127.e2, 2016.

[4] D. Grover, T. J. Li, and C. C. W. Chong, "Intravitreal steroids for macular edema in diabetes," *Cochrane Database of Systematic Reviews*, vol. 17, article CD005656, 2008.

[5] S. Bonnin, O. Sandali, S. Bonnel, C. Monin, and M. El Sanharawi, "Vitrectomy with internal limiting membrane peeling for tractional and nontractional diabetic macular edema: long-term results of a comparative study," *Retina*, vol. 35, no. 5, pp. 921–928, 2015.

[6] R. J. Van Geest, S. Y. Lesnik-Oberstein, H. Stevie Tan et al., "A shift in the balance of vascular endothelial growth factor and connective tissue growth factor by bevacizumab causes the angiofibrotic switch in proliferative diabetic retinopathy," *British Journal of Ophthalmology*, vol. 96, no. 4, pp. 587–590, 2012.

[7] Diabetic Retinopathy Clinical Research Network Writing Committee, J. A. Haller, H. Qin et al., "Vitrectomy outcomes in eyes with diabetic macular edema and vitreomacular traction," *Ophthalmology*, vol. 117, no. 6, pp. 1087–1093.e3, 2010.

[8] P. Massin, G. Duguid, A. Erginay, B. Haouchine, and A. Gaudric, "Optical coherence tomography for evaluating diabetic macular edema before and after vitrectomy," *American Journal of Ophthalmology*, vol. 135, no. 2, pp. 169–177, 2003.

[9] T. Yamamoto, K. Hitani, I. Tsukahara et al., "Early postoperative retinal thickness changes and complications after vitrectomy for diabetic macular edema," *American Journal of Ophthalmology*, vol. 135, no. 1, pp. 14–19, 2003.

[10] U. Stolba, S. Binder, D. Gruber, I. Krebs, T. Aggermann, and B. Neumaier, "Vitrectomy for persistent diffuse diabetic macular edema," *American Journal of Ophthalmology*, vol. 140, no. 2, pp. 295–301, 2005.

[11] A. Yanyali, F. Horozoglu, E. Celik, and A. F. Nohutcu, "Long-term outcomes of pars plana vitrectomy with internal limiting membrane removal in diabetic macular edema," *Retina*, vol. 27, no. 5, pp. 557–566, 2007.

[12] S. J. Song, J. H. Sohn, and K. H. Park, "Evaluation of the efficacy of vitrectomy for persistent diabetic macular edema and associated factors predicting outcome," *Korean Journal of Ophthalmology*, vol. 21, no. 3, pp. 146–150, 2007.

[13] A. Sakamoto, K. Nishijima, M. Kita, H. Oh, A. Tsujikawa, and N. Yoshimura, "Association between foveal photoreceptor status and visual acuity after resolution of diabetic macular edema by pars plana vitrectomy," *Graefe's Archive for Clinical and Experimental Ophthalmology*, vol. 247, no. 10, pp. 1325–1330, 2009.

[14] A. Yanyali, K. T. Bozkurt, A. Macin, F. Horozoglu, and A. F. Nohutcu, "Quantitative assessment of photoreceptor layer in eyes with resolved edema after pars plana vitrectomy with internal limiting membrane removal for diabetic macular edema," *Ophthalmologica*, vol. 226, no. 2, pp. 57–63, 2011.

[15] Y. Morizane, S. Kimura, M. Hosokawa et al., "Planned foveal detachment technique for the resolution of diffuse diabetic macular edema," *Japanese Journal of Ophthalmology*, vol. 59, no. 5, pp. 279–287, 2015.

[16] S. Toshima, Y. Morizane, S. Kimura, and F. Shiraga, "Planned foveal detachment technique for the resolution of diabetic macular edema resistant to anti-vascular endothelial growth factor therapy," *Retina*, 2017.

[17] T. Okanouchi, S. Toshima, S. Kimura, Y. Morizane, and F. Shiraga, "Novel technique for subretinal injection using local removal of the internal limiting membrane," *Retina*, vol. 36, no. 5, pp. 1035–1038, 2016.

[18] J. W. Harbour, W. E. Smiddy, H. W. Flynn Jr, and P. E. Rubsamen, "Vitrectomy for diabetic macular edema associated with a thickened and taut posterior hyaloid membrane," *American Journal of Ophthalmology*, vol. 121, no. 4, pp. 405–413, 1996.

[19] J. N. Ulrich, "Pars plana vitrectomy with internal limiting membrane peeling for nontractional diabetic macular edema," *The Open Ophthalmology Journal*, vol. 11, no. 1, pp. 5–10, 2017.

[20] Y. Okamoto, F. Okamoto, T. Hiraoka, and T. Oshika, "Vision-related quality of life and visual function following intravitreal bevacizumab injection for persistent diabetic macular edema after vitrectomy," *Japanese Journal of Ophthalmology*, vol. 58, no. 4, pp. 369–374, 2014.

[21] R. Grigorian, N. Bhagat, P. Lanzetta, A. Tutela, and M. Zarbin, "Pars plana vitrectomy for refractory diabetic macular edema," *Seminars in Ophthalmology*, vol. 18, no. 3, pp. 116–120, 2003.

[22] J. K. Chhablani, J. S. Kim, L. Cheng, I. Kozak, and W. Freeman, "External limiting membrane as a predictor of visual improvement in diabetic macular edema after pars plana vitrectomy," *Graefe's Archive for Clinical and Experimental Ophthalmology*, vol. 250, no. 10, pp. 1415–1420, 2012.

Permissions

The contributors of this book come from diverse backgrounds, making this book a truly international effort. This book will bring forth new frontiers with its revolutionizing research information and detailed analysis of the nascent developments around the world.

We would like to thank all the contributing authors for lending their expertise to make the book truly unique. They have played a crucial role in the development of this book. Without their invaluable contributions this book wouldn't have been possible. They have made vital efforts to compile up to date information on the varied aspects of this subject to make this book a valuable addition to the collection of many professionals and students.

This book was conceptualized with the vision of imparting up-to-date information and advanced data in this field. To ensure the same, a matchless editorial board was set up. Every individual on the board went through rigorous rounds of assessment to prove their worth. After which they invested a large part of their time researching and compiling the most relevant data for our readers.

The editorial board has been involved in producing this book since its inception. They have spent rigorous hours researching and exploring the diverse topics which have resulted in the successful publishing of this book. They have passed on their knowledge of decades through this book. To expedite this challenging task, the publisher supported the team at every step. A small team of assistant editors was also appointed to further simplify the editing procedure and attain best results for the readers.

Apart from the editorial board, the designing team has also invested a significant amount of their time in understanding the subject and creating the most relevant covers. They scrutinized every image to scout for the most suitable representation of the subject and create an appropriate cover for the book.

The publishing team has been an ardent support to the editorial, designing and production team. Their endless efforts to recruit the best for this project, has resulted in the accomplishment of this book. They are a veteran in the field of academics and their pool of knowledge is as vast as their experience in printing. Their expertise and guidance has proved useful at every step. Their uncompromising quality standards have made this book an exceptional effort. Their encouragement from time to time has been an inspiration for everyone.

The publisher and the editorial board hope that this book will prove to be a valuable piece of knowledge for researchers, students, practitioners and scholars across the globe.

List of Contributors

Kazuyuki Hirooka, Kaori Ukegawa and Eri Nitta
Department of Ophthalmology, Kagawa University Faculty of Medicine, 1750-1 Ikenobe, Miki, Kagawa 761-0793, Japan

Nobufumi Ueda, Yushi Hayashida, Hiromi Hirama, Rikiya Taoka, Yuma Sakura, Mari Yamasaki, Hiroyuki Tsunemori, Mikio Sugimoto and Yoshiyuki Kakehi
Department of Urology, Kagawa University Faculty of Medicine, 1750-1 Ikenobe, Miki, Kagawa 761-0793, Japan

Chia-Ling Lee, Li-Yi Chiu and Tzu-En Kao
Department of Ophthalmology, Kaohsiung Medical University Hospital, Kaohsiung 80708, Taiwan

Kwou-Yeung Wu and Wen-Chuan Wu
Department of Ophthalmology, Kaohsiung Medical University Hospital, Kaohsiung 80708, Taiwan
Department of Ophthalmology, School of Medicine, Kaohsiung Medical University, Kaohsiung 80708, Taiwan

Yo-Chen Chang
Department of Ophthalmology, Kaohsiung Medical University Hospital, Kaohsiung 80708, Taiwan
Department of Ophthalmology, School of Medicine, Kaohsiung Medical University, Kaohsiung 80708, Taiwan
Department of Ophthalmology, Kaohsiung Municipal Hsiao-Kang Hospital, Kaohsiung Medical University, Kaohsiung 81267, Taiwan

Pei-Kang Liu
Department of Ophthalmology, Kaohsiung Medical University Hospital, Kaohsiung 80708, Taiwan
Department of Ophthalmology, Yuan's General Hospital, Kaohsiung, Taiwan

Kuo-Jen Chen
Department of Ophthalmology, Kaohsiung Municipal Hsiao-Kang Hospital, Kaohsiung Medical University, Kaohsiung 81267, Taiwan

Apostolos G. Anagnostopoulos, Nilufer Yesilirmak, Florence Cabot, Daniel P. Waren, Terrence P. O'Brien, Sonia H. Yoo and Kendall E. Donaldson
Bascom Palmer Eye Institute, University of Miami Miller School of Medicine, Miami, FL, USA

Vasilios F. Diakonis
Bascom Palmer Eye Institute, University of Miami Miller School of Medicine, Miami, FL, USA
The Eye Institute of West Florida, Largo, FL, USA

Angeliki Moutsiopoulou
Department of Chemistry, University of Miami, Miami, FL, USA

Robert J. Weinstock
The Eye Institute of West Florida, Largo, FL, USA

Andrea E. Laubichler, Daniel Zapp and Lukas Reznicek
Department of Ophthalmology, Technical University of Munich, Munich, Germany

Christian S. Mayer
Department of Ophthalmology, Technical University of Munich, Munich, Germany
Department of Ophthalmology, University of Heidelberg, Heidelberg, Germany

Ramin Khoramnia and Tamer Tandogan
Department of Ophthalmology, University of Heidelberg, Heidelberg, Germany

Philipp Prahs
Department of Ophthalmology, University of Regensburg, Regensburg, Germany

Dilek Yaşa and Alper Ağca
Beyoğlu Eye Research and Training Hospital, Bereketzade Mah, No. 2, Beyoglu, Istanbul, Turkey

Chul Hee Lee, Min Woo Lee, Eun Young Choi and Min Kim
Department of Ophthalmology, Institute of Vision Research, Gangnam Severance Hospital, Yonsei University College of Medicine, Seoul, Republic of Korea

Suk Ho Byeon, Sung Soo Kim, Hyoung Jun Koh and Sung Chul Lee
Department of Ophthalmology, Institute of Vision Research, Severance Hospital, Yonsei University College of Medicine, Seoul, Republic of Korea

F. Di Renzo, D. Di Taranto, G. Coclite, S. Zaccaria and S. De Turris
Department of Medicine and Health Science, University of Molise, Campobasso, Italy

F. Cifariello
Department of Medicine and Health Science, University of Molise, Campobasso, Italy
Casa di Cura "Villa Maria", Campobasso, Italy

C. Costagliola
Department of Medicine and Health Science, University of Molise, Campobasso, Italy
Casa di Cura "Villa Maria", Campobasso, Italy
I.R.C.S.S. Neuromed, Pozzilli, Isernia, Italy

M. Minicucci
I.R.C.S.S. Neuromed, Pozzilli, Isernia, Italy

Katarzyna Krysik and Anita Lyssek-Boron
Department of Ophthalmology with Paediatric Unit, St. Barbara Hospital, Trauma Center, Medykow Square 1, 41-200 Sosnowiec, Poland

Dariusz Dobrowolski
Department of Ophthalmology with Paediatric Unit, St. Barbara Hospital, Trauma Center, Medykow Square 1, 41-200 Sosnowiec, Poland
Chair and Clinical Department of Ophthalmology, School of Medicine with the Division of Dentistry in Zabrze, Medical University of Silesia in Katowice, Panewnicka 65 St., 40-760 Katowice, Poland
Department of Ophthalmology, District Railway Hospital, Panewnicka 65 St., 40-760 Katowice, Poland

Edward Wylegala
Chair and Clinical Department of Ophthalmology, School of Medicine with the Division of Dentistry in Zabrze, Medical University of Silesia in Katowice, Panewnicka 65 St., 40-760 Katowice, Poland
Department of Ophthalmology, District Railway Hospital, Panewnicka 65 St., 40-760 Katowice, Poland
Hebei Provincial Eye Hospital, Xingtai, China

Ewa Wroblewska-Czajka
Department of Ophthalmology, District Railway Hospital, Panewnicka 65 St., 40-760 Katowice, Poland

Satoru Kase, Kan Ishijima, Kousuke Noda and Susumu Ishida
Department of Ophthalmology, Faculty of Medicine and Graduate School of Medicine, Hokkaido University, Sapporo, Japan

Atsushi Tanaka
Department of Ophthalmology, Faculty of Medicine and Graduate School of Medicine, Hokkaido University, Sapporo, Japan
Enoki Eye Clinic, Sayama, Japan

Wataru Saito
Department of Ophthalmology, Faculty of Medicine and Graduate School of Medicine, Hokkaido University, Sapporo, Japan
Kaimeido Eye and Dental Clinic, Sapporo, Japan

Jiao Lyu, Qi Zhang, Haiying Jin, Tingyi Liang and Peiquan Zhao
Department of Ophthalmology, Xinhua Hospital, School of Medicine, Shanghai Jiao Tong University, Shanghai, China

Jili Chen
Shibei Hospital, Jing'an District, Shanghai, China

Sang Beom Han
Department of Ophthalmology, Kangwon National University Hospital, Kangwon National University, Chuncheon, Republic of Korea

Yu-Chi Liu and Jodhbir S. Mehta
Singapore National Eye Centre, Singapore
Singapore Eye Research Institute, Singapore
Department of Ophthalmology, Yong Loo Lin School of Medicine, National University of Singapore, Singapore

Karim Mohamed-Noriega
Department of Ophthalmology, Faculty of Medicine, University Hospital "Jose E. Gonzalez", Autonomous University of Nuevo Leon, Monterrey, NL, Mexico

Ting Zhang, Hong Zhuang, Keyan Wang and Gezhi Xu
Department of Ophthalmology, Eye, Ear, Nose and roat Hospital, Fudan University, Shanghai 200031, China
Shanghai Key Laboratory of Visual Impairment and Restoration, Eye, Ear, Nose and roat Hospital, Fudan University, Shanghai 200031, China

Norihiro Yamada and Naoko Kato
Department of Ophthalmology, Saitama Medical University Hospital, Saitama, Japan

Takahiko Hayashi
Department of Ophthalmology, Saitama Medical University Hospital, Saitama, Japan
Department of Ophthalmology, Yokohama City University Hospital, Yokohama, Japan
Department of Ophthalmology, Yokohama Minami Kyosai Hospital, Yokohama, Japan
Kikuna Yuda Eye Clinic, Yokohama, Japan
Department of Ophthalmology, Jichi Medical University, Tochigi, Japan

Toshiki Shimizu
Department of Ophthalmology, Yokohama City University Hospital, Yokohama, Japan
Department of Ophthalmology, Yokohama Minami Kyosai Hospital, Yokohama, Japan

Kentaro Yuda
Department of Ophthalmology, Yokohama City University Hospital, Yokohama, Japan
Department of Ophthalmology, Yokohama Minami Kyosai Hospital, Yokohama, Japan
Kikuna Yuda Eye Clinic, Yokohama, Japan

Hidenori Takahashi
Department of Ophthalmology, Jichi Medical University, Tochigi, Japan

Itaru Oyakawa
Department of Ophthalmology, Heart Life Hospital, Okinawa, Japan

Xin Wang and Sai Zhang
Qingdao University, Qingdao 266071, China
Shandong Eye Hospital, Shandong Eye Institute, Shandong Academy of Medical Sciences, Jinan 250021, China

Xiaolin Qi, Suxia Li, Weiyun Shi and Hua Gao
Shandong Eye Hospital, Shandong Eye Institute, Shandong Academy of Medical Sciences, Jinan 250021, China

Ting Liu
Qingdao Eye Hospital, Shandong Eye Institute, Shandong Academy of Medical Sciences, Qingdao 266071, China

Xiaolin Qi, Miaolin Wang, Xiaofeng Li, Yanni Jia, Suxia Li, Weiyun Shi and Hua Gao
Shandong Eye Hospital, Shandong Eye Institute, Shandong Academy of Medical Sciences, Jinan, China

Xiang Chen, Yi Yao, Xiaolu Hao, Xiaocui Liu and Tiecheng Liu
Department of Ophthalmology, e Chinese PLA General Hospital, No. 28 Fuxing Road, Haidian District, Beijing 100853, China

Myrsini Petrelli, Konstantinos Andreanos and Chrysanthi Koutsandrea
First Department of Ophthalmology, National and Kapodistrian University of Athens, General Hospital "G. Gennimatas", Athens, Greece

Konstantinos Droutsas and Apostolos Lazaridis
First Department of Ophthalmology, National and Kapodistrian University of Athens, General Hospital "G. Gennimatas", Athens, Greece
Department of Ophthalmology, Philipps University, Marburg, Germany

George Kymionis
First Department of Ophthalmology, National and Kapodistrian University of Athens, General Hospital "G. Gennimatas", Athens, Greece

Jules Gonin Eye Hospital, Faculty of Biology and Medicine, University of Lausanne, Lausanne, Switzerland

Dimitrios Miltsakakis and Anastasia Karagianni
State Ophthalmology Clinic, General Hospital "G. Gennimatas", Athens, Greece

Abdelhamid Elhofi and Hany Ahmed Helaly
Ophthalmology Department, Faculty of Medicine, Alexandria University, Egypt

Peng-peng Zhao, Nan Liu, Zhi-min Shu and Jin-song Zhao
Department of Ophthalmology, The Second Hospital of Jilin University, Changchun, China

Shuang Wang
Department of Ophthalmology, The Third People's Hospital of Chengdu, Chengdu, China

Keiko Otsuka, Hisanori Imai, Ayaka Fujii, Akiko Miki and Makoto Nakamura
Division of Ophthalmology, Department of Organ erapeutics, Kobe University Graduate School of Medicine, 7-5-2 Kusunoki-cho, Chuo-ku, Kobe 650-0017, Japan

Mizuki Tagami and Atsushi Azumi
Department of Ophthalmology, Kobe Kaisei Hospital, 3-11-15 Shinoharakitamati, Nada-ku, Kobe 657-0068, Japan

Kenji Kashiwagi and Mio Matsubara
Department of Ophthalmology, University of Yamanashi Faculty of Medicine, Chuo, Yamanashi, Japan

Kaijian Chen, Zongli Hu, Jihan Zhou, Ting Yu, Jie Xu, Ji Bai and Jian Ye
Department of Ophthalmology, Research Institute of Surgery and Daping Hospital, Army Medical University, Chongqing, China

Ilias Georgalas, Klio Chatzistefanou, Marilita M. Moschos and Chryssanthi Koutsandrea
First Department of Ophthalmology, National and Kapodistrian University of Athens, Athens, Greece

Konstantinos Droutsas and Apostolos Lazaridis
First Department of Ophthalmology, National and Kapodistrian University of Athens, Athens, Greece
Department of Ophthalmology, Philipps University, Marburg, Germany

Georgios Kymionis
First Department of Ophthalmology, National and Kapodistrian University of Athens, Athens, Greece Jules Gonin Eye Hospital, University of Lausanne, Lausanne, Switzerland

Georgios Bagikos and Dimitrios Miltsakakis
State Ophthalmology Clinic, General Hospital "G. Gennimatas", Athens, Greece

Heba A. El Gendy
Professor of Ophthalmology, Faculty of Medicine, Cairo University, Cairo, Egypt

Noha M. Khalil and Iman M. Eissa
Associate Professor of Ophthalmology, Faculty of Medicine, Cairo University, Cairo, Egypt

Shireen MA. Shousha
Lecturer of Ophthalmology, Faculty of Medicine, Cairo University, Cairo, Egypt

Dilek Yaşa, Zeynep Gizem Erdem, Ufuk ¨Urdem, G¨okhan Demir, Ali Demircan and Zeynep Alkın
Department of Ophthalmology, Beyŏglu Eye Research and Training Hospital, No. 2, Beyoglu, 34421 Istanbul, Turkey

Jie Li, Bo Zhao, Sanmei Liu, Fang Li, Wentao Dong and Jie Zhong
Department of Ophthalmology, Sichuan Academy of Medical Science and Sichuan Provincial People's Hospital, School of Medicine, University of Electronic Science and Technology of China, Chengdu, China

Abdulrahman Mohammed Al-Amri
College of Medicine, King Khalid University, Abha, Saudi Arabia

Ahmed M. Abdel Hadi
Ophthalmology, Faculty of Medicine, Alexandria University, Alexandria, Egypt

Index

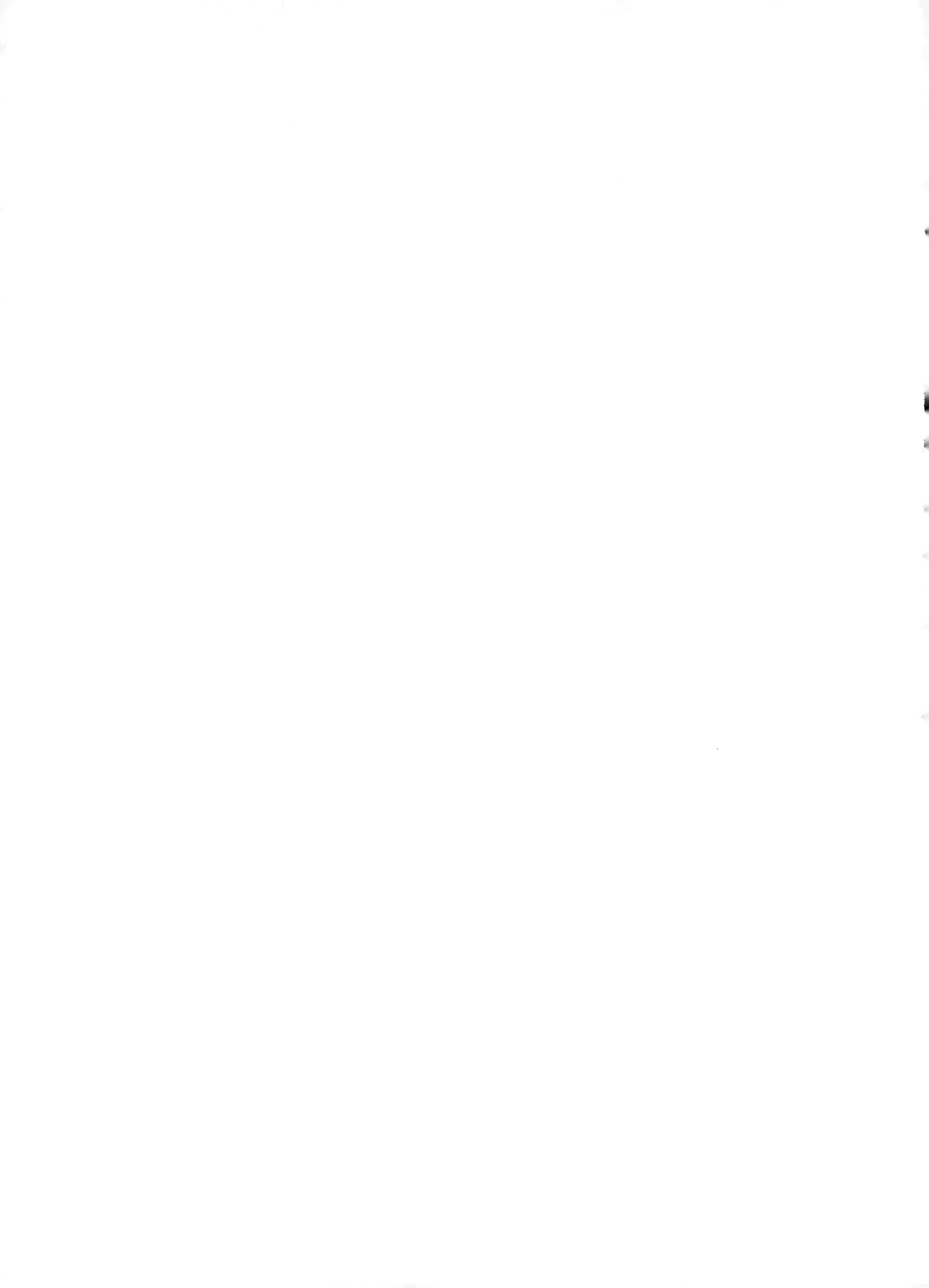